Bioarchaeological Studies of Life
in the Age of Agriculture

Bioarchaeological Studies of Life in the Age of Agriculture

A View from the Southeast

Edited by

Patricia M. Lambert

THE UNIVERSITY OF ALABAMA PRESS

Tuscaloosa and London

1 2 3 4 5 6 / 05 04 03 02 01 00

Cover design by Carleton J. Giles

∞

The paper on which this book is printed meets the minimum require-
ments of American National Standard for Information Science-
Permanence of Paper for Printed Library Materials,
ANSI Z39.48-1984.

Library of Congress Cataloging-in-Publication Data

Bioarchaeological studies of life in the age of agriculture :
a view from the Southeast / edited by Patricia M. Lambert.
    p. cm.
    Includes bibliographical references and index.

    ISBN 0-8173-1007-X (alk. paper)
    1. Indians of North America—Southern States— Antiquities
Congresses. 2. Indians of North America—Health and hygiene—
Southern States Congresses. 3. Indians of North America—Anthro-
pometry—Southern States Congresses. 4. Mississippian culture
Congresses. 5. Southern States—Antiquities Congresses.
I. Lambert, Patricia M., 1958–
    E78.S65B55 2000
    614.4′275—dc21
                                                                99-6777
British Library Cataloguing-in-Publication Data available

In memory of Patricia S. Bridges

Contents

Figures and Tables

TABLES

Acknowledgments

I would like to thank all of the authors for their patience and good cheer as I figured out the intricacies of the editorial process; your hard work and courteous, timely responses were greatly appreciated. Judith Knight, Acquisitions Editor at The University of Alabama Press, was brilliant at keeping the volume on track without ever seeming to push or prod. Clark Spencer Larsen and two anonymous reviewers provided excellent commentary on the volume, and the final product is greatly improved as a result of their efforts. Thanks are also due to Sonia Evans, Tim Evans, and Amanda Larsen for their assistance with the assembly of references. Finally, I would like to thank my former academic adviser, Phillip L. Walker, who served as the discussant at the AAPA symposium on which this volume is based, and who continues to serve in a much appreciated advisory capacity.

I   Introduction

Patricia M. Lambert

This edited volume had its origins in a symposium of the same name organized for the 65th Annual Meeting of the American Association of Physical Anthropologists in Durham, North Carolina. The purpose of the symposium was to move a step beyond studies emphasizing the health consequences of the shift from foraging to farming, to focus instead on variability within societies and regions that had already made this economic transition. Bioarchaeological studies of cultural transitions have provided a wealth of information on the biological costs and consequences of certain lifestyles and lifestyle transitions (e.g., Cohen and Armelagos 1984; Larsen 1987, 1995, 1997). They have commonly documented the deleterious consequences of a heavy dependence on maize and other storable seed cultigens (see Cohen and Armelagos 1984) but have also demonstrated the human capacity to adapt to new ecological situations (e.g., Cook and Buikstra 1979; Rose et al. 1984). The focus on subsistence has sometimes led to unilinear explanations invoking maize as the ultimate culprit in changing patterns of health in prehistoric New World populations, but as Cook (1984:262) cautioned back in the 1980s, "the complicated array of variables—both cultural and ecological—that are linked to subsistence must be understood before we have an adequate context in which to evaluate health changes." Indeed, those societies encompassed in the Southeast cultural tradition broadly defined as Mississippian based on shared participation in cleared field agriculture, hierarchical social organization, and religion were actually quite variable politically and economically (C. Scarry 1993b; J. Scarry 1996). Bioarchaeological research has further shown that the human condition varied considerably in accordance with this diversity (Buikstra 1991). Nonetheless, a stage-like economic progression associated with a concomitant and predictable health decline remains a prominent view of human existence. In this volume, the contributing authors take a closer look at populations commonly lumped into a single cultural category, in this case subsistence agriculturalists, in order to explore variation in the diet, health, and behavior of late prehistoric and early historic peoples of the southeastern United States.

Although most of the chapters in this volume focus on the age of intensive maize cultivation, which had its inception in the last millennium, agricultural production in the Southeast can actually be traced back some 4000 years to the appearance of native domesticates (e.g., cucurbits and sumpweed) in midcontinental Archaic sites (Smith 1992; Yarnell 1993). Maize, a tropical import that figured importantly as a dietary staple only in the last few centuries before European contact, appeared in the region about 2000 years later (Fritz 1993) and did not seriously displace native seed crops until after A.D. 1000 (Yarnell 1993). With the intensification of maize agriculture came the development of the large and well-known political centers at Cahokia, Moundville, and Etowah. Because of their impressive size and monumental architecture, these polities have often been the focus of discussions on late prehistoric developments in the Southeast. However, many smaller polities existed conterminously with these great centers (Rogers and Smith 1995; J. Scarry 1996), varying in size, scale, and economy in accordance with the diverse environments in which cultural developments took place (J. Scarry 1996). This variability is an increasing focus of Southeastern archaeologists as they grapple with the problem of cultural evolution in the late prehistory of this region (e.g., Rogers and Smith 1995).

The purpose of this volume is twofold: to take a closer look at variability in those cultural parameters that lend themselves to osteological investigation (e.g., subsistence practices, warfare, ethnic identity) and to examine the relationship of disease, environment, and lifeways. The results are not always as envisioned. Epidemiological considerations might lead one to predict, for example, that infectious disease would be more of a problem in a populous setting such as Moundville than in a rural village on the North Carolina piedmont because large host populations are more likely to maintain infectious pathogens and to foster conditions conducive to their spread. But it is not unreasonable to assume that benefits to living in large centers might translate into healthier and safer living conditions. Large polities such as

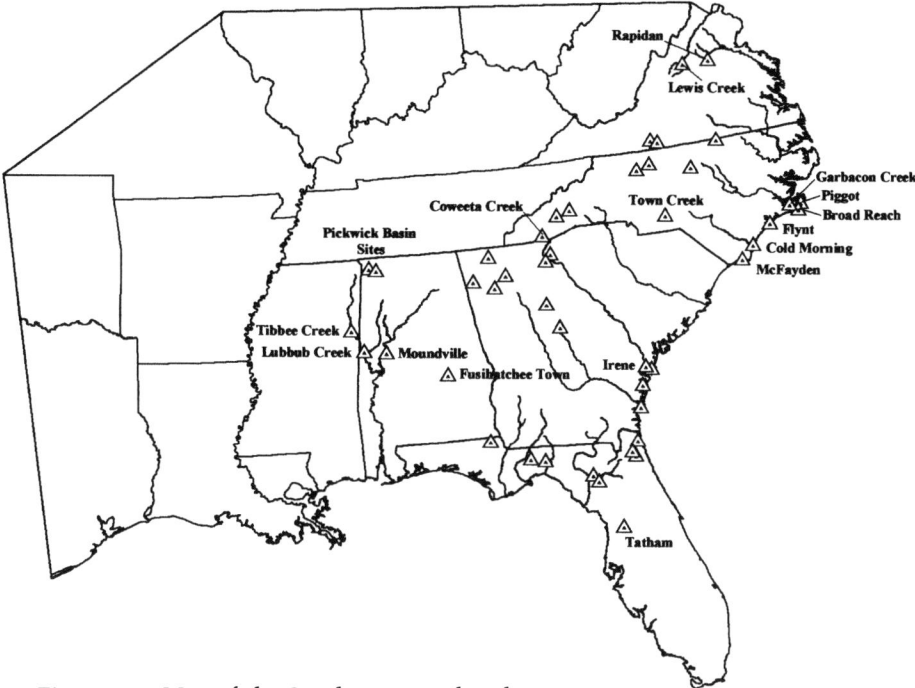

Figure 1-1. Map of the Southeast. For details on site
location, see individual chapters (Map generated by Timothy E. King).

Moundville tended to form in rich bottomland environments, where
resources were abundant, predictable, and transferrable (C. Scarry
1993a; J. Scarry 1996), and an adequate food supply can help to mitigate
the impact of infectious disease. This is just one of the many related
issues explored by papers that span the entire Southeast region, from
Texas in the west to North Carolina and Virginia in the east (Figure
1-1). Chapters are organized by geographic region, beginning in the
Middle Mississippian heartland and ending in Virginia just beyond the
Mississippian cultural periphery.

The volume begins with a contribution by Mary Lucas Powell on
the epidemiology of treponematosis and tuberculosis in the age of agriculture. This synthesis covers both historical and current clinical
thinking on these two infectious diseases, and uses data from fifteen
Southeast states to reconstruct their prehistoric prevalence and distribution. The broad geographic coverage reveals epidemiologically significant patterns in the visibility of these diseases reminiscent of but
also distinct from those of modern strains and provides a basis for understanding ancient pathogenicity.

The next three chapters pertain to Moundville and other settlements in Alabama. In Chapter 3, Patricia S. Bridges, Keith P. Jacobi,

and Mary Lucas Powell review the osteological evidence for violent trauma in aboriginal populations of west-central and northwest Alabama. Their study explores the demographic correlates of warfare in the late prehistory of this region and documents a clear relationship between settlement size and the risk of violent injury. Isotopic evidence for the collapse of the Moundville chiefdom are explored by Margaret J. Schoeninger, Lisa Sattenspiel, and Mark R. Schurr in Chapter 4. Bringing ceramic, botanical, isotopic, and paleopathological evidence to bear on the problem of cultural terminations, the authors propose a biological explanation for the demise of this once populous chiefdom. In Chapter 5, Marianne Reeves compares the health of the contact-period population of Fusihatchee Town with that of the Mississippian period population of Moundville in order to assess the effects of European contact on the native population of Alabama. Focusing on two dental indicators of health, Reeves finds that the consequences of European contact were very different for indigenous residents of Fusihatchee Town, despite their participation in the deerskin trade, than they were for contemporaneous mission Indians of the Georgia Bight.

The following three chapters focus on diet and health in prehistoric and contact-period agriculturalists of Florida and Georgia. Dietary diversity is the subject of Chapter 6 by Dale L. Hutchinson, Clark Spencer Larsen, Lynette Norr, and Margaret J. Schoeninger. Appealing to stable carbon and nitrogen isotopes from human bones, these researchers document a lack of homogeneity in subsistence strategies across this region that appears to correlate with the availability of natural resources and the agricultural potential of the land. In Chapter 7, Clark S. Larsen and Leslie E. Sering examine the health consequences of European contact and missionization on island populations of the Georgia Bight by tracking porotic hyperostosis frequencies in precontact and postcontact agriculturalists. Drawing on worldwide bioarchaeological and clinical studies of iron-deficiency anemia, their data reveal a disturbing picture of life for the missionized native populace. The final study from this region (Chapter 8) by Matthew A. Williamson considers the influence of topography on patterns of arthritis in late prehistoric farmers from interior and coastal Georgia. In a contribution that presages the potential of map data for understanding biological diversity, the author reports some notable differences between upland and coastal dwellers in the severity of degenerative joint disease that suggest an intimate and telling link between surface topography and joint pathology.

The last three chapters in the volume focus on regions at or beyond the Mississippian periphery. In Chapter 9, Elizabeth I. Monahan and David S. Weaver approach the problem of Late Woodland subsistence on the North Carolina coast through an examination of dental, iso-topic, and archaeological evidence. The importance of maize to coastal dwellers of North Carolina is not well understood, and these researchers go a long ways toward resolving the issue of dietary composition in this region. In the following chapter (Chapter 10), Patricia M. Lambert examines health in late prehistoric and contact-period agricultural populations of interior North Carolina and Virginia. Looking for temporal and geographic variability in the frequency of five disease-related skeletal lesions, the author finds evidence for variability in both parameters and argues that local environmental conditions, settlement patterns, and unique cultural practices may all have influenced health in these Southeast farming communities. The volume concludes with a bioarchaeological analysis of mortuary variability in late prehistoric Virginia (Chapter 11). Appealing to skeletal indices of diet and disease, Debra L. Gold refutes a number of hypotheses that have been proposed to explain variability in burial practices, and she offers a different and provocative explanation for the maintenance of diversity in mortuary behavior in this mid-Atlantic state.

The contributed chapters in this volume present new data and offer new perspectives on human biocultural adaptation to the various geographic and cultural landscapes that compose the Southeast culture area. As a compilation of southeastern studies, the volume is intended to build on previous efforts (e.g., Powell et al. 1991) to provide regional archaeologists and bioarchaeologists with new data and insights on life in indigenous communities of this region. Beyond this goal, the chapters in this volume probe new territory in the realm of causation that should broaden its appeal to scholars of human biocultural adaptation and stimulate researchers to have a new look at some old data.

2 Ancient Diseases, Modern Perspectives: Treponematosis and Tuberculosis in the Age of Agriculture

Mary Lucas Powell

Major changes in patterns of Native American mortality, health, and disease accompanied the gradual transition from the Archaic hunter-gatherer lifeway, prevalent before 3,000 years B.P. throughout the Eastern Woodlands, to the sedentary agriculturally dependent late prehistoric lifeway described by the first Europeans to enter the Southeast in the early sixteenth century. The focus of this chapter is the natural history of two infectious diseases present before 1492 in the Eastern Woodlands: treponematosis and tuberculosis. The first produced abundant morbidity (mostly in older adults) but probably had little direct effect on fertility or mortality in populations where it was endemic. The second was far more dangerous: it possessed the ability to wipe out entire small communities in acute epidemics. Both diseases could be maintained indefinitely at the macro-population level despite relatively small individual group sizes.

New perspectives on *when, why,* and *how* these diseases established themselves in Eastern North American indicate that the initial evidence for treponematosis apparently predates that for tuberculosis by almost a millennium. Both diseases show their highest prevalence in late prehistoric (post-A.D. 1000) high-density sedentary villages. Although both have been identified in numerous archaeological population samples through careful comparisons of observed skeletal lesion patterns with key clinical and epidemiological features of modern tuberculosis and treponemal syndromes, the prehistoric and modern disease profiles are not absolutely identical. The burdens on morbidity and mortality levied by the prehistoric New World forms of these diseases may have been substantially different from the disastrous impact of the Old World forms of the same diseases introduced after 1492 by European and African contacts because of two factors: (a) long-term New World prehistoric host/pathogen coadaptation and (b) *relatively* superior prehistoric levels of general population health prior to the devastating cultural and biological impact of European conquest.

Recent methodological and theoretical advances in the identification of these two infectious diseases in human skeletal remains from archaeological excavations clearly demonstrate the transformation of paleopathology over the past century from a harmless pastime of scholarly physicians into a scientific discipline based on objective data interpreted within appropriate cultural and biological contexts. Brief overviews of these advances as regards each disease will be presented in this chapter, followed by summaries of the bioarchaeological evidence for their presence in skeletal series from Alabama, Arkansas, Florida, Georgia, Illinois, Kentucky, Louisiana, Ohio, Oklahoma, Mississippi, North Carolina, South Carolina, Tennessee, and Texas.

TREPONEMATOSIS: ONE DISEASE OR MANY?

The ongoing debate about the nature of treponemal disease in the Eastern Woodlands of North America before 1492 (Baker and Armelagos 1988; Crosby 1969; Desowitz 1997; El-Najjar 1979; Hudson 1968; Powell 1994b, 1998) was complicated at the outset by the limited nature of the clinically derived diagnostic models available to nineteenth-century physicians interested in investigating prehistoric patterns of disease. In 1876, the noted Civil War physician Dr. Joseph Jones published a description of "syphilis" in skeletons excavated from a series of stone box graves from late prehistoric Native American sites in the Nashville Basin region of central Tennessee (Jones 1876). Jones based his diagnosis on distinctive lytic and osteoblastic lesions in the crania and long bone shafts, which in his opinion closely resembled the skeletal pathology characteristic of cases of advanced venereal syphilis, a disease familiar in nineteenth-century clinical practice. In living patients, these bone lesions often underlay contiguous ulcerous gummas of the scalp, forearms, and shins and were accompanied by deep bone pain (ostalgia) and significant soft tissue destruction.

This diagnosis was soon echoed in the reports by other physicians of pathological specimens recovered from prehistoric contexts throughout the Southeast. When Dr. D. S. Lamb of the United States Army Medical Museum in Washington, D.C. examined skeletal material sent to him "from mounds in Moundville, Ala., contributed by Mr.

Clarence B. Moore," he reported, "Of these 70 [bones], fifty show the usual conditions found in bone-syphilis, such as periosteal nodes, especially along the crest of the tibia, irregular erosions, scleroses and necroses of long bones [and] erosions of calvarium [sic] as from gummata. . . . I do not think that there can be any doubt that these bones are from cases of syphilis" (Moore 1907:339–340).

This same diagnosis was reached independently two decades later by the physicians W. L. Haltom and A. R. Shands, who were apparently unfamiliar with Dr. Lamb's earlier study, after examining additional material excavated from Moundville. They concluded, "There appears to be sufficient evidence in these twenty-four bone specimens to prove that syphilis existed in the Mound Builders four centuries before the discovery of America by Columbus" (Haltom and Shands 1938:242). However, they also noted as "interesting" the conspicuous absence of the dental stigmata of congenital syphilis: "despite the examination of many thousands of well-preserved teeth none were found which could be called Hutchinson's incisors" (Haltom and Shands 1938:232).

In his review of the archaeological evidence for pre-Columbian American "syphilis" (Williams 1927, 1932, 1936), the physician H. U. Williams noted the diagnoses by Jones (1876) for Tennessee skeletons and by Ales Hrdlička (1922) for skeletal material from sites in Florida, as well as his own observations from additional material from those two states and from Ohio. In 1944 pathological specimens from various Adena sites in northern Kentucky sent by Charles Snow to Dr. William McKee German for examination elicited a surprised diagnosis. Noting "the numerous sabre shin bones," Dr. German opined, "May not the evidence be adding up to a point where we might consider them evidence of syphilis?" (Webb and Snow 1945:275).

These diagnoses of pre-Columbian "syphilis" published over a period of seventy years by clinically experienced North American physicians who seemed (with the exception of Williams) largely unaware of each others' paleopathological research were all based on venereal syphilis, the only form of treponemal disease that was well known through the medical literature of the time. European physicians stationed at colonial outposts in Africa and Asia also frequently mistook various forms of nonvenereal treponematoses with venereal syphilis, often with disastrous consequences for social policies of disease control (Vaughn 1992).

Drawing on Butler's (1936) provocative "unitarian" thesis of multiple related but nonidentical treponemal syndromes, alternate diagnostic models began to appear in the 1950s written by physicians with extensive clinical knowledge of other forms of this Protean disease: yaws in tropical Africa (Hackett 1951) and endemic syphilis in Iraq (Hudson 1958), Africa (Grin 1956; Murray et al. 1956), and Bosnia

(Grin 1953). A fourth treponemal syndrome called "pinta" had been identified in certain parts of Mexico and Central America (Ash and Spitz 1945). Because pinta does not typically produce bone lesions, it will not be discussed at length here.

Each syndrome is associated in the clinical literature with a particular bacterial spirochete of the genus *Treponema*: *T. pallidum* (venereal and endemic syphilis), *T. pertenue* (yaws), and *T. carateum* (pinta). Hudson (1965) argued that these variations represent different *strains* of *T. pallidum* rather than different *species* of the genus *Treponema* because organisms cultured from lesions of the different syndromes are not distinguishable by classic immunological or microscopic techniques (Turner and Hollander 1957). However, recent comparisons of DNA sequences within and between different pathogenic *Treponema* organisms (e.g., Hardham et al. 1997, and others) have revealed microvariations that may affect pathogenicity. This vast family of related bacteria includes a number of free-ranging saprophytic treponemal spirochetes, whose earlier forms may have given rise to treponemal pathogens infecting primates and, eventually, *Homo sapiens* (Cockburn 1963).

The four modern syndromes "produce a pathological gradient extending from the cutaneous manifestations of pinta to the ulcers of yaws involving both skin and bone, to similar lesions of endemic syphilis affecting the skin, bone, and cardiovascular system, and finally to the lesions of venereal syphilis affecting all of the organs just mentioned in addition to the nervous system" (Steinbock 1976:92). The syndromes are associated with different epidemiological contexts, including variations in cultural factors.

The three endemic treponemal syndromes (endemic syphilis, yaws, and pinta) are typically contracted in early childhood through direct skin-to-skin contact with infectious skin lesions, not through sexual intercourse (Hudson 1965; Kiple 1994; Musher and Knox 1983). Prevalence levels in endemic areas approach 100 percent, and bone involvement of some sort (minor in most cases) occurs in up to 50 percent of late cases, resulting from hyperallergic response by sensitized hosts (Hackett 1951). Invasion of major organ systems is rare, in contrast to the well-known effects of venereal syphilis on the cardiovascular system, the brain, and the motor nerves.

Untreated venereal syphilis severely dampens human fertility through miscarriages and stillbirths of infected fetuses. Because of an important epidemiological characteristic, however, congenital cases are very rarely reported in areas where yaws and nonvenereal syphilis are endemic. Most conceptions occur in women who acquired the endemic infection at least a decade prior to menarche: as a result, the very low level of spirochetes present in their bodies greatly reduces the likelihood of passage through the placenta to infect the fetus. In contrast, because venereal syphilis is most typically transmitted to women through the same behavioral act that results in pregnancy, a woman may literally become pregnant and syphilitic at the same moment, thus exposing her fetus to very high levels of pathogens circulating through the maternal bloodstream (Grin 1956).

Bone lesions of treponematosis may be either nonspecific (periostitis, osteitis, and more rarely, osteomyelitis) or pathognomonic (gummateous osteoperiostitis and *caries sicca*) (Grin 1953, 1956; Hackett 1951, 1976; Hudson 1958). They do not appear during the primary stage of disease but may appear along with skin and muco-cutaneous lesions late in the secondary stage. Tertiary stage lesions may recur intermittently throughout life in ca. 30–50 percent of untreated individuals, often producing significant destruction of oral/nasal tissues (called *gangosa* in tertiary yaws) and distortion of long bone shafts from repeated episodes of periostitis (most notably, the characteristic "sabre shin" tibiae). The direct impact of the endemic syndromes on mortality is negligible because they do not invade vital organ systems, but the gummateous skin lesions invite superinfection by bacterial and mycotic agents and so may invite death by secondary effect. Bones lying close underneath the skin (e.g., the cranial vault, the superior aspect of the clavicle, and the anterior crest of the tibia) are readily affected through spread of infection from adjacent skin lesions.

Hackett (1951:13) remarked apropos of the yaws cases he studied in Uganda, "The patients showing these bone lesions were not severely ill, although they suffered considerable discomfort." Hudson (1961:3) echoed this evaluation in his description of "nature's prognosis" for untreated cases of endemic syphilis: "discomfort and pain, deformity and mutilation, a shortened life perhaps, but little [direct] mortality . . . per se."

Since Jones's 1870s explorations, many prehistoric sites in the Midwest and Southeast have yielded Native American skeletons with grossly distorted tibia shafts (Figure 2-1), such as this specimen from the Mississippian site of Moundville in Alabama, which resembles the classic "sabre shins" seen in modern yaws in tropical regions. Other skeletal individuals from these regions exhibit distinctive osteolytic lesions of the cranial vault, as seen on this cranium from the Mississippian site of Upper Nodena in northeast Arkansas (Figure 2-2), which resemble osseous sequellae of the gummateous scalp ulcerations seen in modern yaws and both forms of syphilis. Still other individuals show destruction of oral and nasal structures, like the extensively remodeled nasal margin on this cranium from Irene Mound (Figure 2-3), sometimes accompanied by localized necrosis of the bony palate suggestive of the hideous mutilations called "gangosa" in modern yaws

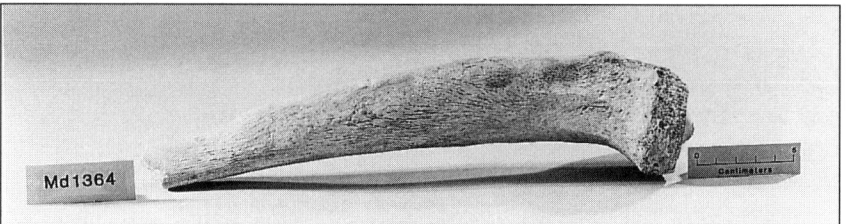

Figure 2-1. "Sabre" Tibia (right) of Young Adult Male. Burial 1364, Moundville, Alabama. (Photograph by Polly Futato)

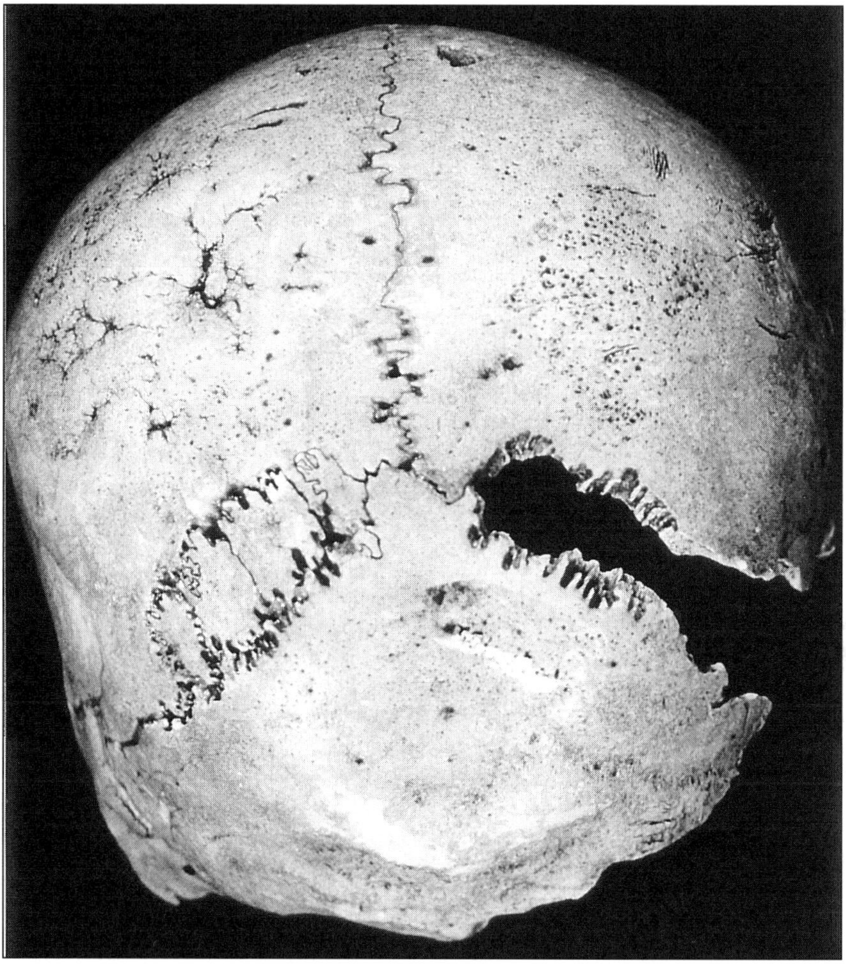

Figure 2-2. Remodeled Caries Sicca Lesions on Posterior Cranial Vault of an Adult Female. AMNH 432, Upper Nodena, Arkansas. (Photograph by Keith Jacobi)

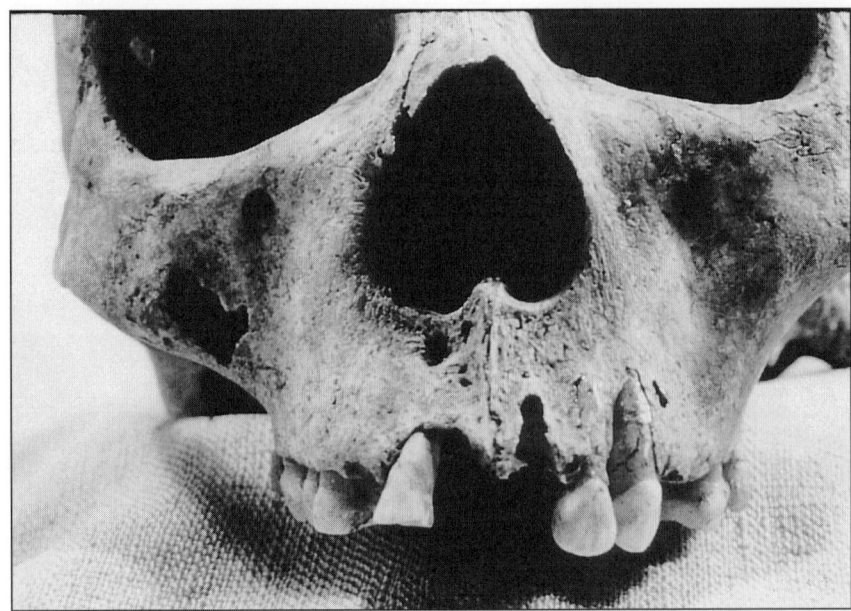

Figure 2-3. Treponemal Lesions of Right Nasal Margin and Right Maxilla of a Young Adult Female. NMNH 385540, Irene Mound, Georgia. (Photograph by Mary Lucas Powell)

and endemic syphilis. The presence of some form(s) of treponemal *disease* in the Eastern Woodlands before 1492 is now generally accepted by paleopathologists and archaeologists (Baker and Armelagos 1988; Larsen 1997; Ortner and Putschar 1981; Powell 1988, 1994b, 1998; Steinbock 1976). This acceptance, based on interpretations of skeletal lesions, has been given additional support by the recent identification of biochemical markers of treponemal infection through antigen-antibody assay (Ortner et al. 1992). But the manifestations of the prehistoric disease throughout Native American populations of the Eastern Woodlands vary across time periods and ecological zones, as we shall see below.

TREPONEMATOSIS IN THE EASTERN WOODLANDS

Before the Age of Agriculture

Treponematosis probably first appeared in the Southeastern Woodlands during the Late Archaic period, some 3,000–4,000 years B.P. The early evidence is not abundant, however. Snow's (1948) identification of three cases from the Late Archaic Indian Knoll site on the Green River in west-central Kentucky has been supported by other researchers who have identified additional cases in that series (Brothwell 1970; Brothwell and Burleigh 1975; Cassidy 1972; Kelley 1980). Several cases have also been tentatively identified from other Late Archaic sites in the same region: Barrett (Sandford et al. 1998; Weaver et al. 1998) and Carlson Annis (Mensforth n.d.). Diagnoses of treponematosis in hunter-gatherer population samples from the Gulf of Mexico and Florida have invoked identifications with all of the modern syndromes that produce bone lesions. At the Callo del Osso site in downtown Corpus Christi, Texas, Jackson and coauthors (1986) interpreted the pattern of widespread prevalence of moderate-to-severe "sabre shin tibia" as evidence of an endemic syndrome perhaps resembling modern nonvenereal syphilis. Dockall and Steele (1995) drew the same conclusions in their analysis of burials from ten hunter-gatherer series located along the western margin of the Gulf coast. Both sets of researchers suggested that the disease could have been maintained on a regional level through the social mechanism of seasonal aggregations, despite the hypothesized small size of the individual hunter-gatherer groups. These interpretations include explicit epidemiological analogies based on observations of endemic treponematosis in historic hunter-gatherer populations in Australia and South Africa (Hudson 1963).

At Morton Shell Mound in southern Louisiana, Robbins (1978) hypothesized that the subtropical ecological setting fostered instead a "yaws-like" treponemal syndrome among the hunter-gatherers who inhabited this marshy region. Bullen's (1972) interpretation of skeletal pathology at the Tick Island Archaic site, however, was clearly guided by her explicit mandate: "What we are now looking for in the archaeological record is incontestable evidence of the *presence* of syphilis in Florida in pre-Columbian times" (Bullen 1972:133). Regarding Bullen's convictions, it should be noted that no cases of congenital transmission were suggested in any of these early Gulf coast series.

Woodland Gardeners and Late Prehistoric Farmers

Treponematosis has been reported from several Woodland-period skeletal series in the Midwest. Examining skeletal remains from Ozark Bluffdweller sites representing Woodland cultures in northwestern Arkansas, Wakefield and Dellinger (1940:457) "were impressed by a number of tibias . . . of increased density and a marked deformity over the anterior aspects [consisting] of a rounded anterior surface. Occasionally this deformity was great enough to give the impression that the bone was bowed anteriorly."

Pathological specimens from various Woodland-period Adena sites in northern Kentucky submitted in 1944 by Charles Snow to a clinical pathologist, Dr. William McKee German, for examination, elicited a surprised diagnosis: "I am struck with the increasing volume of lesions which could by explained by syphilis—the numerous sabre shin bones—" (Webb and Snow 1945:275). Recent reexaminations of the Robbins and Wright Mounds series by George Milner and this author have confirmed a treponemal diagnosis, although not necessarily identical to venereal syphilis (G. Milner, personal communication 1998).

Cook's identification of treponematosis in Middle and Late Woodland village horticulturalists of the Lower Illinois River Valley (1976, 1984) is a superb model of epidemiological differential diagnosis. The abundance of post-cranial skeletal evidence versus the rarity of cranial lesions, the preponderance of healed versus active lesions, the increase in prevalence by age within her population samples, and the absence of dental or skeletal lesions indicative of congenital transmission all suggested some nonvenereal form of the disease, endemic throughout the region and well adapted to its host population.

The presence of pre-Columbian treponematosis becomes increasingly visible throughout the Eastern Woodlands after A.D. 1000. Changes in population density and settlement pattern undoubtedly played a major role in this transition. Sedentary community life conferred on ill persons the benefit of reduced demands for periodic mobility, but this benefit was counterbalanced by the increased danger from abundant pathogens within the confines of crowded villages contaminated with human wastes, insect vectors, and zoonoses carried by domesticated dogs. Increasing population size meant not only more people living within paramount Mississippian communities but also regular interactions with regional villages, hamlets, and farmsteads linked with those central sites.

Endemic treponematosis is not, strictly speaking, a "density-dependent" disease such as the acute viral and bacterial infections so common in industrialized cities. Nevertheless, during the highly infectious primary and secondary stages of the disease, lasting from a few months to several years, individuals may inadvertently spread the disease through shared eating and drinking utensils, clothing, bedding, and nonsexual physical contact. In the modern "yaws belts" of tropical Africa and Asia, the large numbers of young children in crowded villages and towns provide greater densities of both *highly infectious cases* and *previously uninfected individuals*, particularly in ecological and cultural contexts where clothing is minimal throughout most seasons.

Hudson (1965:893) noted that the rise of sedentary villages provided a more congenial setting for endemic treponemal disease than did the hunter-gatherer nomadic lifeway: "The propagation of treponematosis was enhanced in the village by [the] increase in the number of children, and by the increased frequency and intimacy of childhood contacts amid the crowded and unhygienic conditions of village life.

The internal environment was so well suited to the endemic spread of treponematosis that the villages of the world became its citadel and their children the reservoir of yaws and endemic syphilis; they remain so to this day."

The apparent increased prevalence of treponematosis in the Age of Agriculture in the Southeast is typified in Cassidy's (1972, 1984) comparison of the disease at Indian Knoll (2–3 percent of the series) and at the Fort Ancient site called Hardin Village in northern Kentucky, where 31 percent of the series showed the "disseminated periostitis syndrome," which she suggested represented an endemic treponematosis. The same pathology was observed by the present author in a smaller contemporaneous series from the Buckner site north of Lexington. Brothwell identified "at least 9 individuals [with] vault changes that might indicate treponematosis" in a series consisting mostly of adult crania from the slightly earlier May's Lick site not far from Hardin Village, dated to the fourteenth century A.D. (Brothwell and Burleigh 1975:394).

Skeletal pathology diagnostic of treponemal disease is far more common in late prehistoric Caddo maize farmers in Oklahoma and Texas than in Archaic or Woodland hunter-gatherer peoples from this area (Brues 1957, 1958, 1959; Goldstein 1957; Lee 1997; Mires 1982; Powell and Rogers 1980; Robey 1995; Rose and Harmon 1989; Wilson 1998). As Rose and Harmon (1989) note, the reported prevalence rates for skeletal pathology are not always strictly comparable between studies because of differing methodologies employed by the analysts, but inflammatory/infectious reactions definitely increase through time, as do descriptions of individual cases that include treponemal criteria.

At Dickson Mounds in Illinois, the prevalence of an unidentified "inflammatory osseous reaction" affecting mainly the lower limbs of adults increased dramatically from Late Woodland to Middle Mississippian times (Lallo 1973). The paleopathologist who analyzed this series did not conduct a differential diagnosis aimed at identification of specific infectious disease(s). Nevertheless, his descriptions of the predominant forms of osteoblastic lesions, focusing on numerous examples of severely distorted tibiae and other long bones, are strongly suggestive of the endemic treponemal syndromes identified by Cook (1976) in Woodland populations in the Lower Illinois Valley and also by Cassidy (1972, 1984) in her Fort Ancient sample from Kentucky. Lallo observed that only 20.2 percent (24/119) of adult tibiae were affected by this pathological process in the Late Woodland portion of his series; this prevalence rose to 27.4 percent (64/234) during the transition to the Mississippian lifeway and peaked at 84.0 percent (163/194) during the Middle Mississippian era (Lallo 1973:208).

Lesions highly characteristic of treponematosis affecting at least

Table 2-1. Cultural Features That Promote Different Modes of Treponemal
Transmission

Nonvenereal	Venereal

Climate and Clothing

| Climate and social mores promote patterns of dress that minimize physical barriers to frequent nonsexual contact among individuals of all ages. | Clothing for both sexes and all ages typically cover much of the body most of the time. Non-sexual skin-on-skin contact is infrequent. |

Domestic Items

| Regular communal use of eating and drinking utensils by family and/or community members. Sharing of unwashed clothing and bedding is the common pattern. | Individual use of eating and drinking utensils replaces shared pattern. Sleeping areas become more private, less communal. |

Hygiene and Sanitation

| Personal hygiene is poor, due to low availability of hot water and soap for bathing and washing. Inadequate community sanitation promotes insects that serve as mechanical vectors for pathogens. | Personal cleanliness is improved due to better facilities for washing. Improved waste disposal diminishes abundance of many insect vectors of disease. |

Medical Practices

| Weak concepts of contagion and lack of germ theory do not promote isolation of infectious individuals. No medical services are available to eradicate disease, though remedies to alleviate symptoms may be known. | Advanced medical theory may recognize importance of isolation of diseased persons. Medical therapies that actually eliminate pathogens may be available. |

Sexual Customs

| Childhood exposure to endemic treponemes provides some degree of adult immunity to later reinfection, regardless of patterns of adult sexual activity. | Prostitution and general promiscuity encourage the spread of venereal disease in nonimmune adults. |

Sources: Cockburn 1963; Hackett 1963; Hudson 1946, 1958, 1965; Hulton 1984;
Willcox 1972

10 percent of adults (with additional adults and a few subadults showing less specific degrees of pathological involvement) have been reported in late prehistoric horticultural and agricultural population
samples from Alabama (Powell 1988, 1991a, 1998), Arkansas (Powell
1991a), Florida (Hutchinson 1993a, 1993b; Hutchinson et al. 1998;
Iscan and Miller-Shaivitz 1985), Georgia (Hutchinson et al. 1998;
Powell 1991a, 1992a), Illinois (Cook 1976, 1984, 1998; Milner 1983,
1992), Ohio (Orton 1905), Kentucky (Cassidy 1972, 1984; Garten 1997),
North Carolina (Bogdan and Weaver 1992; Reichs 1989; Sandford et
al. 1994, 1998; Weaver et al. 1998), and Tennessee (Eisenberg 1986;
Powell and Eisenberg 1998). However, both the pathological evidence
(lesion form and patterning within individuals, the absence of pathognomonic congenital pathology [Cook 1990, 1994]) and the epidemiological contexts of these populations (Tables 2-1 and 2-2) argue strongly
against interpretation of this disease as analogous to modern venereal
syphilis.

If the latter had been present as a typical form, we would expect to
see in the paleopathological record numerous examples of the distinctive developmental malformations affecting the maxillary incisors and
the first mandibular molars ("Hutchinson's incisors" and "Moon's"
or "mulberry" molars), whose prevalence in congenitally transmitted
cases of venereal syphilis has been estimated at ca. 30 percent in modern clinical samples (Cook 1994; Jacobi et al. 1992). These malformations render the defective dental enamel of these teeth more subject to
damage after eruption; however, such defects have been reported in historic population samples known to have been afflicted with venereal
syphilis and whose general rates of tooth wear were similar to those
typical of most late prehistoric populations (Jacobi et al. 1992).

Arguments pro and contra a New World origin for venereal syphilis
were debated anew at a recent International Congress on the origins
of venereal syphilis in Europe (Dutour et al. 1994). From the extensive
evidence presented at this lively scientific venue, the pre-Columbian
presence of *some form(s)* of treponemal disease is more clearly apparent in the American bioarchaeological record than in its European
counterpart. It seems possible that the introduction of New World treponematosis, fundamentally endemic in its native form and acquired
through variable means from Native American contacts, into the quite
different epidemiological context of late-fifteenth-century European
populations may have resulted in a *venereally spread* outbreak of a
"new" disease. Alfred Crosby (1969:122–164) noted that the New
World was identified by several medical authorities as the source of the
terrible new disease, spread by venereal contact, which swept western
Europe in the late 1490s. Among them was the Spanish physician Ruy
Diaz de Isla, who stated in 1539 that "the disease had its origin and

Table 2–2. Pre-1492 Southeastern Native American Life: Cultural Features
Affecting Transmission of Treponematosis

Specific Cultural Features That Would Promote One Mode Over the Other	MODE	
	Endemic	Venereal
Clothing Young children often were unclothed until they reached puberty. Adults' garments often left the arms and legs bare.	Yes	No
Shared Domestic Items Common family use of eating utensils was typical. Domestic interior space was closely shared, including bedding.	Yes	No
Hygiene and Sanitation Bathing was common in streams, but bactericidal soap was unknown. Sweat lodge treatments might have killed some treponemes in open lesions. The abundant flies served as mechanical vectors of pathogen transmission.	Yes	No
Medical Practices Isolation of ill individuals was not typical. Minor lesions were usually left uncovered. Herbal medicines could treat disease symptoms but not eliminate them.	Yes	Yes
Numerous early European accounts comment on apparent absence of venereal diseases.	Yes	No
Effect of Sexual Customs Variable among different groups, but no institutionalized prostitution.	Variable	

Sources: Hudson 1976; Lawson 1709; Swanton 1946; Vogel 1970

birth from always in the island which is now named 'Espanola.'" Furthermore, if Old World forms of treponematosis were indeed as rare in western European populations as they appear in the bioarchaeological record, perhaps because they had been very recently introduced from tropical Africa or the Near East, it is possible that these populations' immunological vulnerability may have contributed to the savage virulence of the new disease as reported in contemporary medical accounts of the first decades of its appearance (Quetel 1990). At the present time, then, regarding the nature of treponematosis in the Eastern Woodlands before 1492, it still seems prudent to say, "Why call it syphilis?"

TUBERCULOSIS

The modern disease known as tuberculosis is most often caused in humans by the gram-negative microorganism *Mycobacterium tuberculosis* or (in areas where bovine tuberculosis is still prevalent) *Mycobacterium bovis*, although immuno-compromised individuals may fall prey to other atypical mycobacteria (Clark et al. 1987; Schlossberg 1994). In endemic contexts, most people in each generation are initially infected in early childhood, most frequently from inhalation of pathogen-laden droplets exhaled from individuals with active pulmonary lesions. If general levels of health are good, more than half of those infected will never develop any clinical symptoms of disease, but individuals with faulty immune response (because of poor nutrition or other infections) may develop primary lesions in their lungs or hilar lymph nodes.

If death does not ensue, the mycobacteria may be walled up within fibrous capsules in the body, halting further progression of the disease. The microorganisms can remain viable for decades, however, even today with superior medical therapy, and severe systemic stress in later life may reactivate the disease process. Localized foci may rupture and spread mycobacteria via direct or hematogenous dissemination throughout the body, producing lesions in all types of tissue, including bone, and infecting new victims (Hoeprich 1977; Myers 1951; Schlossberg 1994). In longstanding cases, overstimulation of immune responses in hypersensitized tissues may result in such proliferation of granulomatous tissue within the lungs that pulmonary capacity is compromised and death follows.

Because of the extremely long viability of the encapsulated organisms, tuberculosis may be passed from one generation to the next in very small populations even if reinfection from outside sources is rare (Myers 1951). Tuberculosis was a major cause of death in children, adolescents, and young adults before the development of effective surgical and antibiotic therapies; the mortality from pulmonary tuberculosis ranged from 111 to 289 per 100,000 people in Europe and the United States in the first years of the twentieth century (Ortner and Putschar 1981).

Within the skeleton, the thoracic and lumbar vertebrae, ribs, and sternum are at high risk of hematogenous infection from active pulmonary lesions because of the pathogen's affinity for cancellous bone containing hemopoetic (red) marrow. Cavitation of vertebral bodies leads to spinal collapse, the anterior kyphosis that characterizes Pott's disease. Very little perifocal reactive bone formation accompanies localized cavitations in long bone epiphyses or metaphyses, and periosteal reaction is also rare. The hip and knee joints are often affected in tuberculous infants, children, and adolescents, with adult onset rare (Ortner and Putschar 1981; Schlossberg 1994).

In general, the disease process leads predominantly to destruction of existing bone tissue, rather than to proliferation of new bone tissue, a pattern with important implications for paleopathological diagnoses in curated archaeological series. The bones predominantly affected are fragile and prone to poor preservation and often not systematically collected in archaeological excavations. Skeletal lesions occur in only a small minority of cases with estimated prevalence rates ranging from 3 to 7 percent by most authorities (Ortner and Putschar 1981; Steinbock 1976), though Kelley and Micozzi (1984) have suggested that rib lesions may occur twice as frequently in pulmonary tuberculosis, which composes 90 percent of human cases.

Recent advances in molecular analysis of ancient amplified DNA and other organic materials have provided independent verification of previous paleopathological diagnoses of tuberculosis in human remains from New and Old World archaeological sites. DNA fingerprinting is used successfully to identify index cases in modern localized outbreaks of antibiotic-resistant tuberculosis by comparing different strains of *Mycobacterium tuberculosis* pathogens (Alland et al. 1994), and recovery protocols of DNA from ancient human tissues have been standardized. Comparisons of prehistoric mycobacterial DNA recovered from preserved individuals in Germany (Baron et al. 1996), England (Roberts and Dixon 1993; Taylor et al. 1996), Scotland, and Turkey (Spigelman and Lemma 1993) with DNA profiles of members of the modern *M. tuberculosis* complex (principally *M. tuberculosis* and *M. bovis*, the two species that most commonly infect mammalian hosts) suggest that tuberculosis has an exceedingly ancient pedigree as a human disease.

Most of these molecular studies have focused on a 123 base-pair segment of DNA, known as *IS6110*, unique to the *M. tuberculosis* complex (Salo et al. 1994). At the 1997 International Congress with the title "The Evolution and Palaeopathology of Tuberculosis," held in Szeged, Hungary, discussions of mycobacterial DNA and RNA were featured in seventeen of the eighty-six papers presented, a rate of almost 20 percent. Nine papers presented molecular aspects of modern mycobacteria in the United States, Guadeloupe, France, Hungary, Slovakia, and Austria. Eight other presentations summarized analyses of ancient mycobacterial DNA in human remains from Egypt, the Middle East, Borneo, Moravia, Lithuania, the Midwestern and Southwestern United States, Ontario, Peru, and Chile.

Another new molecular technique is based on detection of mycolic acids produced by pathogenic mycobacteria inside infected human hosts. This technique has been successfully applied to bone samples from identified tuberculous patients in a historic hospital cemetery (Newcastle Infirmary) as well as to samples from pathological and non-pathological skeletons from two archaeological sites in England (Child et al. 1997). These fatty acids in the cell walls of the mycobacteria can be readily detected by liquid chromatography (Ramos 1992), and this method has been used for some time in clinical settings for the verification of *M. tuberculosis* complex infection in living patients.

Mycolic acids may be found in tissues distant from the site of tuberculous lesions in ill individuals, and these acids are also detectable in individuals who have been *exposed* to the pathogenic mycobacteria but who have not developed symptoms of clinical disease. The exciting application of this clinical technique to archaeological specimens opens the way for investigations of true *prevalence* of prehistoric tuberculosis, that is, the proportion of *infected to uninfected* individuals in a skeletal sample rather than the mere identification of those few individuals who developed recognizable bone lesions before death. Modern tuberculosis affects bone in fewer than 10 percent of clinically ill patients (Schlossberg 1994), so lesions identifiable by paleopathological criteria represent merely the tip of the tip of the iceberg of tuberculous infection in past populations.

Ancient Tuberculosis in the New World

The first published report describing tuberculosis in prehistoric Native American skeletal material was made by W. F. Whitney (1886), only four years after the initial isolation of the bacillus *Mycobacterium tuberculosis* by Robert Koch in 1882. Throughout most of the twentieth century, paleopathological investigations into the possible prehistoric New World presence of the disease were dominated by views of the physical anthropologist and physician Ales Hrdlička. He had become acquainted with the ravages of the disease in his medical studies of Native American peoples in the Southwestern United States and northern Mexico during the first decade of the century. Hrdlička noted that tuberculosis assumed epidemic proportions on nearly every Indian reservation and concluded that "tuberculosis was rare, if it did exist" before extensive contact with European- or African-born colonizers. He based this diagnosis on careful consideration of a combination of factors, including *medical evidence* (lack of traditional remedies for the disease's prominent symptoms and pathological markers in elderly people), *historic and ethnographic records* (no reference to the disease by writers who reported on the earliest contacts), *oral history* (testimony by elderly Native Americans that the disease was "unknown or seldom seen among them in their early days"), and *archaeological evidence* (the absence of tuberculous human skeletal remains of unquestionably pre-Columbian origin and the extreme rarity of diagnostic pathology "in Indian bones dating from the period of the earliest contact with the whites"). Therefore, he reasonably concluded in his 1909 study, "The Indian presents everywhere a greater susceptibility to the disease than the white man; this means a lesser immunization of his system, indicating the more recent introduction of the infection into his race." He also recognized the significant negative impact of the generally very poor health status of reservation Native Americans, noting "It is to be assumed *on purely logical grounds* that the disease must have been much less frequent among the Indians in former times when they lived a more natural and active life, were better inured to hardships, and with exception of particular localities and periods, were better provided with suitable food" (Hrdlička 1909:1 [italics mine]).

Hrdlička's study included five reservations and one Indian school with high tuberculosis prevalence but differing "conditions of climate, environment, civilization, and contact with the whites." As Jane Buikstra noted in the introduction to her symposium volume, which she dedicated to Hrdlička's memory, this rigorous scholar "attributed paramount importance to cultural and environmental factors, with such oft-cited variables as lack of racial immunity and hereditary weakness assuming lesser importance" (Buikstra 1981:5). So although Hrdlička's investigation of tuberculosis was in some ways characteristic of "the study of bone" during the early and middle twentieth century, his emphasis on *interpretation of disease experience within an epidemiological context* was ahead of his time.

The next eminent physician to consider the question of pre-Columbian tuberculosis, Dr. Dan F. Morse, viewed the question from the perspective of his extensive medical experience at the Peoria Municipal Tuberculosis Sanitarium. In 1961 Morse published a major review of the available evidence from prehistoric Native American remains and artistic representations alleged to represent tuberculosis. His long interest in prehistoric Native American archaeology led him to doubt the pre-Columbian origin of several published specimens. Morse (1967, 1969) developed a set of rigorous criteria, based explicitly on "the careful comparison of observed prehistoric lesion patterns against those which, in his experience, were characteristic of clinically documented cases of tuberculosis" (Buikstra 1981:8). These criteria concentrated primarily on spinal pathology. He also evaluated (and rejected) various artistic images that depicted supposedly tuberculous "hunch-backed" individuals, molded in clay or painted on rock cliffs, but he concluded that other culturally based interpretations were more anthropologically and medically appropriate.

Morse utilized Hrdlička's prevalence data to predict that, if tuberculosis had been indeed present in prehistoric North America, one should expect to see *diagnostic vertebral tuberculosis* in approximately 6.7 of every 1,000 skeletons excavated. This statement disregards an essential difference between clinical and archaeological population samples: the mortality profiles of the latter are affected by cultural factors both intrinsic (mortuary programming) and extrinsic (theories and methods that affect archaeological recovery and curation of human remains) as well as by environmental factors that influence differential preservation of individuals of different ages (and therefore potentially different susceptibilities to specific diseases) (Roberts and Manchester 1995). Morse's predicted archaeological skeletal prevalence, incidentally, is less than one-tenth the reported prevalence of skeletal tuberculosis (8.8 percent = 88 cases per 1,000) cited in a review of the disease in the United States in 1969 and 1973 (Farer et al. 1979). The prehistoric specimens that he found acceptable on medical grounds were far too few, in his opinion, to justify a reasonable diagnosis of a genuinely pre-Columbian New World presence of the disease.

He was joined in this opinion, for some of the same reasons, by a third eminent physician, Dr. Aidan Cockburn, whose clinical experience with the disease fostered his interest in its natural history. He agreed with Hrdlička that the most typical form of Native American involvement, adenitis of the cervical lymph glands or "scrofula," bespoke a relatively recent population history with the disease, and he further noted the absence of any "satisfactory domestic animal [in prehistoric Native American contexts] to serve as an intermediate host or as a reservoir for the disease, a necessary factor as the pathogen spread to a human host" (Cockburn 1963:220–221). In his view, the prehistoric Americas also lacked sufficiently large population concentrations to foster such a communicable disease, and he firmly rejected the possibility of a New World pre-Columbian focus.

In 1973 these carefully considered negative verdicts were convincingly challenged by the first *microbiological* evidence for New World precontact tuberculosis: the report by Marvin Allison and colleagues of identifiable acid-fast bacilli from the body of a mummified child from the Nazca culture of southern Peru, dated around A.D. 700, who exhibited miliary tuberculosis and advanced bone lesions (Allison et al. 1973). Eight years later, in the volume of papers from Buikstra's 1978 symposium (Buikstra 1981) Allison and colleagues reported eleven additional cases from Peru and Chile with bone and/or soft tissue lesions characteristic of tuberculosis, dating from 800 B.C. to A.D. 1600; two of the Chilean cases with cavitary pulmonary lesions yielded acid-fast bacilli.

Buikstra and her fellow authors explored the epidemiology of this dread disease from a dynamic perspective, arguing that sufficient points of similarity existed between bone lesions of modern tuberculosis and those observed in prehistoric peoples throughout the Americas in cultural and ecological contexts that would have permitted maintenance of the disease, to posit the existence of a genuinely New World form of tuberculosis. The oldest cases came from sites in Peru and Chile (Allison et al. 1981), with one specimen dated at 160 B.C. and three others at A.D. 290. Tuberculosis has also been identified in late prehistoric precontact Andean populations (Buikstra 1981), as described for example in Buikstra and Williams's (1991) report on numerous cases of "a tuberculosis-like pathology" from fourteenth-century A.D. Estuquina in southern Peru. The discovery of ancient mycobacteria closely resembling modern *M. tuberculosis* within lung and lymph node lesions in mummified Andean bodies (Allison et al. 1973, 1981) supported the diagnosis based on pathognomonic tuberculous skeletal lesions in those same individuals.

These remarkable discoveries shifted paleopathological investigations of New World tuberculosis from the realm of the *theoretical* (does it seem plausible that the disease existed, given the constraints of population size, lack of suitable animal reservoirs, and paucity of skeletal evidence?) to the realm of the *verifiable* (can the ancient mycobacteria recovered from lesions be identified as pathogenic for tuberculosis?). In the 1990s molecular analyses of ancient pathogens and metabolites recovered from diseased bodies joined the investigative armamentarium focused on the question of indigenous New World tuberculosis. The 1994 report by Salo and colleagues on their identification of *M. tuberculosis* DNA in lesions from a Peruvian mummy dated around A.D. 1000 drew widespread attention to the research potential of this molecular approach and elevated the biological characterization of ancient New World pathogenic *Mycobacteria* spp. to a higher level.

In the Eastern Woodlands little evidence of this disease predates the Middle Woodland period. The oldest case reported is by Rathbun and coworkers (1980) in their description of an individual with vertebral and pelvic lesions suggestive of tuberculosis from Daw's Island on the South Carolina coast (3,300–3,700 B.C.). No pre-Woodland period skeletal evidence of tuberculosis has been reported during intensive searches of several large Middle and Late Archaic skeletal series from Indian Knoll and other sites in the Green River region of Kentucky; these searches included some 3,000 skeletal individuals (V. Haskins, personal communication 1998; Kelley 1980; R. Mensforth, personal communication 1998; Powell 1996a; M. Sandford, personal communication 1998). Similar studies of numerous Archaic skeletal series from

Tennessee (M. O. Smith, personal communication 1998) or Alabama (P. Bridges, personal communication 1998) show the same results.

In the Midwest and Southeast after 1000 A.D., however, the disease appeared at sites in Illinois (Buikstra and Cook 1978, 1981; Milner 1982, 1983, 1992; Milner and Smith 1990), Ohio (Katzenberg 1977; Widmer and Perzigian 1981), Kentucky (Cassidy 1972; Garten 1997), Tennessee (Kelley and Eisenberg 1987; Widmer and Perzigian 1981), Arkansas (Murray 1989), Georgia (Blakely 1978; Blakely and Mathews 1986; Powell 1991a, 1992a), Alabama (Powell 1988, 1991a, 1992a), and North Carolina (Lambert, this volume).

A computer simulation constructed by McGrath (1988) incorporated pathological and epidemiological features of modern tuberculosis to model the course of the disease over 100 years given different levels of population density and interaction in Woodland and Mississippian communities in the Lower Illinois River Valley. Her results suggested that the disease could not have been maintained for long periods without disappearing or causing the extinction of its human host populations. Buikstra and Cook (1981) had convincingly identified the disease at one of the sites (Schild) included by McGrath, and Milner (1992) described several cases from the Norris Farms #36 site, a small fourteenth-century Oneota frontier outpost in the same region. The most likely explanation for this apparent contradiction between the paleopathological, molecular, and epidemiological evidence is that the prehistoric Midwestern form of the disease did not produce the high levels of mortality associated with untreated modern tuberculosis.

Fort Ancient populations in Ohio (Turpin) and Kentucky (Hardin Village) also suffered from the insidious killer (Cassidy 1972; Garten 1997; Widmer and Perzigian 1981), as did the Mississippian communities of Arnold (Widmer and Perzigian 1981) and Averbuch (Kelley and Eisenberg 1987) in Tennessee. In Georgia, several individuals at the Mississippian Irene Mound site display lesions of vertebrae (Figure 2-4) or the sacroiliac joint (Figure 2-5) characteristic of tuberculosis (Powell 1991a, 1992a). Blakely and Mathews (1986) describe one case of spinal tuberculosis (a female in her early twenties) from the precontact Savannah II phase at the Beaverdam site (A.D. 1400–1600) in northeast Georgia. At the nearby contemporaneous Mississippian site of Etowah the skeletal evidence for this disease was more equivocal, the patterning of resorptive lesions suggesting either tuberculosis or North American blastomycosis (Blakely 1978).

At Moundville, the paramount community of a Mississippian chiefdom in west-central Alabama, no Early Mississippian individuals display lesions suggestive of tuberculosis. Nevertheless, during Moundville II (1250–1400 A.D.) several cases appear: the severely deformed

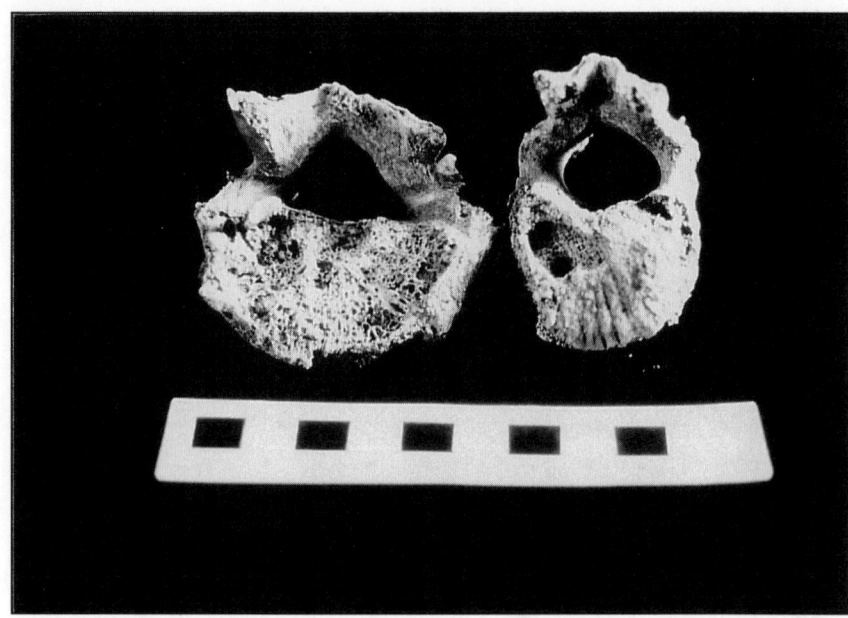

Figure 2-4. Two Vertebrae of a Young Adult Female Showing Tuberculous Lesions. NMNH 385562, Irene Mound, Georgia. (Photograph by Mary Lucas Powell)

spine of a young adult male (Figure 2-6) closely resembles radiographs and pathological descriptions of modern cases of spinal tuberculosis, known as "Potts' disease" (Myers 1951). Several other adults display less severe vertebral damage, and others exhibit osteoblastic rib lesions strongly suggestive of pleural tuberculosis (Roberts et al. 1994). The smaller Mississippian community of Lubbub Creek, located some 70 km to the west of Moundville, showed no evidence of the disease (Powell 1988), nor did the small Mississippian cemetery on Koger's Island in the Tennessee River in northwest Alabama (Powell 1996b).

At several of the late prehistoric sites mentioned above, high levels of skeletal and dental markers of stress, including porotic hyperostosis and cribra orbitalia, which indicate severe chronic iron-deficiency anemia, and frequent evidence of traumatic injuries characteristic of warfare suggest that the natural immunocompetence of the inhabitants was severely stressed. Two of the sites noted above, Norris Farms #36 in northern Illinois and Averbuch in central Tennessee, display high prevalences of multiple markers of severe skeletal stress. Norris Farms #36 was apparently an Oneota frontier settlement established within hostile territory, to judge from the extremely high levels of mortal injuries and mutilations (Milner and Smith 1990). Numerous wounded

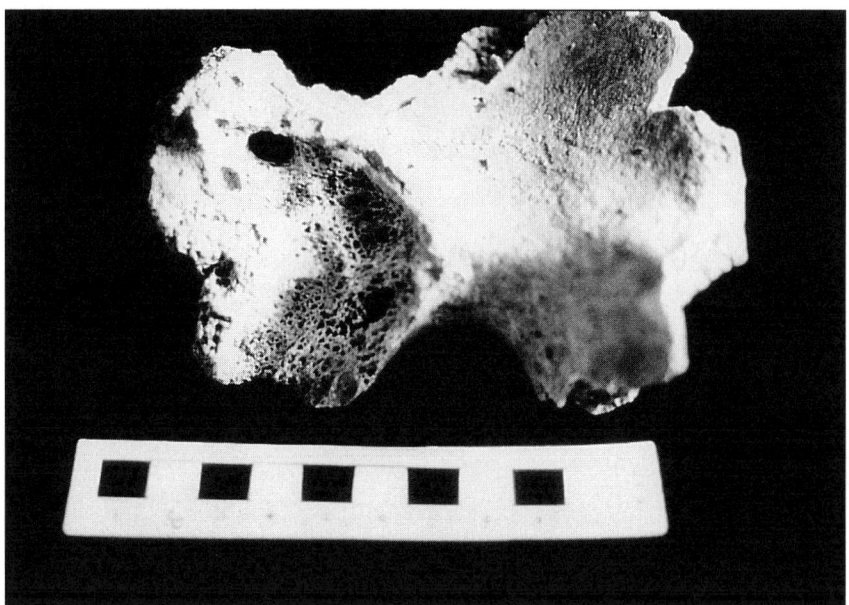

Figure 2-5. Left Ilium of Adult Female with Tuberculous Destruction of Sacroiliac Auricular Surface. NMNH 385411, Irene Mound, Georgia. (Photograph by Mary Lucas Powell)

individuals displayed debilitating skeletal lesions from treponemal disease and/or tuberculosis that would have limited their ability to flee or defend themselves against assault. A similarly high level of multiple stressors appears in the Averbuch series from Tennessee (Eisenberg 1986; Kelley and Eisenberg 1987), another site that shows abundant evidence of intergroup conflict.

Current applications of molecular analyses to human skeletal material from the Eastern Woodlands are expected to shed further light on the nature of this regional prehistoric form of the disease. The successful analysis by Braun and coworkers (1998) of amplified ancient DNA from fragments of mycobacterial pathogens lodged within skeletal lesions from the Schild site in Illinois and the Iroquois ossuary at Uxbridge in southern Ontario has supported the earlier paleopathological diagnosis of tuberculosis at these two sites (Buikstra and Cook 1981; Pfeiffer 1984). Bone samples from two sites in Kentucky, Indian Knoll (Archaic) and Hardin Village (late prehistoric), have been submitted by the W. S. Webb Museum of Anthropology, University of Kentucky, for mycolic acid analysis at the University of Newcastle. Tuberculosis, the disease, had not been definitely identified at the earlier Kentucky site, but the presence of several skeletal individuals with am-

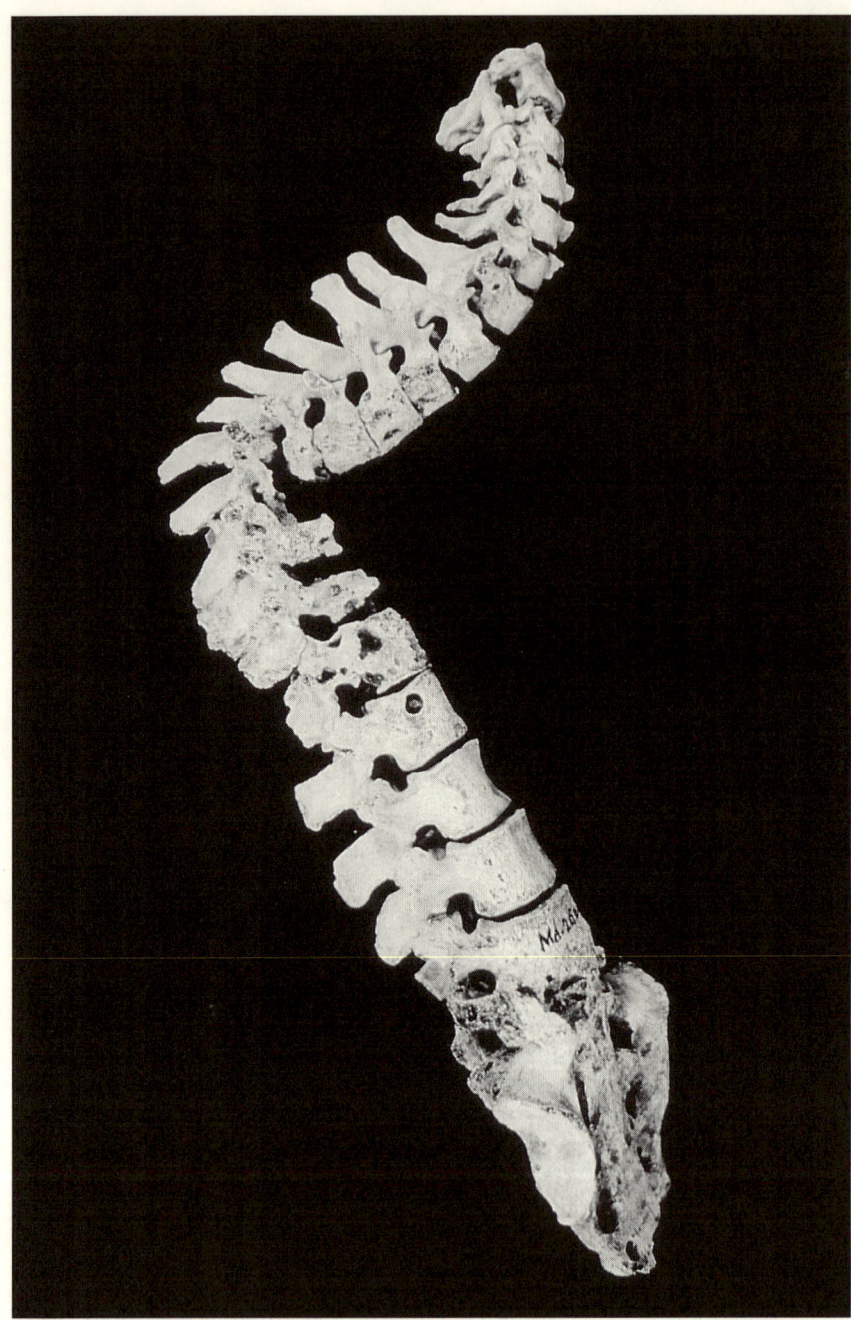

Figure 2-6. Vertebral Column of a Young Adult Male with Pott's Disease (Spinal Tuberculosis). Burial 2150, Moundville, Alabama. (Photograph by Keith Jacobi)

biguous spinal lesions suggested that molecular analysis might be useful. The two individuals sampled from the later site displayed vertebral lesions strongly suggestive of the disease (Garten 1997).

SUMMARY

Because all living organisms possess the capacity to evolve via genetic mutations, some of which will be maintained by natural selective pressures, paleopathologists who study patterns of ancient infectious diseases can never assume that ancient and modern forms of the same diseases are identical in their effects on their human hosts. Prehistoric American tuberculosis may have been less lethal than its modern analog, as suggested by McGrath's computer simulations, but this conclusion is by no means certain nor are the possible reasons to support it well understood. Differential virulence of modern strains of *Mycobacterium tuberculosis* has been well documented (Schlossberg 1994), and molecular comparisons of precontact and modern strains may eventually reveal similar variations. In the first decade of the twentieth century, Hrdlička (1909) recognized the disastrous impact of enforced reservation settlement on patterns of morbidity and mortality in Native Americans, particularly as regards tuberculosis, an opportunistic disease par excellence. As William Johnson notes in his survey of tuberculosis, "Perhaps no other disease better illustrate[s] the principle of multifactorial causation: The tubercle bacillus is a necessary but not the only condition. In addition, the host and the host's environment contribute numerous other causes central to its pathogenesis" (Johnson, in Kiple 1994:1059).

It seems more clearly evident that prehistoric American treponematosis, being essentially endemic in form, did carry less dreadful consequences for its victims than does modern venereal syphilis, for three reasons.

1. Because it was an endemic disease contracted by virtually everyone in childhood, it would not have borne the taint of illicit sex that stigmatizes our contemporary STDs, thus sparing its victims social ostracization.

2. Because it was an endemic disease contracted by virtually everyone in childhood, most girls by menarche had passed through the primary and secondary stages of the disease most dangerous to a developing fetus because of high maternal bloodstream levels of treponemal pathogens capable of crossing the placenta. The lack of congenital cases reported in modern endemic treponematosis has been attributed to this aspect of its epidemiology by certain medical specialists in the disease (Grin 1953, 1956; Murray et al. 1956). And this feature prob-

ably explains the extreme rarity of convincing evidence for congenital transmission in the Eastern Woodlands paleopathological record.

3. The modern endemic treponemal syndromes may drastically affect skin, mucous membranes, and bone, but they apparently do not affect essential organ systems as does tertiary-stage modern venereal syphilis: the cardiovascular system, the central nervous system, and the viscera. The near-absence of treponemes in these late-stage lesions argues to some clinicians that the destruction of tissues owes more to unregulated hyper-immune response evoked by decades of sensitization to the pathogens than to any direct action of the treponemes themselves. Whatever the mechanism, venereal syphilis in the pre-penicillin era could significantly limit population growth by increasing the prevalence of miscarriages, stillbirths, and neonatal deaths and could maim and kill many adults through cerebral paresis, tabes dorsalis, aortic aneurysms, and uncontrollable osteomyelitis. It seems likely that pre-Columbian victims of American treponematosis were spared these worst consequences, though some individuals in each generation clearly suffered some tertiary-stage disability.

At some late prehistoric sites, various individuals appear to have been affected simultaneously by treponematosis *and* tuberculosis, not a surprising situation considering the opportunistic nature of the latter disease. The two diseases display, in a sense, mirror images of each other in the bioarchaeological record because of their contrasting morbid and mortal effects (summarized in Table 2-3). Tuberculosis is far less visible than endemic treponematosis in archaeological series, for the following reasons.

1. Most otherwise healthy individuals who become infected with tuberculosis do not develop clinical disease; those who do often die from pulmonary or gastrointestinal lesions before adjacent skeletal regions are affected. By contrast, virtually 100 percent of individuals infected by treponemal syndromes will display some degree of *morbidity*, often with chronic recurrence but without associated premature *mortality*.

2. In older curated archaeological collections, spinal elements tend to be less well represented than long bones because vertebrae are more prone to postmortem destruction and many field projects neglected to collect them systematically. For example, in the Moundville series, fewer than 40 percent of the individuals were represented by thoracic and/or lumbar vertebrae, the most common sites of tubercular bone lesions. By contrast, more than 70 percent were represented by the postcranial bones most characteristically affected by treponemal infection.

3. The nature of the lesions produced by the different diseases also plays a role in affecting favorably or unfavorably the chances for post-

Table 2-3. Tuberculosis and Endemic Treponematosis: Morbid and Mortal Effects

	Tuberculosis	*Endemic Treponematosis*
I. <u>Epidemiology</u>		
Causative Organism	*Mycobacterium tuberculosis, Mycobacterium bovis*	*Treponema pallidum, Treponema pertenue*
Mode of Infection	Respiration, ingestion	Skin lesions
Modal age at exposure	Childhood	Childhood
Modal age at onset of clinical disease	Young adulthood	Childhood
Duration of infectious period	Decades	5-10 years
Viability of pathogen in environment	Extended periods	Brief periods
II. <u>Pathology</u>		
Initial lesions	Lungs, hilar lymph nodes	Mucocutaneous tissues
Subsequent lesions	Any organ system	Mucocutaneous tissues, bone
Prevalence of disease in endemic contexts	10-50 percent	25-100 percent
Radiographic prevalence of bone lesions	3-7 percent	5-15 percent
Predominant skeletal response	Osteolytic, minor osteoblastic	Osteoblastic, minor osteolytic
Skeletal regions typically affected	Spinal column, ribs, sternum, hip and knee joints	Tibia, fibula, ulna, radius, humerus, clavicle, cranial vault and oral/nasal region
Potential for lethal effect	Moderate to high	Low

Sources: Hackett 1951; Hoeprich 1977; Hudson 1946; Kelley and Micozzi 1984; Myers 1951; Ortner and Putschar 1981

mortem preservation. The osteolytic lesions characteristic of tuberculosis destroy bone tissue and weaken the fabric of affected skeletal elements. By contrast, the osteoblastic lesions characteristic of endemic treponematosis produce additional bone, thickening the cortex of affected long bones and rendering them more resistant to dissolution.

Therefore, paleopathologists investigating the presence of these two diseases must keep in mind that the *less* visible one (tuberculosis) may have killed far more people than did the one whose presence is easier to verify (treponematosis), although the latter may have in fact produced more widespread pain and transient disability in the population.

We do not yet know the *true* origins of these two diseases in the New World: whether in some form they crossed the Bering Strait with the ancestors of Native Americans or whether they arose in situ from indigenous saprophytic organisms (a possibility for treponematosis, given the broad range of environmental spirochetes) or zoonotic disease (for tuberculosis). The possibility of a zoonotic origin for New World tuberculosis has been neglected, primarily (I believe) because of Morse's and Cockburn's reservations about the absence of "any satisfactory domestic animal" reservoir (but see Klepinger 1982). The appearance of Old World tuberculosis in the Middle East 8,000 to 4,000 years ago has been linked with the domestication of cattle, and so domesticated bovids have long been considered the exemplary domesticated reservoir of the disease because human infection by *Microbacterium bovis* has been abundantly documented worldwide. Ingestion of milk from tubercular cows was the predominant mode of infection. Nevertheless, human infection via aerosolized bacilli has also been reported (Grange and Yates 1994) and apparently accounts for the persistence of human cases of *M. bovis* tuberculosis in rural districts in Europe years after pasteurization of milk was legally mandated. Recent cases of *M. bovis* tuberculosis have been reported in individuals born in southeast England decades before the effective eradication of bovine tuberculosis in domesticated cattle herds; these cases appear to represent endogenous reactivation of earlier untreated pulmonary infections, which may be then spread to other humans via the typical aerosol route (Grange and Yates 1994).

Infection by *M. bovis* can cause pathological symptoms in a wide range of domesticated and feral mammalian species, however, ranging from badgers to seals to camelids to American bison (Lignereux 1997). Humans may be infected in the course of such nonalimentary activities as herding, butchering, and even training infected animals (Grange and Yates 1994; Aufderheide and Rodriguez-Martin 1998). The association may be more causal than fortuitous between (a) the domestication of camelids by Native Americans in Peru and Chile and (b) the subsequent appearance *in those same populations* of pathological soft tissue and skeletal lesions that contain mycobacterial organisms very similar (some would say, identical) to the two major members of the modern *M. tuberculosis* complex, *M. tuberculosis* and *M. bovis*, that cause tuberculosis in humans and other mammals. In the Eastern Woodlands of North America potential animal reservoirs would minimally include two major Native American prey species, white-tailed deer (*Odocoileus virginianus*) and American bison (*Bison bison*), and probably other species as well. Future research on the origin(s) of indigenous New World human tuberculosis should incorporate available information from the extensive veterinary literature on *M. bovis* infections, as well as examinations of appropriate faunal remains for molecular evidence and pathological lesions associated with this ubiquitous pathogen, in order to verify its possible precontact presence in the Americas.

Nor do we know exactly how these two native diseases were "swamped" by the Old World forms introduced after A.D. 1492 by Europeans and Africans. Reexposure of hosts previously infected with treponematosis or with tuberculosis carries very different implications. In the modern treponematoses, immunity to reinfection gradually develops during the course of untreated disease; this immunity also confers protection against later infection by the same or another treponemal syndrome (Chulay 1990; Tramont 1990). In untreated cases, the individual is most infectious early in the disease (particularly during the first year), but because of the gradual reduction of the level of pathogens in the host's body, infectivity naturally wanes and is typically nullified by the fourth year (Tramont 1990). A Native American exposed first to New World treponematosis (whatever its form), typically in childhood, and then later exposed to either venereal syphilis (from Europe) or yaws (from tropical Africa) would probably have exhibited a sufficiently strong immune response (if the general level of health was good) to avoid a new disease episode, unless New and Old World strains had diverged in cross-immunity during their millennia of separation.

The situation with tuberculosis was likely just the opposite, however, because individuals with silent, untreated infections may develop clinical disease if challenged immunologically by reexposure to tuberculous pathogens (Dannenberg 1994). Therefore, a Native American with normal immunocompetence who was infected early in life by the pathogenic agents of New World tuberculosis might have experienced no clinical disease at all until reexposed to either New or Old World strains at a time when concomitant physiological stresses from other diseases, malnutrition, or even psychosocial distress had reduced host immunologic capacities. But the consequences would most likely have been mortal.

In reality, we are now just *beginning* to chart the temporal and spatial distributions of the pathogenic agents, from their earliest appearances among Archaic hunter-gatherers and Woodland villagers to their fulmination in densely occupied late prehistoric townspeople. A symposium titled "North American Treponematosis: A Natural History," organized by Mary Lucas Powell and Della C. Cook for the 1998 meetings of the American Association of Physical Anthropologists, focused on delineation of the various expressions of indigenous treponematosis observed in skeletal remains dating from Archaic times to the centuries immediately preceding extensive Native American contacts with European and African invaders. The interested reader is referred to the publication of that symposium's proceedings and to Buikstra's masterly summary of indigenous American tuberculosis presented at the 1997 Szeged Congress.

3 Warfare-Related Trauma in the Late Prehistory of Alabama

Patricia S. Bridges
Keith P. Jacobi
Mary Lucas Powell

The widespread extent of warfare or raiding in native societies in North America has been known for many years. Besides historic accounts, skeletal remains have yielded ample evidence of the frequency of indigenous warfare. These accounts include numerous examples of death caused by arrows or spearpoints and cases of perimortem mutilation, such as decapitation, dismemberment of limbs, and scalping cutmarks (for example, Bridges 1996; Hoyme and Bass 1962; Jurmain 1991; Miller 1994; Milner 1995; Milner et al. 1991; Neumann 1940; O'Shea and Bridges 1989; Owsley 1994; Owsley et al. 1977; Owsley and Berryman 1975; Owsley and Bruweldheide 1997; Smith 1995; Snow 1941, 1942; Webb and DeJarnette 1942; Willey and Emerson 1993). These data clearly show the important role that interpersonal conflict played in earlier societies. Nevertheless, skeletal remains have not been widely used to assess differences in the impact of aggressive encounters and in the nature of injuries associated with them.

This chapter surveys information on skeletal remains from a variety of archaeological sites in northern and western Alabama in order to examine how the nature of interpersonal conflicts evolved over time and how they varied at sites of different sizes and for cultures of different degrees of complexity. These data suggest not only that warfare became more important in late prehistory but also that it is possible to trace changes in techniques and weaponry from different types of traumatic injuries.

The Archaeological Record of Interpersonal Conflict in Alabama

Evidence for interpersonal conflict is widespread at a variety of sites in the Deep South as early as Middle Archaic times (Smith 1995; Webb and DeJarnette 1942). This chapter concentrates on two regions lying largely in Alabama: the Pickwick Basin of the Middle Tennessee River Valley of northwestern Alabama and the Tombigbee and Black Warrior drainages in west-central Alabama and eastern Mississippi. A large sample of skeletal remains from the Archaic and Mississippian periods is present from the Pickwick Basin. In west-central Alabama skeletal collections come primarily from Woodland and Mississippian contexts. Examining these two regions reveals several different themes to be explored: change in level and type of interpersonal aggression over time in Alabama, the impact of the introduction of the bow in the Late Woodland period, and responses by Mississippian societies to bow warfare in terms of fortifications and methods of waging war.

Pickwick Basin, Northwestern Alabama

Skeletal samples from the Pickwick Basin largely date from the Archaic and Mississippian periods. Although there are Middle Woodland (Copena) sites in the region, they are not represented by well-preserved skeletal remains. Interpersonal conflict is evident in the earliest relatively large skeletal samples in this region, which date to the Middle Archaic period, about 6000–4000 B.C. (Walthall 1980). One site from this period is Mulberry Creek (1Ct27), a shell mound from which 134 skeletons were excavated by the W.P.A. in the late 1930s. Among the burials was a multiple grave of three adult males with a number of embedded Morrow Mountain dartpoints (Webb and DeJarnette 1942). This burial was found near the bottom of the shell mound and probably dates to the early part of the Middle Archaic period or close to 6000 B.C. (Walthall 1980). Another male single burial from this site also had an embedded point in the spinal column, suggesting that death caused by interpersonal conflict was not an isolated incident.

An Archaic site in the Pickwick Basin, the Perry site (1Lu25), also preserves evidence for interpersonal violence. Largely a late Archaic shell mound (4000–1000 B.C.), the Perry site yielded over 1,000 skeletons when excavated by the W.P.A. in the 1930s (Webb and DeJarnette 1942, 1948a). The original researchers noted that 7 of 256 individuals (later identified as Archaic—see below) had embedded spearpoints. In this case, the victims were almost equally divided between males and females, with four males and three females having embedded points. One individual survived the injury. Skeleton 1Lu25-2 (a female) showed complete healing around a dartpoint embedded in the right humerus. Others (for example, 1Lu25-903, noted as having a point lodged in the right orbit) clearly did not survive. Not all Archaic sites in the Pickwick Basin contain examples of individuals with embedded points, however. Little Bear Creek, located near Mulberry Creek, shows no evidence for interpersonal conflict in the known Archaic sample (N = at least 23 adults: Bridges 1985, 1989; Webb and DeJarnette 1948b). In short, variation does seem to exist in the level of interpersonal aggression at Archaic sites in the region, but it is clear that aggression was by no means exceptionally rare.

The next cultural period that has well-represented skeletal remains in the Pickwick Basin dates to Mississippian times (ca. A.D. 1050–1500). Koger's Island, the Mississippian center in this region, provides much more striking evidence for warfare-related mortality. The location of the site—which was on an island in the Tennessee River—was probably chosen for defensive purposes. No fortifications were discovered at the site; however, the excavations were primarily limited to the cemetery.

As part of the same series of W.P.A. excavations mentioned above, the Mississippian cemetery at Koger's Island was explored in the late 1930s (Webb and DeJarnette 1942). Of the 108 individuals recovered, 22 (or 20 percent) came from four mass burials holding from five to eight individuals each. These burials were not at first recognized to result from violent death: no points were embedded in bone, associated grave offerings characteristic of Mississippian burials were present, and the bodies were laid out neatly and not mutilated in any obvious way. Later analysis, however, revealed the presence of cranial cutmarks resulting from scalping on six individuals from the multiple burials. In addition, one skeleton from a mass grave had an unhealed cranial fracture. In short, the bodies in the larger interments seem likely to have been the victims of violent encounters. In addition to the mass graves, one individual from a single interment also preserves scalping cutmarks, making a total of 7 (of 108) individuals at the site who were scalped around the time of death (Bridges 1996).

Mississippian skeletons are also commonly found as intrusive burials in Archaic shell mounds in the Pickwick Basin, but so far these have not been systematically examined for evidence of perimortem injuries. However, a skull of probable Mississippian age from the Perry site has recently been described as preserving a partially healed scalping, much like one seen at Moundville (Jacobi et al. 1996), suggesting that Koger's Island is not the only Mississippian site in the Pickwick Basin affected by aggression. Certainly, there is abundant evidence that warfare was a primary concern of the local population in late prehistory.

West-Central Alabama

West-central Alabama also provides information on changes in interpersonal violence over time. Here skeletal samples are best represented by Late Woodland and Mississippian sites. During the Late Woodland period (A.D. 600–1050), the bow was introduced into the region. At the end of the Late Woodland, maize agriculture was adopted. These two events fundamentally changed the local economy and the nature of interpersonal conflict in the region.

The Late Woodland site 1Pi61 (Jenkins and Ensor 1981) is testimony to the fact that mortality related to interpersonal violence was rampant in the area. Eight (of 96) individuals had projectile points either embedded in or in close proximity to vital organs; five of these were found in multiple burials of three individuals each. One of the three single interments with an embedded point was decapitated and placed face down in the burial pit. The position of the arms and legs suggested that the body had been bound, implying this may have represented a captive (Hill 1981).

The small River Cut #1 site (22Lo860) in eastern Mississippi is also of Late Woodland age. Only four burials were found at this site, one of whom had been killed. This young male had projectile point tips embedded in the left humerus and right hip and cuts consistent with points in several of the right ribs (Turner 1986).

To the east of this region is one additional site that provides intriguing evidence for the importance of warfare during the Late Woodland–Mississippian transition in Alabama. Pinson Cave, dated to approximately A.D. 1040 ± 80 years, contained an ossuary of perhaps as many as 100 burials (Walthall 1980). Only part of the cave was excavated, yielding a minimum of 44 individuals. Seven Hamilton-like arrowpoints, which are similar to both late Woodland and early Mississippian types from Alabama, were found embedded in bone. Fifty of these points were found scattered among the excavated remains, suggesting that most of the interments had been killed and later deposited in the cave (Oakley 1971). Arrowpoints constituted the majority of the artifact assemblage; in contrast to other sites of the same age, only a few small potsherds were associated with the site.

Evidence for warfare continues into the Mississippian period in the Tombigbee River Valley region. The small Tibbee Creek farmstead in eastern Mississippi is typical, with one of nine Mississippian burials preserving a point lodged in the shoulder. This burial, as was the case for the Late Woodland River Cut #1 victim, is of a young male (O'Hear and Larsen 1981).

The midsize Mississippian formal cemetery (1Pi33) at the Lubbub Creek site in western Alabama also contains examples of individuals dying violently. Only one of the 36 skeletons in this sample has an embedded point, but this figure may be misleading, inasmuch as this individual was part of a multiple burial. In this grave, two complete extended males were placed one on top of the other in the burial pit. The lower skeleton, associated with a copper plate depicting a raptorial bird, is presumed to have been the principal interment. There is no direct evidence as to cause of death for this individual. Lying over this individual was a skeleton with a point in the rib cage, which has been interpreted as a sacrificial victim. Also in the grave were articulated arms, legs, and feet representing from one to two individuals. These are assumed to be trophies of war (Hill 1981). None of the additional 33 Mississippians (Summerville I-III) and only one of the 64 protohistoric (Summerville IV) individuals buried elsewhere at the site displayed trauma indicative of interpersonal violence; the latter was an adult female in the large ossuary and had a healed depressed cranial fracture (Powell 1983).

The importance of warfare in west-central Alabama during Mississippian times is further strengthened by the palisade seen at the associated village of Lubbub Creek. No fortifications are currently known from Late Woodland sites in this region, but they are common in Mississippian contexts (Rafferty 1986). Parts of up to six palisades and a circular ditch thought to be a dry moat were found at Lubbub Creek (Cole and Allbright 1983). The most massive part of the fortifications was an extensive "outer palisade" constructed early in the Mississippian occupation. The excavated section of this defensive structure was located at the northwestern edge of the community. This section contained six bastions, which would have offered protection for archers. Assuming that the palisade would have enclosed the entire bend, it must have been at least 600 m long. Because the palisade enclosed not only the village but also what appears to have been "vacant" land, it may have surrounded some maize fields as well (Blitz 1993).

A final defensive structure—a ditch or dry moat averaging 1.3 m in depth—was dug during protohistoric times and formed a rough circle around the community estimated at 230 m in length (Peebles 1983). Given the small resident population size of Lubbub Creek during the Mississippian occupation—estimated at 90 people at its height and often considerably smaller—it is clear that the community and probably its nearby neighbors invested a great deal of energy in defense.

The final western Alabama site to be considered is the Mississippian center of Moundville located along the Black Warrior River to the east of the Tombigbee drainage discussed above. Evidence for warfare at Moundville is largely indirect. The extensive palisade and bastion system, which was rebuilt several times, provides evidence that defense of the site was crucial to its inhabitants (Vogel and Allan 1985). A palisade, believed to have run for 5 km, enclosed Moundville within a rough circle running to the banks of the Black Warrior River on each side. Similar to the Lubbub structure, it contained bastions at intervals of 35–40 m.

Recent excavations aimed at stabilizing the eroding riverbank at Moundville have yielded additional information and radiocarbon dates of a small part of the palisade system (Scarry 1995). In this section, two distinct palisade systems were present. The more northerly palisade was first built in the middle of the Moundville I period (A.D. 1050–1250). It was rebuilt or altered at least six times, probably over a period of 60 or more years. This palisade was later removed and was replaced by one to the south during the early part of the Moundville II period (A.D. 1250–1400). This segment was probably repaired at least once and may have been in place from 20 to 40 years (Scarry 1995).

There is no preserved skeletal evidence that any individual at Moundville died violently. Nevertheless, there are two specimens that do provide information on the effect of warfare on Moundville's inhabitants. The healed scalping described by Snow (1941) and another example recently discovered in the collection (Jacobi et al. 1996) document at least the short-term survival of two individuals at the site after being attacked and scalped.

In summary, various sites in northern and western Alabama provide archaeological evidence of conflict and interpersonal violence, including embedded dart- or arrowpoints, unhealed cranial fractures, scalping cutmarks, trophy body parts buried with complete individuals, mass interments, and defensive structures such as palisades, bastions, and moats. Archaeological evidence for violent death is present during all time periods, but there is a greater range of activities associated with interpersonal aggression in late prehistory. Next, this chapter will consider in more detail the bioarchaeological data and what these data can add to archaeological evidence: specifically, the number of individuals dying violently and the nature of injuries both healed and unhealed. Differences in these variables may tell us something about the level and types of interpersonal violence in each of these societies.

Materials and Methods

Osteological data are primarily drawn from four sites with relatively large cemetery samples of approximately 100 or more individuals. Two are from northwest Alabama (the Perry [1Lu25] and Koger's Island [1Lu92] sites), and the remaining two are located in west-central Alabama (1Pi61 and Moundville). As described above, all four sites record instances of interpersonal violence, although the nature of these conflicts is highly variable. Several smaller Mississippian sites from west-central Alabama and eastern Mississippi also preserve cases of interpersonal aggression, including Lubbub Creek (1Pi33) and Tibbee Creek (22Lo600) (Hill 1981; O'Hear and Larsen 1981). The burial samples from these sites are too small to be included in the overall comparisons of traumatic injuries; however, instances of violent death are noted when present.

The Perry site (1Lu25) is a large Archaic shell mound from which over 1,000 skeletons were excavated by the W.P.A. in the late 1930s. Besides Archaic skeletons, later Mississippian (and possibly Woodland) remains have been intruded into the mound. Only the first four (of five) units excavated (which included a total of 708 burials) have been published (Webb and DeJarnette 1942, 1948a). As is usual for large, multicomponent shell mounds, the stratigraphy is complex, and many skeletons cannot be easily assigned to a time period.

In preparation for an earlier study (Bridges 1985), 256 burials at the site were assessed as Archaic in age, based on either burial inclusions or depth below pottery-bearing levels. For this sample, information on embedded points was taken from notes on file at the Laboratory for Human Osteology in Tuscaloosa, Alabama. These data were collected by workers under the direction of Marshall T. Newman and Charles E. Snow. Only part of their findings has been published (Newman and Snow 1942); therefore this information largely derives from unpublished notes. Data on traumatic injuries for Archaic individuals at the Perry site are taken from a different set of unpublished records, in which a subset of the Archaic sample (N = 94) was examined under the supervision of Keith Jacobi.

Koger's Island (1Lu92) from the same region is a Mississippian cemetery, which was also excavated by the W.P.A. during the 1930s, before the construction of Pickwick Reservoir. Although a village midden was present at the site, it was not excavated, so our understanding of the site is confined to the burials and their contents. The burials are arranged in a series of five rows and form a distinct cemetery (Peebles 1971). Recent laboratory analysis has revealed the presence of 108 individuals in this sample. All skeletons were sexed and aged by the senior author as part of an earlier study (Bridges 1996). For the current study, a broad range of traumatic injuries was coded, including fractures, perimortem mutilation, such as scalping cutmarks, and evidence of violent death (i.e., unhealed cranial fractures).

The Late Woodland cemetery, 1Pi61, in west-central Alabama was excavated by the University of Alabama Office of Archaeological Research (now called the Division of Archaeology) (Jenkins and Ensor

1981). Although designated a cemetery, the burials show no formal organization and are often placed in used storage pits or beneath the floors of houses. The data on skeletal remains (including age, sex, and traumatic injuries) discussed here are derived from M. C. Hill's (1981) analysis of the burials. There were 96 individuals excavated at 1Pi61.

Because of its prominence, excavations have been carried out at Moundville for over 150 years, with varying degrees of professionalism. Although C. B. Moore excavated a large series of skeletal remains in 1905 and 1906, the present location of this collection is unknown, except for a few pathological specimens sent to the Army Medical Museum. The known skeletal material at Moundville derives primarily from excavations carried out from 1932 to 1941. Unlike the case for the other sites mentioned above, the skeletons now available for study (about 1,500) do not represent the total number of burials excavated (which was 2,222). Poor preservation explains only part of the disparity between these figures. Many skeletons seem not to have been removed from the ground unless they were "interesting" (in terms of pathology, grave inclusions, or cranial type) or were well preserved. In addition, it seems clear that other "interesting" specimens were later removed from the remaining collection, making it probable that the prevalence of traumatic injuries, among other pathologies, is underrepresented. In short, the sample from Moundville is not by any means complete (Powell 1988).

All data on age, sex, status, and frequencies of fractures from this site come from Powell's (1988) study. The general inventory of the entire collection, maintained by the Laboratory for Human Osteology in Tuscaloosa, however, contains some examples of craniofacial injuries not found in Powell's subset of the sample. When present, these are also noted. In addition, recent work has reexamined evidence of healed scalping injuries in this collection (Jacobi et al. 1996; see also Snow 1941, 1942).

BIOARCHAEOLOGICAL EVIDENCE FOR INTERPERSONAL CONFLICTS

Mortality

Perhaps the simplest measure of the impact of interpersonal conflict on societies is a comparison of the mortality that can be attributed directly to violence. Evidence for violent death is taken from several sources. First, earlier researchers' reporting of embedded points (unhealed) is taken to indicate mortality (Hill 1981; Oakley 1971; Turner 1986; Webb and DeJarnette 1942, 1948a). Second, perimortem fractures and partially healed scalpings are also assumed to indicate death re-

Table 3-1. Summary Distribution of Injury Type

	Archaic	Late Woodland	Mississippian	
	1Lu25	1Pi61	Moundville	1Lu92
Embedded points	2%[1]	8%	0%	0%
Scalping cuts	0%	0%	0%[2]	5%
Cranial fractures	0%	0%	1%	5%
Other upper body fractures	6%	25%	10%	46%
Lower body fractures	12%	16%	6%	22%

[1]Unhealed lesions only. If healed injuries are included, this rises to just under 3 percent.

[2]No unhealed scalping cutmarks have been identified at Moundville, but partially healed scalpings are present.

sulting directly or indirectly from aggressive acts (Bridges 1996; Jacobi et al. 1996). Finally, mass graves containing at least one individual with a perimortem injury or embedded points are thought to be an indirect reflection of violent death. For example, although several of the associated skeletons in the mass graves at Koger's Island show no conclusive skeletal evidence for cause of death, it is probable that they too were victims of warfare (see Bridges 1996).

Mortality resulting from interpersonal conflicts varies widely at the sites considered here. Approximately 2 percent of the Archaic skeletons at the Perry site have embedded points that show no signs of healing (Table 3-1). When individuals associated with those skeletons in multiple graves are included, this percentage rises to just over 4 percent, largely due to a mass grave of five individuals. Other Archaic sites in the Pickwick Basin region of northwestern Alabama show percentages of skeletons with embedded points ranging from 0 to 3 percent. At the nearby Mississippian site of Koger's Island, however, 21 percent of the individuals show perimortem injuries or are buried in mass graves with those who do. This is by far the highest level of mortality seen at any site examined for this study.

Moving to the west-central Alabama region, the Late Woodland 1Pi61 is intermediate in the level of mortality from conflict, at 13 percent of individuals having embedded points or being closely associated with them. Later Mississippian cemeteries show some variation in mortality from violence in this region. The large center of Moundville has no recorded instances of deaths occurring as a direct result of aggression, although the partly healed scalpings from that site suggest that infections resulting from these injuries eventually caused the individuals' demise (Jacobi et al. 1996).

The two other Mississippian cemeteries mentioned above—the farmstead of Tibbee Creek (22Lo600) and the single-mound, palisaded site at Lubbub Creek (1Pi33)—both show frequencies of violent death at around 11 percent, essentially equivalent to the earlier 1Pi61. With the exception of Moundville, sites of Late Woodland or Mississippian age in western Alabama tend to have mortality rates from violence of just over 10 percent. Mortality is roughly three times higher or even greater in Late Woodland and Mississippian sites (with the exception of Moundville) than in Archaic sites from northwestern Alabama.

Sex Differences in Mortality. The sex ratio of deaths from aggressive encounters also changes over time. The Mulberry Creek Middle Archaic site has only males killed by dartpoints; however, the sex ratio at the mostly Late Archaic Perry site is more evenly divided. Four of seven individuals with embedded points are males, whereas the other three are females. One of the females at the Perry site survived the wound, but the risk of dying violently is still roughly equivalent for the two sexes, at 11 percent for males and 8 percent for females. At the Late Woodland 1Pi61, the sexes also have a similar rate of violent death (as assessed by embedded points or inclusion in a multiple burial with other individuals with embedded points) of 19 percent for adult males and 18 percent for females. Nevertheless, the Mississippian sites show that males tend to be the primary victims of interpersonal conflict. At Koger's Island, 37 percent of all adult males and 23 percent of females died violently. And at Mississippian sites in west-central Alabama, only males and no females were killed, although mortality overall is lower there than at Koger's Island. In general, there seems to be an increase in male mortality in the Mississippian period both in northwestern and west-central Alabama. This pattern of higher adult male (versus female) mortality from violent trauma has been reported both for archaeological series throughout eastern North America and for intergroup conflicts within historically and ethnographically documented small-scale societies (Milner 1998:79).

Age Differences in Mortality. At all sites, adults are more frequently subject to violent death than are subadults. At the Archaic Perry site, no subadults have embedded points, although one juvenile is associated with a mass grave of five individuals, otherwise consisting of adult females. Only one of 11 possible victims at this site (or 9 percent) is a juvenile. At the Mississippian Koger's Island in the same region, three of 23 (13 percent) of individuals dying violently are subadult. Of all juveniles at the site, 8 percent are victims.

At the Late Woodland 1Pi61 site, three of 12 victims (25 percent) are juvenile. However, there is a high percentage of subadults buried at this site (40/96 or 42 percent), so this frequency may be misleading. Of all subadults at 1Pi61, about 8 percent are found in multiple graves associated with victims of embedded points, a frequency equivalent to that at Koger's Island. Only one juvenile—an adolescent, possibly male—has an embedded point. The smaller Mississippian site of Lubbub Creek has only adults in contexts associated with warfare. The hamlet of Tibbee Creek has a young male (15–17) with an embedded antler tine point.

Several conclusions may be drawn from these data. As noted above, juveniles are much less likely to die in warfare than are adults of either sex. They are not immune to the effects of violence, however, even in Archaic contexts. In addition, subadults rarely show any direct evidence of violent death; rather they are usually found associated with adults who preserve embedded points. The only subadults with embedded points are male adolescents, who were probably regarded differently than were younger children or adolescent girls. In virtually all cases in which mortality from warfare may be assumed, juveniles (other than adolescent males) are found in mass graves consisting primarily of females and other subadults.[1] There seems to be a dichotomy, then, between mass burial contexts owing to violence when the victims are either primarily adult males or, less often, females and children. This pattern remains fairly constant across all time periods examined here. There are also no significant differences over time in numbers of juveniles dying as a result of interpersonal violence; the frequencies are relatively low for all periods. Higher adult than juvenile mortality from violent trauma has been noted elsewhere (Milner 1995, 1998) for archaeological series throughout eastern North America.

Traumatic Injuries

Patterns of traumatic injuries may reflect in varying degree the influences of both environmental and cultural factors, including levels of interpersonal violence. First to be considered are the frequencies of healed and unhealed fractures. Second, fracture distribution (or where injuries occur) will be discussed. Finally, evidence for perimortem mutilation, specifically scalping, will be described.

At the Perry site, 19 percent of a sample of Archaic skeletons have healed fractures. Nearly all of these individuals have a single injury, and none has more than two. Koger's Island, situated in the same environmental setting, has the much higher frequency of 43.5 percent, more than twice that at the Perry site. Moreover, the 47 individuals at Koger's Island with injuries have, on average, 1.6 fractures each (Table 3-2). This average is raised by six individuals who have three or more fractures each. One of these, a female, has six healed fractures, including injuries to her facial bones. At both sites, nearly all fractures occur

Table 3–2. Traumatic Injuries at Koger's Island (1Lu92)

Specimen Number	Sex	Age	Burial Size	Traumatic Injuries
1	–	3		
2	–	10–14		
3	–	7–8		
4	Male	20–24		
5	Female	20–24		R rib
6	Male	25–29		R clavicle, L metatarsals 3,4
7	–	11–12		
8	–	9–12 mos.		
9	Female	18–19		
10	Female	40–49		
11	Male	35–39		
12	–	9–10		
13	Male	35–39		R rib, R fibula, L femur
14	Female?	20–24		R metatarsal 3, L talus
15	Male	40–44		L wrist
16	Female	40–44		RL clavicle, L fibula
17	Male	40–49		
18	–	0–6 mos.		
19	–	6–18 mos.		
20	Male	30–39		R rib 2, R fibula
21	Male	30–34		R metacarpal 5
22	Male	30–39		
23	Male	30–39		R ulna
24	Female	25–29		R frontal, L fibula
25	Female	15–19		
26	Female	35–39		
27	–	13–14	–5, with	
28	–	9 mos.	101–102	
29	–	2–3		
30	Female	15–19		
31	Male	40–44		Rib
32	Male	35–39	–5	
33	Male	25–35		Scalping
34	Male	30–34		Scalping
35	Male	40–44		Scalping
36	Male	20–24		Scalping, R ulna
37	Female	50+	–5	Rib
38	Male	40–49		Scalping, L clavicle
39	Male	30–39		Hand phalanges
40	Male	20–24		L fibula, L metatarsal 5

Table 3–2. continued

40A	Female	15–19		
41	Male	35–44	⎫	R rib
42	Female	30–39	⎬ –3	R rib, R metacarpal 1
43	Female	45–55	⎪	L ankle
44	–	fetus	⎭	
45	Female	50–59		L radius, L ulna
46	Female	40–49	⎫ –2	L humerus
47	Female	45–49	⎭	L ulna
48	(no bones into lab)			
49	Female?	14		
50	(no bones into lab)			
51	Female	15–19		
52	Female	40–49		
53	Female	20–29		
54	Female	30–39		
55	–	9 mos.		
56	–	12–13		
57	Female	35–39		R lower rib, L parietal
58	–	2		
59	Male	25–29		R metatarsal 5, L humerus
60	Male	40–44	⎫ –2	R humerus, L rib
61	Male	40–49	⎭	R foot phalanx
62	–	9 mos		
63	–	newborn		
64	Female?	30–39		
65	Female	15–19		
66	Male	35–39		R parietal, R tibia/fibula, 7th cervical vertebra
66A	–	0–1		
67	Female	30–39		L ulna
68	–	1–2		
68A	–	2–3		
69	–	2–3		metacarpal or metatarsal
70	Male	30–39		R rib 2
71	–	6–9 mos.		
72	Female	17–19		Scalping, L ulna
73	Female	40–49		R radius
74	Male	40–44		
75	Male	50–59		R clavicle, L fibula, rib
76	–	6 mos		
77	–	9 mos?		

Table 3-2 continued on next page

Table 3–2. continued

Specimen Number	Sex	Age	Burial Size	Traumatic Injuries
78	Female	20–29		L rib
79	Male	30–39		R rib, 1st thoracic vertebra
80	–	0–6 mos		
80A	–	2–3		
81	Female	25–29		R fibula, L ulna, L tibia
81A	–	9–12 mos		
82	–	0–3 mos		
83	Female	20–27		fused sacrum to coccygeal 1–2
84	–	3–4		
84A	Male	35–45		L metatarsal 2?
84B	–	6–9 mos		
84C	–	6 mos		
85	Male?	30–35		L pubis
86	–	10		
87	Female	30–50		R radius
88	(no bones into lab)			
89	Female	20–27		R fibula
90	Male	35–39		R hand phalanx
91	Female	40–49		L rib 1
92	Male	30–39	–8	L rib?
93	Male	25–35		R ulna
94	Male	35–45		Unhealed – frontal
95	Male	30–34		
96	(no bones into lab)			
97	–	6–12 mos		
98	–	7–8		
98A	–	7–8		
99	–	9–12 mos		
100	Female?	30–50		
100A	–	fetus		
100B	–	10–11		
101	Female	30–39	–5 with 26–28	Scalping, R clavicle, R tibia/ fibula, L zygomatic, L humerus, L rib
102	–	3–4		

Burial size refers to the number of individuals in a single grave.

in adults. When we consider adults alone, the fracture rate at Koger's Island rises to 68 percent. For the Perry site, this figure is 27 percent.

At the Perry site, 20 percent of females and 38 percent of males preserve healed fractures. Therefore, males are nearly twice as likely as females to suffer from injuries, although their risk of violent death is roughly equivalent. The two sexes at Koger's Island have much more similar fracture rates than those at the Perry site, with 71 percent of males and 62 percent of females showing traumatic injuries. Both frequencies are substantially higher than for either sex at the earlier Archaic site.

At the Late Woodland 1Pi61 site in west-central Alabama, 23 percent of the 96 individuals show a total of 40 fractures. Although this implies that most individuals with fractures have approximately two each, five skeletons (three males and two females) with at least three fractures account for many of the injuries. The largest number of individual fractures (N = 7) occurs in a female. As at the Pickwick Basin sites, most injuries are in adults, 39 percent of whom have at least one healed fracture. At 1Pi61, as at Koger's Island, males have slightly greater fracture rates than females, but this difference is not a significant one; 46 percent of males and 36 percent of females have at least one healed injury.

Moundville shows by far the least fractures of any of the sites in this study, with only 37 cases in the 564 individuals examined (<7 percent). As discussed above, the removal of certain pathological elements from this sample has reduced the overall numbers of healed injuries present. Nevertheless, any curational bias should not have affected the sex ratio of injuries or their anatomical distribution. Males are nearly twice as likely as females (19:10) to have healed traumatic injuries (Powell 1988).

The overall fracture rate, in some respects, follows the mortality rate at these sites, with Koger's Island highest, followed by 1Pi61, the Perry site, and Moundville. The sex ratio of those with fractures varies from that of the violent deaths, however. Males have approximately two times as many fractures as females at the Archaic Perry site in northwest Alabama, whereas the sex ratio is nearly equivalent at Koger's Island. This situation is reversed for mortality rates at these two sites, with the Perry site having a similar sex ratio in violent deaths, while at Koger's Island, males clearly outnumber females in the mass graves. In west-central Alabama, the Late Woodland cemetery 1Pi61 has only slightly elevated numbers of injuries in males, making it similar to Koger's Island. However, Moundville has many more fractures in males than in females. An examination of the sex ratios suggests that healed fractures and aggression are not so strongly linked in these populations as the overall figures would suggest.

Table 3–3. Distribution of Fractures

| | Archaic | Late Woodland | Mississippian | |
	1Lu25	1Pi61	Moundville	1Lu92[1]
Cranium	0	0	3	5
Vertebrae	0	0	2	3
Ribs	1	1	8	16
Clavicle	0	5	4	6
Humerus	0	2	3	4
Ulna	2	6	15	8
Radius	1	5	12	3
Wrist/Hand	2	5	7	5
Pelvis	1	0	6	1
Femur	3	1	2	1
Tibia	1	1	3	3
Fibula	4	5	10	11
Ankle/Foot	2	8	11	8
TOTAL N	94	96	564	108

[1]There is one additional fracture from Koger's Island, which is either of a metacarpal or metatarsal, belonging to an infant.

Although more males have fractures than do females, at both 1Pi61 and Koger's Island it is a female who has the most fractures (seven and six respectively). This circumstance suggests the question of whether aggression against women may have raised the fracture rate in later prehistoric societies. The six fractures on the Koger's Island female include one to the zygomatic bone; cranial and facial fractures are generally assumed to result more often from interpersonal violence (Roberts and Manchester 1995). The female from 1Pi61, however, has no observable head or facial injuries. Certainly, there does not seem to be the widespread patterning of violence against females in the Southeast that has been documented in other regions of North America (Smith 1996a; Wilkinson and Van Wagenen 1993).

Anatomical Distribution of Fractures

The two earlier sites (the Archaic 1Lu25 and Late Woodland 1Pi61) have the greatest number of fractures in lower limbs, and secondarily, upper limbs (Tables 3-1, 3-3). Specifically, 1Lu25 shows most fractures in the fibula, followed by the femur, and then the ankle/foot, wrist/hand, and ulna. The Late Woodland 1Pi61 has the most fractures in the ankle/foot region, followed by the ulna, and then the fibula, wrist/hand, radius and clavicle. The Mississippian sites, however, tend to show the greatest number of fractures in the upper body. They also are the only sites that preserve cranial and vertebral fractures. Moundville has more fractures of the ulna than any other bone, followed by the radius and then the ankle/foot. Koger's Island has more rib fractures, then fibula, and ankle/foot injuries. In short, although all sites show relatively high frequencies of lower leg and foot fractures, only the Mississippian samples preserve uniformly high numbers of upper body injuries.

Of course, many of these fractures are no doubt caused by accidents and not by warfare-related wounds. It may be possible in part to distinguish between these types of injuries. In the past it has been frequently suggested that "parry fractures" of the ulna were the result of blocking a blow from an attacker (Angel 1974; Wood-Jones 1910). However, medical studies of this subject (for example, Schultz 1972) suggest that many ulnar fractures are the result of accidents rather than of violence. Therefore, parry fractures cannot be used alone as a simple measure of interpersonal aggression. Cranial fractures are much less likely to occur from accidents than from violent encounters, however, and they may be a better indicator of interpersonal conflict (Roberts and Manchester 1995; Walker 1989).

As noted above, only the two Mississippian sites in this sample contain individuals with cranial injuries. At Koger's Island, five individuals have some sort of injury to their crania.[2] One is an unhealed depressed lesion on the frontal, obviously occurring around the time of death. The rest are healed. Two are found on the parietals, one is on the frontal, and the fourth is a well-healed fracture of the zygomatic bone. Two of the injuries are to males (including the unhealed fracture); the remaining three are in adult females.

Powell (1988) found no cranial fractures in her subset of the Moundville skeletons but discovered two instances of cutting marks on the calvarium. However, the complete collection contains several individuals with cranial fractures. One, a child of age 6–7, preserves a small circular depressed region near the sagittal suture. Another (aged 17) possesses a healed fracture of the left mandible in the molar region. Finally, an adult female also has a healed injury on her frontal bone. In short, the only sites to preserve individuals with cranial injuries are Mississippian in age; earlier sites show no instances of these types of fractures. It should be noted that cranial injuries have been seen in Archaic skeletons from Kentucky (Smith 1996b). Mississippian sites also have large numbers of rib and vertebral fractures. Although these have not been linked directly to interpersonal aggression, it is plausible to suggest that increased amounts of upper body injuries might be due to violent encounters.

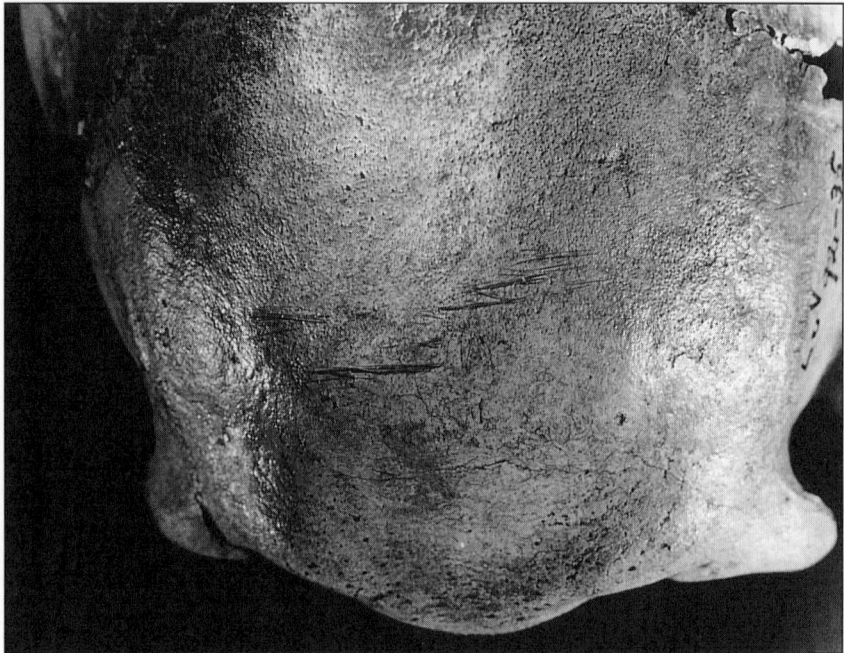

Figure 3-1. Perimortem Cutmarks on Individual from Koger's Island (1Lu92—Burial 35).

Although it might be assumed that upper body fractures, if associated with warfare, would be more frequent in males, this is not always the case. At Koger's Island, 21 of 39 adult males (54 percent) and 18 of 34 adult females (53 percent) have at least one upper body fracture. At Moundville, however, males have more than twice as many upper body fractures (0.7 percent of all bones) as females (0.3 percent). This largely corresponds to the overall sex ratio of fractures at this site. Male participation in warfare therefore cannot alone explain the high frequency of upper body injuries, especially at Koger's Island. An additional possibility is female-directed violence. An elevated prevalence of upper body and facial fractures in females from Plains archaeological sites has been suggested to be due to domestic violence (Owsley and Bruweldheide 1997).

Scalping Marks

Two kinds of lesions related to scalping are present on crania from the samples examined here: perimortem cutmarks (Figure 3-1) and infectious lesions circumscribing the vault that indicate survival of the victim for weeks or months after the encounter (Figure 3-2). The only

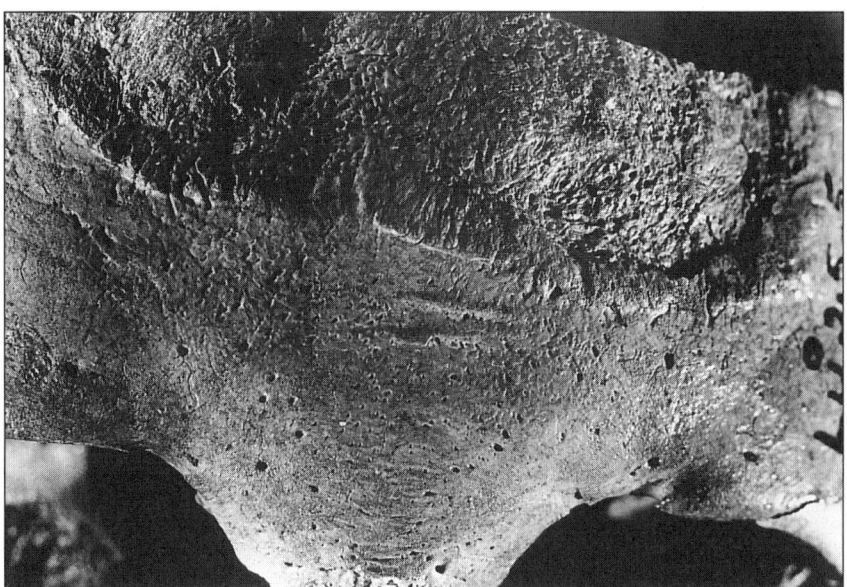

Figure 3-2. Individual from the Perry Site (1Lu25—Burial 5) Who Survived for a Time after Scalping. There has been healing on the cranial vault.

perimortem scalping cuts found to date in these samples are from the site of Koger's Island (Bridges 1996). Nevertheless, it should be noted that this is the only site that has been intensively examined for the presence of these marks, and given their small, somewhat insignificant appearance, it is not surprising that they might not yet be noticed at other sites.

As discussed elsewhere (Bridges 1996), seven individuals from Koger's Island (five males, two females) have unhealed cranial cutmarks caused by scalping (Table 3-1). Six of the seven were found in the four mass graves at the site; one came from a single interment. No children were scalped, even though one of the multiple burials contained three subadults, along with two adult females (one of which had been scalped). At this site, 14 percent of the males and 6 percent of the females show these cuts, figures that parallel the sex ratio of deaths caused by violence (37 percent:21 percent).

The infectious lesions associated with partially healed scalpings are more visible than the cutmarks and therefore more easily identifiable. Although Snow noted the first example of these lesions over 50 years ago (1941, 1942), additional specimens from the region have only recently been discovered, at Moundville and in northwestern Alabama in an intrusive burial at the Perry site (Jacobi et al. 1996). All dated skeletons with partially healed scalpings (as well as the unhealed

wounds) are of Mississippian age. However, scalping cutmarks have
been identified on Archaic remains from the Kentucky Lake Reservoir
to the north (Smith 1995).

Status and Traumatic Injury

Status can be assessed for the Mississippian sites in this sample
(Koger's Island and Moundville). Powell's (1988) study of the Moundville remains found no significant differences in traumatic injuries due
to status. She notes however that the highest-level elite skeletons are
missing from the sample there.

Six of the burials at Koger's Island are associated with items similar to those which are thought to confer high status at Moundville. Five
of the six are males. Of all six, five individuals (80 percent) had at least
one fracture as compared to 39/67 low-status adults from the site (58
percent). The number of fractures per person is slightly greater in high-
status individuals: 9/5 (1.8) versus 64/39 (1.6) in lower-status burials.

The major difference between status rankings is related to mortality from violence and scalping cutmarks. None of the individuals ac-
corded a high status burial shows signs of death from aggression or
scalping cutmarks; these are confined to lower-status interments. The
ages of the high-status individuals are not, as might be expected, different (or older) than the others. Of the five males, one was 20–29, three
30–39, and one 40–49, similar to male mortality at the site as a whole,
including the mass graves (Bridges 1996).

Although historically males gained status through exploits in warfare, there is no clear evidence from the osteological data presented
here that the same was true in prehistory. There are slightly elevated
fracture rates, possibly due to warfare or the ball game, in the high-
status individuals from Koger's Island, but these are not much different
from those in lower-status burials. This confirms Powell's findings at
Moundville (1988). None of the higher status skeletons has a cranial
fracture, the type most often associated with aggression; however, all
of those with fractures have at least one in the upper body (clavicle,
rib, ulna, and thoracic vertebra). Nevertheless, the same is true of the
majority of the lower-status individuals, and the sample sizes are so
small that this difference may not be meaningful.

There are several potential reasons for the apparent lower status of
the individuals in the mass graves. For one, the fact that these individuals were buried together suggests a lack of time or energy to invest
in single interments, probably as a direct result of the depredations
of the raid causing the deaths. Also, their society may have formally
ascribed a lower—or different—status to those dying in warfare. It
should be emphasized, however, that the skeletons in the mass graves
are neatly laid out, and most contain burial offerings, so there is no

obvious difference between them and the majority of the single interments from the site, except for the number of individuals and their injuries. Of course, achieving high status through exploits in raiding
would have come only if the individual was victorious; dying would
not be considered a success. Finally, we must remember that the victims probably were defending their home or caught away from it at the
time of the raid. They were not necessarily the foremost warriors but
may be more representative of the society as a whole. Certainly, death
in warfare did not confer status, but it is still possible that success did.
If so, it is not associated with longer life expectancy, however, nor with
a greatly increased prevalence of fractures.

DISCUSSION

Mortality

What do these findings tell us about changes in interpersonal violence
over time? First, they affirm that conflicts between individuals are a
common factor in human societies, despite variable demographic and
subsistence conditions. Regardless of the cultural period, there are examples of aggression leading to injury or death. The scope of these conflicts varies over time, however. At most of the Archaic sites in the
Pickwick Basin, there is a low level of mortality from violence. Most
examples involve a single individual and probably result from interpersonal disagreements that culminated in violent encounters, rather than
raiding or warfare. The multiple burial at Mulberry Creek suggests at
least a larger number of involved individuals. In addition, one of the
skeletons from that burial is missing the hands and forearms, which
may have been taken as trophies (Webb and DeJarnette 1942). This
practice is usually associated with more organized raiding or warfare,
rather than simple interindividual conflicts (Mensforth 1996).

Certainly, scattered Archaic sites in Tennessee and Kentucky provide evidence for periods of more organized warfare between groups.
The Cherry site in Tennessee, for example, contains a mass grave that
probably holds the victims of a small massacre. Mortality from violence at the rest of the Cherry site was about 10 percent, much higher
than other Archaic sites in the region. In addition, several examples of
perimortem mutilation (trophy taking or scalping) are also known from
the Kentucky and Tennessee Archaic sample (Mensforth 1996; Smith
1995, 1996b).

Clearly, what were generally small-scale interpersonal conflicts
may have erupted at times during the Archaic period into more widespread and organized raiding. Nevertheless, a more significant and lasting change seems to have coincided with the introduction of the bow

and arrow in the Eastern Woodlands during the Late Woodland period (Blitz 1988). Adoption of the bow is associated with a tremendous increase in mortality, which can be seen in the numbers of individuals with embedded points from this period. In Alabama, the low levels of mortality seen in the Archaic period (0–3 percent in the Pickwick Basin sites), rise to over 10 percent in the Late Woodland 1Pi61. The technological superiority of the bow is clearly tied to the increase in raiding at this time.

As a response to bow warfare, later Mississippian communities began to incorporate defensive features, including fortifications with bastions, as well as the placement of villages on islands with water barriers. In addition, population nucleation at this time would have enhanced defensibility, as well as enlarged the labor force engaged in palisade construction. These defensive strategies resulted in changes in mortality and injuries, which can be seen in the skeletal samples examined in this study.

During the Mississippian period, both mortality from violent injuries and the predominant types of injuries themselves become more variable among sites. The greatest mortality is seen at smaller and mid-sized sites; Moundville has no preserved instances of mortality occurring directly as a result of violence. Within the smaller and mid-sized sites, cause of death varies according to site size and defensibility. Small, undefended hamlets like Tibbee Creek contain individuals with embedded arrowpoints, a pattern identical to that seen in the Late Woodland period. Mid-sized sites with defensive features (Lubbub Creek, Koger's Island) also show high mortality from violence but rarely from embedded arrowpoints. Bow warfare at palisaded sites would be less certain than at small, undefended farmsteads. Individuals at the mid-sized and larger Mississippian sites, then, are largely protected from the bow, but they may still be susceptible to other types of warfare. The largest and best-defended sites, such as Moundville, would have presented an overwhelmingly formidable face to invaders and would be largely secure from warfare except under unusual circumstances.

The sex ratio of violence-related mortality changes over time, although there is little apparent difference in age ratios. Juveniles are always less subject to mortality from violence than are adults, although they are not immune to it. In the Archaic and Late Woodland periods, males and females generally die in roughly comparable numbers from interpersonal aggression. During the Mississippian period males become more common in contexts associated with violent death. They are never the exclusive victims, however: all the mass graves at Koger's Island contain at least one adult female. Nonetheless, the role of males in warfare clearly became more important in Mississippian times, leading to a dramatic increase in early male mortality at the Koger's Island site (Bridges 1996).

Fracture Rates

The Archaic hunter-gatherers at the Perry site may have been more prone to accidental trauma than later groups. The sex ratio of injuries is highest at the Perry site, with males having three times as many injuries as females. One explanation is that male hunting activities, especially with a spear rather than a bow, would result in a higher frequency of accidental trauma simply because it was necessary to get close to game animals in order to kill them.

The extremely high fracture rates at 1Pi61 and Koger's Island require an alternative explanation. It is not simply their subsistence activities that led to high accident rates, since Moundville, with presumably a similar subsistence economy to Koger's Island, has so few fractures. (Powell's subset of the Moundville collection has only 1/10th the number of fractures that are at Koger's Island.) Similarly, the high percentages of fractures at the Late Woodland 1Pi61 and Mississippian Koger's Island cannot result from their living in dangerous environments, inasmuch as other societies in the same regions show fewer injuries. It seems most likely that the high fracture rates at these sites are tied at least partially to the high levels of mortality in warfare.

Other Mississippian activities could be responsible for these fractures as well. Specifically, the ball game, played largely by males, was renowned for the often-spectacular injuries (including death) associated with it. For example, in a historic Creek game during the late 1800s, one person was killed during play, three died later, and fifteen individuals took at least a month to recover (Tuggle 1973). Teams often intentionally tried to cripple skilled players on the opposite side (Adair 1930; Mooney 1890). The ball game, like warfare, was an avenue by which males gained status in Mississippian and historic Southeastern societies. Indeed, the ball game was often called the "little brother of war" (Hudson 1976; Swanton 1928).

Nevertheless, the sex ratio of injuries at Koger's Island argues against warfare and the ball game as the primary causes of traumatic injuries. The sex ratio of mortalities (not injuries) is skewed somewhat to males at Koger's Island. Injuries occur at nearly the same rate in males as in females there (53:47). Obviously, females have more traumatic injuries than would be predicted from their lower participation in warfare, as seen in mortality rates. Perhaps Mississippian females had a higher rate of accidental injuries at this site when compared to Moundville, associated with their greater participation in subsistence chores related to agriculture. Another explanation may be that females were actively engaged in defense of the site—and therefore subject to similar injuries as were the males—but simply were not killed as often, possibly because women were sought as captives. Another possibility is violence against women.

Maria Smith (1996b) notes that female-directed violence has been identified in the Plains, Southwest, and Midwest, as seen by craniofacial trauma, but not so far in the Southeast. Several female skeletons from the Late Woodland and Mississippian periods of Alabama may represent female-directed violence, however, or possibly violence against war captives. The two individuals with the largest number of healed traumatic injuries are both female: one from 1Pi61 with seven fractures and another from Koger's Island with six fractures and unhealed scalping cutmarks. The individual from 1Pi61 has no cranial fractures, so it is not possible to identify these positively as nonaccidental. The Koger's Island female has a healed zygomatic injury, which is likely to be due to violence. In addition, two other females from Koger's Island preserve healed cranial fractures. Although it is clear that females were at times involved in warfare—they are certainly represented in the mass graves and are among the scalping victims—some injuries could also have resulted from female-directed violence. If so, it is infrequent and does not exhibit the clear patterning seen at sites in the Midwest and Southwest (Smith 1996a; Wilkinson and Van Wagenen 1993).

Fracture Types

In terms of fractures, the Late Woodland 1Pi61 and the Mississippian Koger's Island were similar, both having high frequencies. The Archaic Perry site and Moundville had fewer numbers of fractures, which as discussed above, may be tied to their lower participation in interpersonal conflicts. One might expect therefore that types of fractures would be similar at 1Pi61 and Koger's Island and distinguish them from the other two sites. This expectation was not upheld; instead, the two Mississippian sites had the most similar kinds of fractures. The earlier sites were dramatically different, in lacking certain types of injuries.

The types of traumatic injuries seen at each site may be important in helping to determine the nature of interpersonal conflict there. For example, cranial injuries have been linked to interpersonal aggression, whereas many other fractures may be accidental. None of the two earlier sites examined here showed any examples of cranial trauma, but the two Mississippian sites had multiple cases. In addition, the two Mississippian sites preserved individuals with vertebral fractures (lacking in the earlier sites) and relatively high numbers of rib fractures. In short, upper body injuries were far more common in the later, rather than in the earlier, sites.

At Koger's Island, four cranial injuries are healed and one unhealed, suggesting that at least one individual was killed as a result of this type of wound. As discussed in Bridges (1996), two of the healed vault lesions appear to have been caused by a thin bladed instrument, similar in shape to the historic tomahawk. Prehistorically, this weapon would probably have been a ground stone axe.

Two other fractures (one healed, one unhealed) were clearly caused by a different kind of weapon, one that included a pointed end. Given the deep indentation on the crania caused by these weapons, it is improbable that they were Mississippian arrowpoints, which are small and triangular and unlikely to inflict such damage. More likely is some kind of warclub, and some type that incorporated sharp edges, such as the crowned mace, which is associated with warfare in Mississippian iconography (Allan 1996). An example of a crowned mace is depicted on a carved shell gorget from Sumner County, Tennessee; the mace is shown as held in the left hand of a warrior, who carries a human head in his right (Fundaburk and Foreman 1957:Plate 47). The crowned mace is clublike and ends in a curved blade, which comes to a point at either side.

Although many Mississippian representations of these types of clubs are clearly ceremonial objects, they may symbolize a more functional weapon. For example, a wooden warclub from Key Marco is virtually identical in form to the crowned mace (Cushing 1897). Another possible instrument that could have caused these injuries would be a warclub studded with rocks or one coming to a point; both weapons are described in early historic accounts (Swanton 1946).

The types of cranial injuries that may have been caused by warclubs have been found so far only in the Mississippian sites of Koger's Island and Moundville. These sites lack individuals with embedded points, which are, however, present at earlier Archaic and Woodland and smaller Mississippian sites. There is therefore a dichotomy between types of mortality or injuries and site size and cultural period.

Evolution of Prehistoric Warfare

What do these differences in fracture rates and distribution tell us about warfare in the prehistoric Southeast? First, both mortality rates and traumatic injuries are at their greatest levels in Late Woodland and small to medium Mississippian sites. The largest and best-defended communities, such as Moundville, are protected against such injuries. Second, the type of injury sustained during battle changes over time. At earlier sites, individuals are most often wounded with darts or arrowpoints. No cranial fractures or scalping cutmarks were seen in this sample for individuals of Archaic or Woodland age, although they have been identified elsewhere in the region during the Archaic time period (Smith 1995).

In the Mississippian period, types of injuries vary according to site size and defensibility. Smaller settlements, such as Tibbee Creek and Lubbub Creek, include individuals killed by arrows. Somewhat larger sites with defensive features, such as Koger's Island and Moundville, contain skeletons with cranial fractures, some of which were fatal. Differences in cause of death and types of injuries suggest a change in the style of warfare, from primarily bow-oriented in the Late Woodland period to more hand-to-hand combat using the warclub, especially at more complex Mississippian sites.

Undoubtedly, the rise of hand-to-hand combat was prompted by the construction of palisades around many Mississippian settlements. Fortifications of this type clearly helped defend against bow warfare. The presence of a substantial palisade at Moundville and the location of Koger's Island on an island suggest that both of these sites had defensive features protecting against bow warfare. Small Mississippian farmsteads, such as Tibbee Creek, were probably not fortified and thus would have been more vulnerable to attack with the bow and arrow. The mid-sized site of Lubbub Creek did have a palisade, but fortifications of this sort are not completely invincible and of course are no help if one is caught outside the walls. The one individual with an embedded point at Lubbub Creek has been interpreted as a captive, in which case the palisade would again have been irrelevant. Regardless, larger, better-fortified sites are less vulnerable than smaller, less well-defended ones, but they are not necessarily impregnable.

The data presented here suggest the following scenario. Violent death was present, but infrequent, in Alabama as early as the Middle Archaic period. With the introduction of the bow in the Late Woodland, raiding became endemic in the Deep South. This stage is represented by 1Pi61, which contained a number of individuals with embedded arrowpoints; some of these individuals were buried in mass graves. Later Mississippian societies responded in various ways to both increased levels of violence and to bow warfare. Large fortified sites such as Moundville would have the greatest defensibility and hence the least mortality. Mid-sized sites such as Koger's Island and especially small hamlets (Tibbee Creek) would be more vulnerable to attack; thus they have huge mortality levels.

As new defensive structures and strategies developed, the style of warfare evolved as well. As warfare became more important, its practice became more formalized, including at times large, well-organized war parties (Dye 1990). Trophies denoting success in raids—scalps and body parts—were commonly taken. Male participation in warfare became the norm, with the majority of deaths being males, rather than the more equal sex ratio seen at earlier sites.

In addition to the bow and arrow, the warclub became important as a weapon, but perhaps more so as a symbolic representation of warfare in the Mississippian period (Hudson 1976). The emphasis on clubs and maces, both as depictions in iconography as well as rare ceremonial weapons, suggests that the use of hand-held weapons conferred greater prestige on Mississippian warriors than did use of the bow. The functional use of warclubs in battle may also be seen in woodcut reproductions of Le Moyne's paintings from the 1560s, representing a Timucuan war party (Lorant 1946). As a result of use of the warclub, there is an increase in cranial and upper body fractures during the Mississippian period in Alabama.

In conclusion, skeletal evidence helps demonstrate the growing importance of warfare in the late prehistory of the Deep South and changes in how it was waged. These changes include: (1) an increase in warfare-related mortality in the Mississippian time period, especially at small or mid-sized sites, (2) greater male mortality as a result of interpersonal conflicts, (3) variation in cause of death (ranging from embedded points to hand-to-hand combat), (4) differences in fracture distribution and types, resulting in increased upper body and cranial fractures, especially at larger or better-defended Mississippian sites, and (5) a rise in the incidence of body part trophies, such as scalps. These changes are accompanied by an increasing sophistication in strategy and techniques that may be a factor in the abandonment of the Middle Tennessee River Valley in late prehistory, as Mississippian peoples moved to larger, more defensible centers.

ACKNOWLEDGEMENTS

This work was funded in part by the Professional Staff Congress-CUNY Research Award Program of the City University of New York. The authors thank the Alabama State Museum of Natural History and Eugene Futato of that institution for access to the skeletal collections and assistance in studying them. John Blitz, Warren DeBoer, Maria Smith, and Paul Welch answered numerous questions and provided references.

NOTES

1. Burial 616-620 at the Archaic Perry site consisted of four young females and one child (aged 7). One female had a point embedded in a thoracic vertebra; two others had points lying within their chest cavities. At the Late Woodland 1Pi61 site, two multiple burials contained juveniles. One, 13A-C,

held an infant, a young female, and an adolescent, possibly a male. The female and adolescent were found with points in their chest regions. Burial 61A-C consisted of an adult male, female, and a child aged 7–9. A projectile point was associated with this burial. Finally, at Koger's Island, juveniles were found in one of four mass graves. This burial was the only one of the four to contain only females and children. Both females were in their thirties, and one of them had been scalped around the time of death. The juveniles were aged 9 months, 3–4 years, and 13–14 years.

2. Cranial trauma at Koger's Island is further described in Bridges (1996). That report describes four individuals with cranial fractures. Since that article appeared, another example has been identified in the collection. 1Lu92-94, a female in her late twenties, has a small oval lesion on the right frontal bone, which is deeply indented in the center. This wound probably represents a traumatic injury made with some sort of pointed weapon.

4 Transitions at Moundville: A Question of Collapse

Margaret J. Schoeninger
Lisa Sattenspiel
Mark R. Schurr

The site of Moundville in west-central Alabama is the archaeological remnant of a prehistoric political and ceremonial center that oversaw a regional population of several thousand people between ca. A.D. 1000 and 1500 (Peebles 1987a). At its peak, Moundville was one of the largest such centers in the Southeast and covered about 100 ha on a high terrace overlooking the Black Warrior River. The site was first mapped in the late nineteenth century and first excavated early in the twentieth century; it has been studied intensively over several decades by several generations of excavators (Peebles 1974, 1987a; Peebles and Schoeninger 1981; Steponaitis 1983; Scarry 1986; Powell 1988; Welch 1991; Knight 1992; Knight and Steponaitis 1998a, 1998b). Much still remains to be done in terms of analysis of excavated materials, but the general outlines of the site's history are clear.

The earliest settlement at Moundville apparently occurred around A.D. 1050 and included a single mound some time shortly thereafter. The greatest extent of the site came early in its history, probably between A.D. 1200 and 1250 when multiple large mounds were constructed in a planned pattern (Knight 1994). The site was occupied until the mid-1600s, although the political system of which it was the center had collapsed over 100 years earlier. Most researchers believe that the collapse was the result of an internal disruption (Knight and Steponaitis 1998a); when De Soto's party reached the area in 1540, power in the region was centered away from Moundville (Hudson

Table 4-1. Ceramic Seriation at Moundville

Ceramic Period	Ceramic Descriptor	Dates (A.D.)
West Jefferson	Baytown Plain—a plain ware	950–1050
Moundville I	Serving and Storage: *Low frequency* Cooking: *High frequency*	1050–1250
Moundville II	Serving and Storage: *Proliferate* Cooking: *Decline relative to serving and* *storage*	1250–1400
Moundville III	Serving and Storage *Continue to predominate relative* *to cooking* *Some types vanish late*	1400–1550
Moundville IV	Some stylistic links with Period III New suite of types	1550–1650

Sources: Steponaitis 1983; Welch and Scarry 1995; Knight and Steponaitis 1998a

1997). There is, however, no consensus on the source of disruption within the Moundville polity. One suggestion is that the decline was the result of inherent instability of the type of hierarchical society it exemplified (Hudson et al. 1990). This hypothesis is difficult to evaluate or to test beyond suggesting that individuals react negatively to authority (Knight and Steponaitis 1998a) or by comparing alternative examples of declines (Peebles 1987a; Steponaitis 1991). Recent publications dealing with the region recommend evaluation of alternative hypotheses and reconsideration of previously published carbon stable isotope data (Schurr and Schoeninger 1995; Schoeninger and Schurr 1998). Such is the goal of the present chapter.

Such evaluation requires an accurate chronology of the site as well as an understanding of the relationship between Moundville and the other communities along the Black Warrior River. Work during the 1970s established a ceramic seriation summarized in Table 4-1 (based on Steponaitis 1983; Welch and Scarry 1995; Knight and Steponaitis 1998a). In conjunction with burial goods seriation and radiocarbon dates on various structures within Moundville and the valley, these ceramic data indicate an outline of development (taken from Knight and Steponaitis 1998a) within the valley as a whole (see Table 4-2). Moundville's function and relations within the Black Warrior River changed over time.

Table 4–2. Developmental Periods at Moundville

Ceramic Period	Developmental Period	Developmental Period Dates (A.D.)
West Jefferson	Intensification of local production	900–1050
Early I	Initial centralization	1050–1200
Late I/Early II	Regional consolidation	1200–1300
Late II/Early III	The paramountcy entrenched	1300–1450
Late III/IV	Collapse and reorganization	1450–1650

Source: Knight and Steponaitis 1998a

During the earliest Developmental period (Intensification of Local Production), few if any people lived in the area that was to become Moundville. The population along the Black Warrior River was distributed in large villages supported by maize agriculture supplemented with starchy seeds and other wild resources, particularly acorns and hickory nuts (Scarry 1993b). The shift to field production of corn apparently began during this period, and because the area was sparsely populated (Welch 1991), this shift is thought to have provided a food surplus that allowed support for crafts people (Scarry 1993b). Some Southeastern river valleys show evidence of local overcrowding, subsistence stress, and warfare at this time, and subsequent development within the Black Warrior River Valley is assumed to have been affected by events in other areas of the Southeast (Knight and Steponaitis 1998a).

This development is apparent in the subsequent Developmental period (Initial Centralization), during which a settlement of significant size was established at Moundville. Botanical remains indicate increased dependence on maize and decreased use of nuts relative to the earlier period (Scarry 1997), although stable carbon isotope ratios in human bone collagen indicate that less than half of calories, on average, were derived from maize during Ceramic Period I (see Table 4-3; Schoeninger and Schurr 1998). This is based on a small (n = 4) and highly variable sample (standard deviation = ±4.0‰ compared with ±0.8‰ to ±1.1‰ in the other three Ceramic periods). Most of the variability is due to a single burial that has a $\delta^{13}C$ value (−20.8‰; see Table 4-4) that is isotopically similar to that of terrestrial fauna. A diet of fish, which have quite negative $\delta^{13}C$ values, wild plants foods, and minimal maize would account for the low human value. It is possible that a West Jefferson period burial was incorrectly identified as a Moundville I burial. Fluoride measurements (Schurr 1989) show that the burial (2282WP) with the next lowest $\delta^{13}C$ value (−14.5‰) has a high fluoride content (see Table 4-5; bone was not available for the bur-

Table 4-3. Carbon Isotope Data from Moundville: A Comparison of Ceramic Periods with Developmental Periods

Ceramic Period	δ^{13}C‰±s.d.(n) (PDB)‰	Development Period (Ceramic Period)	δ^{13}C‰±s.d.(n) (PDB)‰
I	−15.1±4.0(4)	Initial centralization (Early I)	−20.8(1)
II	−10.4±1.0(3)	Regional consolidation (Late I/Early II)	−13.7±1.5(4)
III	−10.3±1.1(30)	Entrenched paramountcy (Late II/Early III)	−10.4±0.9(13)
IV	−11.1±0.8(24)	Collapse and reorganization (Late III/IV)	−11.0±1.0(27)
Aquatic Fauna	−23.5±1.2(16)		
Terrestrial Fauna	−20.2±1.5(5)		
Maize	−8.0±0.1(5)		

Data from Schoeninger and Schurr 1998

ial with the lowest δ^{13}C value). Based on previous applications of fluoride dating to the Moundville burials (Haddy and Hanson 1982), high fluoride contents are generally correlated with burials that are chronologically early. Taken in combination, the stable carbon isotope ratios and fluoride contents suggest that maize consumption intensified significantly during the Moundville I period, although more samples from this early period must be analyzed before reaching a conclusion.

The valley's population size is not well known for the Initial Centralization period, but there was enough labor available to build two small platform mounds, one at Moundville and the other in the immediate vicinity (Welch 1997). The majority of the valley's population is thought to have lived in small settlements but with a fairly dense population on the terrace at Moundville itself (Steponaitis 1991). Such a widespread population distribution pattern and a lack of evidence of fortification at Moundville and elsewhere in the valley does not support the intra- or interregional strife assumed in some scenarios of Moundville's development (Knight and Steponaitis 1998a). The appearance of nonlocal raw materials during this period at Moundville (Michals 1998; Steponaitis 1991) suggests that interregional contact took the form of trade rather than aggression. These trade relations continued for nearly 200 years.

During the subsequent Developmental Period of Regional Consolidation (A.D. 1200–1300), Moundville was established as the paramount center of a regional polity that extended nearly 40 km along the river.

Table 4–4. Carbon Isotope Data from Moundville

PERIOD Lab #	FIELD #	AGE	SEX	BONE	% COLLAGEN	C:N	δ^{13}C (PBD‰)
I							
167	2544 WP	A	?	bone	3	3.3	−20.8
143	2282 WP	MA	F	rib	6	3.6	−14.5
118	2042 Rho	YA	F	rib	16	3.3	−12.7
191	2884 RW	OA	M	rib	12	3.7	−12.1
Early II							
183	2687	MA	M	rib	11	4.1	−15.4
Late II							
152	2326	OA	F	humerus	19	3.7	−11.0
88	1748	MA	M	parietal	5	4.1	−10.9
53	1516	A	F	parietal	14	3.0	−9.2
Early III							
135	2166 WP	YA	F	rib		2.9	−11.6
200	1717	OA	?	bone	19	3.3	−11.4
10	1088	OA	M	parietal	14	2.9	−11.2
48	1491 SD	YA	F	rib	7	3.1	−10.6
123	2102	A	?	rib	18	2.8	−10.2
93	1789	YA	F	mandible	11	3.1	−10.2
66	1570	MA	M	rib	5	3.3	−10.0
92	1788	A	?	femur	8	2.9	−10.0
199	1544	?	?	bone	18	3.5	−9.9
60	1539	MA	F	temporal	10	2.9	−8.3
Late III							
158	2417	YA	F	rib	13	3.4	−12.2
17	1183 EE	YA	M	femur	3	2.5	−11.3
16	1181 EE	A	M	rib	8	2.8	−8.5
IV							
222	1 Tu4-M	MA	M	rib	7	3.0	−13.2
210	1 Wx1-1	MA	F	parietal	6	3.6	−12.7
211	1 Wx1-5a	A	F	patella	7	3.2	−11.7
225	1 Tu4-FF	A	F	rib	4	3.7	−11.7
204	1 Ha 19-I	YA	F	parietal	3	3.5	−11.5
224	1 Tu4-Z	YA	M	rib	4	2.7	−11.4
226	1 Tu4-HH	A	M	rib	3	3.2	−11.4
208	1 Ha 19-R	YA	F	parietal	7	3.3	−11.4
209	1 Ha 19-S	OA	F	radius	1	3.8	−11.3

Table 4.4 continued on next page

Table 4–4. continued

PERIOD Lab #	FIELD #	AGE	SEX	BONE	% COLLAGEN	C:N	$\delta^{13}C$ (PDB)‰
217	I Tu4-C	OA	F	fibula	12	3.2	−11.3
212	I Wx1-5b	A	M	patella	4	3.3	−11.3
207	I Ha 19-P	MA	F	rib	7	3.2	−11.1
219	I Tu4-3	YA	F	occipital	4	3.5	−11.1
227	I Tu4-JJ	A	F	parietal	2	3.3	−11.1
216	I Wx1-40	YA	M	rib	8	3.4	−11.0
228	I Tu4-KK	YA	?	rib	1	3.4	−10.9
220	I Tu4-J	OA	M	rib	10	3.3	−10.9
230	I Tu4-MM	YA	F	rib	7	3.8	−10.7
218	I Tu4-D	MA	M	occipital	6	3.3	−10.3
229	I Tu4-LL	YA	F	rib	19	3.0	−10.2
214	I Wx1-12	OA	F	rib	3	3.4	−10.1
221	I Tu4-L	MA	M	parietal	4	3.0	−10.1
202	I Ha19-D	YA	F	occipital	9	3.2	−10.1
215	I Wx1-18	OA	F	rib	3	3.5	−9.3

Table 4–5. Fluoride Content of Moundville Ceramic Period I Burials

Burial	% Fluoride	Std. Dev.	$\delta^{13}C$ (PDB)‰
2544 WP	—	—	−20.8
2282 WP	.244	.012	−14.5
MD2042 Rho	.087	.006	−12.7
MD2284 RW	.165	.004	−12.1

Note: Fluoride measured after Schurr (1989), three replicates per sample. An F-test indicates the results are significantly different, $F(2,6) = 276.2$, $p<.0001$. A least significant difference test found that the fluoride contents of all three samples were significantly different from each other at the 0.05 significance level. Bone was not available from 2544 WP for Fluoride analysis.

Approximately 20 major mounds, surmounted by public buildings, elite residences, and mortuary temples, were situated around a central plaza with east-west bilateral symmetry and with pairing of the residential mounds and mortuary temple mounds (Peebles 1969; Knight and Steponaitis 1998a). A palisade was erected and remained in use with several repairs until the end of the period, suggesting a need to secure the main center from intra- or interregional threats. Nonlocal stone, copper, marine shell, and pottery appear both as grave goods and as raw material in higher frequencies than in the previous Development period (Peebles 1987a; Steponaitis 1991; Knight 1992; Scarry

1998), suggesting increased interregional trade connections over previous times. These trade connections indicate potential lines of contact that may have played a part in subsequent events. The exotic ceramics derive from the lower Mississippi River Valley and southern Alabama to the south of the Black Warrior and also western and central Tennessee to the north and west. Marine shell was traded into Moundville from the Gulf coast. Copper originated in the Great Lakes regions to the north and the Appalachians to the east. Trade implies an outflow of goods balanced by the inflow that is recorded as mortuary items. Processed maize, nutmeats, and deer meat moved from the outlying settlements into Moundville (Scarry and Steponaitis 1992; Welch and Scarry 1995), presumably as tribute (Welch 1991), and these goods, when in surplus, were traded out. Several thousands of people living in single mound centers, farmsteads, and villages up and down the Black Warrior Valley are thought by many to have been controlled by Moundville (Welch 1998).

Moundville itself reached its highest density at around 1,000 people during this period. Elites lived in residences atop mounds and carefully arranged houses between the mounds, and the palisade accommodated nonelite nuclear families. A small number of individuals (n = 4) sampled for stable isotope analysis can be assigned to this Development period. We assume that a $\delta^{13}C$ value of $-20‰$ indicates a diet of 100 percent C_3 (based on the terrestrial fauna) and that $-8‰$ indicates 100 percent C_4 (based on data from Pecos Pueblo maize agriculturists who ate bison meat [Spielmann et al. 1990]). The data suggest that the four individuals from the Period of Regional Consolidation ate between 40 and 65 percent maize supplemented by a significant portion of foods like nuts or deer. If fish provided the majority of dietary protein, these people could have been eating significantly more maize; the negative $\delta^{13}C$ values for aquatic fauna would offset the less negative maize values. It is not known whether people in the outlying communities ate similarly.

Political consolidation continues into the next Development period, The Paramountcy Entrenched (Knight and Steponaitis 1998a), and the function of Moundville appears to have changed (Steponaitis 1991). By early in Ceramic Period III at least eight secondary mound sites were occupied within the valley, although none of them was large. The valley's population was around 10,000, with approximately 300 people at Moundville, small groups at secondary mound sites and the remaining majority living in farmsteads. The economy of Moundville's remaining residents apparently changed. A proliferation of serving vessels appears at the site with a concomitant decrease in cooking vessels, indicating that crafts people and/or elites, removed from basic food production, were provided subsistence (Welch and Scarry 1995). In addi-

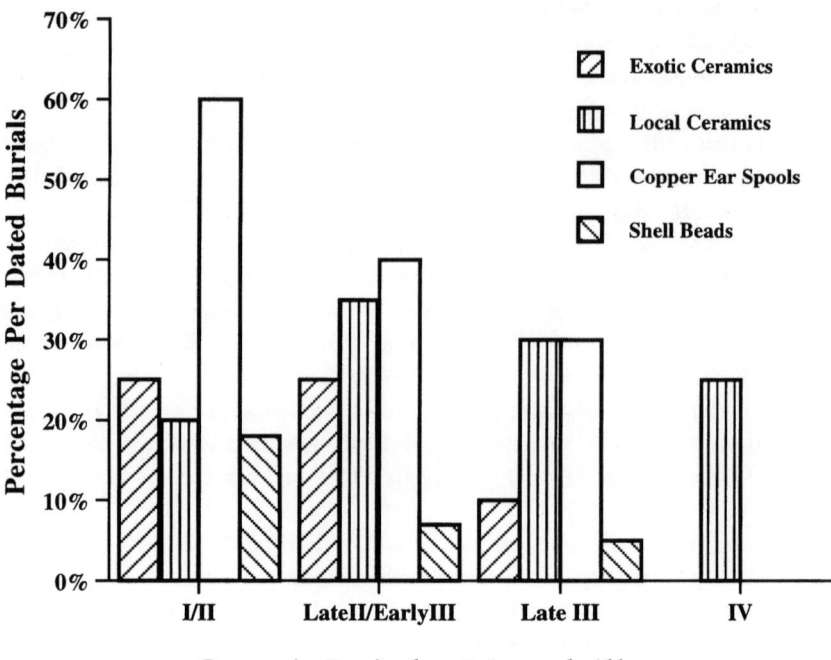

Ceramic Period at Moundville

Figure 4-1. Percent of Burials Accompanied by Specific Categories of Grave Goods in Four Periods of Occupation at Moundville. Changes in frequency serve to indicate changes in the site's function and in interregional trade connections. Shell beads and exotic ceramics were traded from the Gulf coast and other areas to the south. In contrast, copper ornaments originated from the north and east (data from Peebles 1987a; Steponaitis 1991).

tion, the number of burials at Moundville far outnumbers the expected resident population of the site, suggesting that the burials represent residents of the valley as a whole rather than just those at Moundville (Steponaitis 1991). Both elites and nonelites are buried in cemeteries rather than in mounds, as previously. Perhaps food was traded for crafts and/or funeral arrangements. The palisade is no longer present, and this fact in conjunction with the relatively large number of exotic and local prestige items recovered from Moundville (see Figure 4-1; Peebles 1987a) suggests that intra- or interregional strife was less of a concern at the center than in the previous period and that trade was thriving. Overall, the pattern suggests that people moved to be closer to their fields and that there was no reason (warfare or coercion) for doing otherwise (Holl 1993). The individuals in the stable isotope sample from this period ate significantly more maize, on average, than did those from the preceding period. Assuming that these individuals are representative of all valley residents, this suggests an increased reliance on maize in this period throughout the Moundville polity.

Early in the following Development period (Collapse and Reorganization), however, there is evidence of perturbation in the system. Late in Ceramic Period III, there is a decrease in the frequency of items obtained via intra- and interregional trade (see Figure 4-1; Peebles 1987a). The percent of local ceramics deposited drops only slightly relative to early Ceramic Period III, but materials obtained from interregional trade drop significantly. For copper ear spools, 40 percent were deposited early in Period III (Entrenched Paramountcy) in contrast to 30 percent late in Period III (Collapse and Reorganization). Nonlocal ceramics drop from a high of 25 percent to 10 percent, and strings of shell beads, always at low frequency, show an additional decrease late in Period III. This suggests an overall decrease in trade in Early Period III (Knight and Steponaitis 1998a) or Late Period III (Peebles 1987a). Whatever triggered this change also affected Moundville's inhabitants more directly. By the end of Late Period III, only four of the original 20 mounds at Moundville show signs of occupation or construction, and fewer burials were being placed anywhere within the site (Steponaitis 1983). The outlying mound sites with nucleated villages have their own cemeteries at this time (DeJarnette and Peebles 1970; Welch 1991). In addition, although serving and storage vessels continue to predominate relative to cooking vessels, some ceramic types vanish late in Ceramic Period III. Taken together, these changes suggest that control of craft production and mortuary ritual was moving from Moundville to the outlying settlements. The sequential timing of these events supports the interpretation of a perturbation during Period III rather than at the end of the period (A.D. 1500) when De Soto visited the area (Hudson 1997). The carbon stable isotope values from the small number of samples from Late Period III (n = 3) tentatively suggest that a drop in maize consumption had occurred. Two of the three samples have $\delta^{13}C$ values (−12.2‰, −11.3‰) that are close to the average (−11.0±1.0‰, n = 27) for the subsequent Development Period, Collapse and Reorganization.

Along with artifactual evidence for perturbation, there is also an increase in the frequency of skeletal pathologies in individuals buried at Moundville at this time relative to earlier periods, although the overall frequency remains low (Powell 1998). Skeletal evidence for anemia is rare, but the skeletal evidence occurs in higher frequency relative to the previous period. Tuberculosis is apparent in several skeletons, and this evidence suggests that the disease was fairly common within the population (Powell 1992a). Because people suffering from tuberculosis may transmit the disease intermittently for many years (Benenson 1995), the extended survivorship of infected individuals ensured disease transmission within the population and maintenance at endemic levels within the valley as a whole. Treponemal lesions on several skeletons indicate a similarly endemic and chronic level of infection of this disease as well (Powell 1991a, 1992a).

During this same period, several Spanish expeditions contacted the Gulf coast (Walthall 1980; Milanich and Milbrath 1989) and could have introduced new diseases such as measles, smallpox, and influenza into the Southeast. The earliest expeditions were led by Alonso Alvarez de Pineda, whose group spent six weeks in the Mississippi estuary region in 1519. Subsequently, around 1528, the Pánphilo de Narváez expedition landed in Tampa Bay and traveled along the Gulf coast to the Mississippi River. These contacts could have contributed indirectly to the disruption within the Moundville polity by interfering with traditional trade networks to the south. When the De Luna expedition of 1546 disembarked at Pensacola Bay on the Gulf coast of Florida, it was unable to obtain food because of widespread population disruption in the region resulting from Spanish diseases traveling from the Carolina coast. When the De Soto expedition moved through the region near Moundville in 1539–1543, few if any people were living at Moundville (Steponaitis 1983; Hudson 1997).

The pathogens commonly carried by European explorers usually kill too quickly to leave a skeletal signature. Microbiological tests may identify such organisms in skeletal materials in the future, but they are not adequate at present (S. Paabo, personal communication 1996). Even so, there is some justification for considering this alternate hypothesis at this time. An infected trader from the Gulf coast in 1519 could have come directly into Moundville where the first contact would have been with an already weakened elite segment of the polity. If mortality among these elites was high, not only trade but also the entire structure of the chiefdom would have been further disrupted. The risk of mortality would have been extremely high because there was no immunity, and other factors could have enhanced their susceptibility (Milner 1980; Powell 1991a, 1998) even though overall population density was too small to maintain these diseases at endemic levels. The representation of grave goods at Moundville, however, argues against large-scale population disruption in the valley. The frequency of local ceramics in burial contexts declines somewhat over time (see Figure 4-2) but does not completely drop off as expected with large depopulation and a catastrophic collapse. Thus, although it is still possible that acute, epidemic diseases were mitigating factors, they do not appear to be a sole cause of the polity's collapse late in Ceramic Period III.

What is less clear is how the combination of endemic disease, epidemic disease, and other disruptions caused by the Spaniards may have

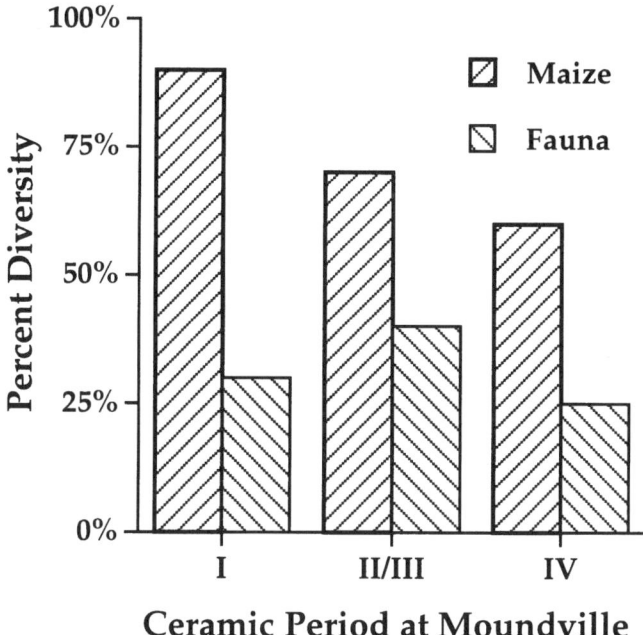

Figure 4-2. Morphological Diversity of Maize and Fauna Recovered from Three Periods of Occupation at Moundville. Whereas faunal diversity remains roughly constant through time, maize diversity drops throughout (data from Scarry 1993a, 1993b).

affected the overall reproductive success of the Moundville population. The long-standing chronic conditions of anemia, tuberculosis, and treponemal infection could have led to the death of a few affected persons, but that outcome was relatively rare. Thus, the original conditions were not likely to be major causes of mortality. Even so, genital tuberculosis has been shown to lead to coital inability, difficulties in conception, and pregnancy loss and is an important cause of subfecundity where tuberculosis is common. Anemia can lead to a higher rate of spontaneous abortions as well as an increased risk of maternal mortality (McFalls and McFalls 1984). In contrast, although venereal syphilis clearly affects reproductive success, the observed skeletal lesions were probably due to nonvenereal treponematosis (Powell 1991a), which would have influenced fertility only indirectly as a consequence of physical disfigurement and potential difficulties finding mates. Tuberculosis and anemia, if exacerbated by adverse nutritional and disease states caused by early indirect Spanish contact, however, may have been important causes of subfecundity in the Moundville population during Late Moundville III. A decrease in population at the end of

Moundville III would have placed the polity at a disadvantage compared to other chiefdoms that may have been militarily competitive (Welch 1991). The prevailing pattern of warfare largely depended on overall group size of fighting men. Lack of military success would negatively influence the Moundville chiefdom elites.

Whether or not this scenario actually took place, assuming that interregional trade is an expression of chiefly roles in external relations, the decline in such trade suggests that these relations had altered. By Ceramic Period IV, life along the Black Warrior was very different (Sheldon 1974). Most of the inhabitants lived in nucleated villages lacking mounds. The disruptive events late in Period III culminated with most of the mound sites in the valley being abandoned by the mid 1500s and with the one at Moundville largely depopulated by the end of the century. Interregional trade to the south (exotic ceramics and shell beads) appears to have stopped almost completely (see Figure 4-1). Ceramic Period IV shows a new suite of pottery types that may indicate unknown influences, even though there are some links to previous periods (see Table 4-1; Knight and Steponaitis 1998a). This is the main portion of the last Development Period, Collapse and Reorganization.

Compared with Period III and throughout Ceramic Period IV, there is a marked increase of skeletal pathologies indicative of anemia (Hill-Clark 1981; Powell 1988; Hill 1996). Although the scoring criteria used for identification are not consistent across studies, the indicators of anemia appear to be more frequent and more extreme in the later period (Hill 1996; Powell, personal communication 1996). An early suggestion proposed that the anemias are iron-deficiency anemias, a result of increased maize ingestion, but the carbon stable isotope data (Schoeninger and Schurr 1998) indicate a decrease in maize consumption rather than an increase (difference in means significant at 0.01 level in a two-tailed test). The $\delta^{13}C$ values indicate an average drop of around 10 percent in Moundville IV as well as in the last Development period overall. But anemias may come about as a result of a high pathogen load (Kent 1992), and it is possible that the chronic infectious diseases combined with other complications may be a factor in the increase in frequency and severity of anemias rather than the diet per se.

Overall these data suggest that the general health of the population within the Black Warrior River Valley continued to decline in the sixteenth century (Hill-Clark 1981; Powell 1998). The decrease in maize consumption that may have begun late in Period III suggests an explanation. Disruption by disease and/or usurpation of maize stores by the Spanish could account for a decrease in use of maize by the people living along the Black Warrior River for a few years at most. The decreased dependence over the longer time from late in Period III and throughout

Period IV suggests that adequate maize was not available for an extended period of time. One possibility is that overpopulation outstripped the carrying capacity of the land, but this seems unlikely based on Spanish accounts (Hudson 1997). Another possibility is that the land itself could no longer produce adequate maize to support the existing population, but this also appears unlikely (Scarry 1993a, 1993b). Most of the Moundville sites are located very close to the river in the floodplain portion of the valley on productive agricultural soils that do not flood during planting or growing seasons (Scarry 1993a, 1993b). Such fields would have been relatively immune to depletion.

Another possibility is that the maize itself became less productive. During the periods of occupation within the Black Warrior Valley, the overall morphological diversity of maize declined, and the number of maize varieties decreased to two (Scarry 1993a, 1993b; see Figure 4-2), suggesting that genetic diversity had declined. An alternative hypothesis is that, with the decrease in maize diversity and in maize strains, the maize itself became more susceptible to failure by diseases that affect maize strains. Loss of or lower productivity in maize harvests as a result of blight would have eliminated a food surplus and would also explain the shift in the last Developmental period for people to include more wild crops in their diets. In addition, nutritional stress caused by limited crop yields would account for the increase in pathologies that have been observed. A lowering of a dependable nutrient source coupled with a chronic pathogen load and Spanish disturbances could have critically affected the polity. This line of reasoning suggests a destabilization of the political system along the Black Warrior largely because of internal biological reasons, and it is necessary to devise biological probes for testing. We are currently investigating the possibility of maize blight in conjunction with climatic variability. In addition, we expect that fluoride dating (Haddy and Hanson 1982; Schurr 1989) will permit us to clarify further the chronology of dietary change.

In summary, the population within the Moundville polity peaks during Period III, and the stable carbon isotope data indicate that maize agriculture intensification increases throughout. Further, although the estimates are uncertain, there is no support for large-scale depopulation of the valley until late in Period IV when Spaniards move into the continental interior. Trade drops off during Ceramic Period III, but the pattern of disruption does not support the massive depopulation expected to result from diseases transmitted from the Gulf coast, which would have been the likely source. There is a significant decline in dietary maize in Period IV that may have begun in Late Period III. It is unlikely that widespread disease explains this pattern of long-term decline in maize dependence. The drop in maize diversity with its potential vulnerability appears the next obvious target for investigation.

Acknowledgments

We thank Svante Paabo and Mary Lucas Powell for discussions related to identification of infectious diseases in human skeletal material. We particularly thank Mary Powell for reading a previous version of the manuscript and for making many excellent comments. Thanks also to Pat Lambert, whose invitation allowed us to explore further the fascinating question of this polity's collapse. Lane Beck prepared many of the samples for analysis. Funding was provided by NSF grant BNS-9004063 to MJS and MRS. We also gratefully acknowledge Christopher S. Peebles, whose early cooperative project first involved many of the individuals currently working on aspects of the Moundville polity.

Notes

1. Samples of human bone representing many of the Ceramic and Developmental periods were obtained from the Alabama Museum of Natural History. Animal bone, attributed to Ceramic Period I, was provided by Lauren Michals. The majority of the samples could not be assigned reliably to a single period, particularly in the case of the earlier periods. Only samples that can be assigned to specific ceramic periods, or in the case of Period III, that can be assigned to early or late within the period, are included here in Table 4-4. All samples were cleaned mechanically of surface debris and then ultrasonicated in double-distilled water. The organic fraction of bone was extracted in several ways and results compared on duplicate samples. Bone was ground, passed through a 0.71mm mesh screen, and demineralized in hydrochloric acid. The resultant organic fraction (mainly the protein, collagen) was dissolved (hydrolyzed) in a weak, hot hydrochloric acid solution (following Longin 1971 with modifications for humic acid removal by DeNiro and Epstein 1981 and Schoeninger and DeNiro 1984). In addition, pieces of bone were demineralized in weak hydrochloric acid (HCl) at room temperature (Sealy 1986). Some samples were demineralized (following Tuross et al. 1988; Schoeninger et al. 1989) in cold ethylenediaminetetraacetic acid, which enhances protein recovery in degraded samples. Comparison of results from samples and controls demineralized both by HCl and EDTA revealed no differences among preparation methods, and in those cases where more than one preparation was made, the average value was used in the calculations presented.

In all cases, dried organic material was weighed into clean quartz tubing with excess cupric oxide, elemental copper, and elemental silver. The tubing was sealed under vacuum, combusted at 800°C, and allowed to cool to room temperature. The resulting H_2O, CO_2, and N_2 were separated cryogenically in a glass vacuum line, and the carbon dioxide and nitrogen gas were analyzed mass spectrometrically. The CO_2 was prepared both at Harvard University and at the University of Wisconsin and was measured in Dr. John Hayes's laboratory at Indiana University and in Schoeninger's laboratory at the University of Wisconsin on Finnegan MAT Delta E mass spectrometers. Duplicate samples indicated nonsystematic variation and were within 0.4‰, on average.

5 Dental Health at Early
Historic Fusihatchee Town:
Biocultural Implications of
Contact in Alabama

Marianne Reeves

The research presented here traces changes in patterns of diet and health stress from the Mississippian period into the historic period in Alabama using a model that compares published data on dental health at the prehistoric Moundville site (ca. A.D. 1050 to 1550) to new research on dental health at early contact period Fusihatchee Town (ca. A.D. 1640 to 1814). Comparisons with Moundville, a major Mississippian civic and ceremonial center in west-central Alabama, can highlight alterations that occurred in health and diet in Alabama along with the change (from ca. A.D. 1400–1600) to social and political egalitarianism (Waselkov et al. 1987), dispersed settlement (Peebles 1987a), and European contact.

Direct ancestry between the historic inhabitants of Fusihatchee and Mississippian peoples at Moundville is not suggested. The two were ethnically distinct and spatially separated by a distance of approximately 150 miles. It has been suggested that the people(s) of Moundville were ancestors of the Choctaw (Little and Curren 1995), whereas the occupants of Fusihatchee Town are well documented historically as Creek Indians. The cultural differences between these groups preclude any suggestion of cultural continuity between Moundville and Fusihatchee peoples. The validity of the comparison, however, lies in its investigation of the general changes in diet and health patterns in light of the shift from large to smaller-scale occupation sites and in conjunction with the consequences of European contact in Alabama. Tracking such shifts can provide a more thorough understanding of the dynamic, complex forces involved in political, social, and economic changes after A.D. 1500 among native peoples, who faced unbridled European expansion into their lands and livelihoods (Waselkov et al. 1987).

The contact period was an extraordinary time of turbulent cultural and biological change in the Eastern Woodlands. Amerindians were enslaved and missionized, removed from their homelands, and relocated by European newcomers (M. Smith 1987). Dependence on maize agriculture in native communities in the Southeast generally increased through the historic period (Larsen 1995). Much of the research on the changes that occurred in health patterns from the prehistoric to historic periods has documented a general decline in dental health, with rates of dental caries and enamel hypoplasia increasing, particularly in the later contact period. With a general framework for the changes in health that occurred with the disintegration of major civic and ceremonial centers, the intensification of agriculture, and European contact in the Southeast as the backdrop, this investigation focuses on the prevalence of dental pathology at two archaeological sites in Alabama, the major Mississippian mound center of Moundville and the early historic town site of Fusihatchee.

HISTORICAL FRAMEWORK FOR THE CONTACT PERIOD

It is widely recognized that a general decline in native health accompanied European contact in the Southeast. Epidemics of smallpox and measles decimated native populations, and venereal and congenital syphilis became widespread. Nonspecific responses to health stressors such as periostitis and enamel hypoplasia are often prevalent in skeletal populations from the contact period as well and are taken to indicate a decrease in health levels from the precontact era (Larsen and Milner 1994). Additionally, the physical hardships of enforced labor and relocation contributed heavily to native mortality rates (M. Smith 1987).

A complicating factor of health stress generally in the historic period was the increasing reliance on maize and other soft foods in the diet. It has been suggested that this gradual dietary change resulted in a decreasingly varied diet and, in some cases, lessened the potential for obtaining all of the dietary vitamins, minerals, and amino acids needed for adequate nutrition. Exactly what constitutes adequate nutrition remains to be defined, and many nutritionists find that what constitutes *malnutrition* is substantially easier to describe (Schoeninger and Moore 1992). For our purposes, the most significant point to keep in mind is that diet and infectious disease work in a synergistic fashion

(Buikstra and Mielke 1985; Schoeninger and Moore 1992; Scrimshaw 1975; Scrimshaw et al. 1968). If the diet is poor, an individual's immune system is less likely to be able to fend off infection; and under infectious disease stress, an individual is less likely to be able to take in (and in some cases, absorb) an adequate level of nutrients. Thus, the contact period for the people of Alabama, as in other parts of the Eastern Woodlands, was a time when all of these stress factors were operational and were, in the end, crucial determinants of health and survivorship rates among Native Americans.

In addition to the cultural and biological stressors associated with European contact in the Southeast, the change in settlement patterns from complex chiefdoms to scattered, small-scale village occupations in the protohistoric period had its own repercussions. In biological terms, a shift from the occupation of a (periodically) densely populated area to widely scattered occupation sites might entail some of the following changes in health status: (1) a general decrease in disease prevalence resulting from less person-to-person contact and more sanitary living conditions and (2) equal distribution of food resources and an improved dietary status for the population as a whole resulting from a more egalitarian political and societal structure. Absent from these considerations of health changes in the Mississippian/Protohistoric and early historic transition is the complicating factor of European contact, however. If the health changes associated with contact are added into the equation, what kind of reconstruction of past health and diet emerges? A reconstruction of contact-period health in central Alabama could be expected to reveal a general decrease in health status relative to late prehistoric complex societies in the Mississippian period. In essence, the assumption is that the consequences of contact in some ways outweigh those of change within and among native groups in the protohistoric and early historic periods. Bioarchaeological analysis of the dental remains from the Fusihatchee Town site, in addition to ethnohistoric and paleoethnobotanical analyses of the site, suggests that this scenario is not likely.

PREVIOUS BIOARCHAEOLOGICAL ANALYSES OF HISTORIC CREEK POPULATIONS

Only a few bioarchaeological analyses of early historic Creek skeletal remains have been conducted. Powell (1994a) has investigated remains from the Lower Creek town of Ocmulgee, recovered from Macon Plateau, a major early Mississippian mound site at Ocmulgee National Monument in central Georgia. Two series of historic period burials were recovered from Macon Plateau. Nine burials found in the vicinity of Mound C were dated to the historic period. An analysis of the skeletal remains revealed neither bone lesions nor dental enamel defects. Remains recovered from 61 burials at the 1690 Trading Post in the Middle Plateau area (to the east of Mound C) yielded no evidence of nutritional deficiencies in the sample, whereas several adults displayed evidence of pathology (healed periosteal lesions indicative of endemic treponematosis). The poor preservation of skeletal material at Ocmulgee town, however, prevents a thorough investigation of the health of its inhabitants (Powell 1994a).

Turner (1984) analyzed the archaeological population from the early historic Upper Creek town of Hoithlewaulee in central Alabama. He concluded that, by the early 1700s, the Creeks had acquired a biological adaptation to smallpox, a highly infectious disease transmitted to native populations through contact with European colonists. Turner describes a complete *absence* of enamel hypoplasia, periosteal lesions, and porotic hyperostosis in the series, and he attributes the absence to this remarkable adaptation. Nevertheless, the evidence for smallpox adaptation is weak at best, and the reason for the absence of dental and skeletal markers of stress in the sample remains unclear.

THE FUSIHATCHEE TOWN SITE

Archaeological Background

The Fusihatchee Town site (1EE191) on the lower Tallapoosa River in Elmore County, Alabama, was first excavated in 1980 by Gregory Waselkov of the University of South Alabama and Craig Sheldon and John Cottier of Auburn University. From 1985 until 1996, salvage excavations were carried out at the site in response to the construction of a gravel quarry sanctioned by the site owners. The investigators believe that Fusihatchee functioned as one of many Upper Creek towns along the Tallapoosa, carrying on an active trading relationship with nearby French and English settlers. The historic component of the Fusihatchee site can be bracketed tightly in time, with occupation from 1640 to 1814, when federal troops under the command of General Andrew Jackson burned the town. Waselkov and coworkers (1987) have identified Atasi and Tallapoosa components at Fusihatchee Town dating to 1680–1700 and 1750–1780, respectively. Diagnostic glass bead types (which have been used at other Creek sites to date human burials), Spanish hoes, sheet brass gorgets, Creek ceramics, as well as later English stoneware and buttons, French faience, and silver artifacts have been recovered from Fusihatchee. The authors further note that burials in the historic Creek town of Hoithlewaulee were often found inside or near houses; the patterning of burials at Fusihatchee Town is similar, with burial pits often occurring within the boundaries of bed post-

Table 5-1. Age Structure of the Historic Fusihatchee Sample

Age Category	N[1]	%
Subadult	93	35.3
Adult	130	49.2
Unknown	41	15.5

[1]Total n = 264

holes inside house structures. Dimmick (1989:8) describes historical accounts of Creek burial practices: "It was not unusual for a warrior to be buried under his wife's house and for her to observe a long mourning period (an enforced period of fidelity) after his death."

Skeletal Population

The skeletal sample from the Fusihatchee Town site is composed of 284 individuals. Twenty of these have been identified as belonging to the Late Woodland period Autauga phase. The remaining 264 individuals are believed to date to the Atasi and Tallapoosa phases of the historic period and include 130 adults, 93 subadults, and 41 individuals for whom a numeric or broad categorical age is indeterminate (see Table 5-1). The collection is poorly preserved, and many individuals are missing more than half of the skeleton. In addition, many of the burials were disturbed by looters in the 1930s. Approximately 41.7 percent of the 223 individuals in the aged sample, defined as adult or subadult, had lived less than 16 years at the time of death (58.3 percent lived to 16 years). The mean age at death in the Fusihatchee Town series is 18 years (median age, 16 years); however, to what extent this figure is a result of the population's fertility, rather than high mortality, is unknown. Table 5-2 summarizes the distribution of the aged sample of 223 individuals into discrete age categories, and it reveals few infants and many young adults. This unusual mortality profile is likely a result of two factors. First, there is an underrepresentation of infants in the sample, a common problem in cemetery samples stemming from poor preservation of infant skeletons and collection strategy bias (see Walker et al. 1988). Second, the young adult mortality hump may be a result of measurement error either in the aging method or in preservation bias, rather than an accurate reflection of high young adult mortality (see Howell 1982).

Dental Analysis

The focus of this analysis is on two pathological conditions of the dentition: dental caries and enamel hypoplasia. All deciduous and permanent teeth were examined for dental caries with the aid of a 16x hand

Table 5–2. Age at Death

Age Category (years)	N[1](D$_x$)[2]	% (d$_x$)
0 – 1.0	6	2.69
1 – 4.9	38	17.04
5 – 9.9	24	10.76
10 – 14.9	17	7.62
15 – 19.9	25	11.21
20 – 24.9	24	10.76
25 – 29.9	22	9.87
30 – 34.9	27	12.11
35 – 39.9	17	7.62
40 – 44.9	13	5.83
45 – 49.9	8	3.59
50+	2	0.90

[1]Total n = 223. [2]D$_x$ denotes absolute number of dead of age x.

lens under oblique fluorescent light; the location of lesions was scored as occlusal or non-occlusal. The labial enamel of deciduous and permanent maxillary central incisors and mandibular canines was also examined for enamel hypoplasia under similar magnification and lighting conditions. Extremely worn or damaged teeth were excluded from the analysis. Enamel surfaces of intact teeth were given the "fingernail" test to determine presence or absence of significant grooving of the surface. Conventional methods for scoring enamel hypoplasia have recently been criticized by Ensor and Irish (1995) and by Berti and Mahaney (1995). For the purposes of this study, however, only lesions that passed the "fingernail" test (tactile detection of a groove or pit in the enamel) were scored as hypoplastic. It is possible that the frequency of enamel hypoplasia in the Fusihatchee sample has been underrepresented by this scoring method. Powell (1988) describes hypoplastic lesions as pitted and grooved defects and uses macroobservation, as well as comparison to other affected tooth types, to define a defect. Although not identical, the major criteria for defining defects in Powell's study were also used in the Fusihatchee Town study (macroobservation of pitted and grooved defects), minimizing the potential for interobserver error, particularly when the comparative analysis is limited to prevalence by individual rather than by tooth type or number of lesions.

Dental Pathology

Dental caries. Dental caries prevalence is an important source of information in evaluating relative levels of health and nutrition in past

Table 5–3. Carious Lesions in Deciduous and Permanent Teeth

		Deciduous	Permanent	Total Teeth
All Tooth Types	N	19/263	252/1463	271/1726
	%	7.22	17.23	15.70
Molars	N	14/151	168/524	182/675
	%	9.27	32.06	26.96
Premolars	N	–	43/412	43/412
	%	–	10.44	10.44
Canines	N	0/47	15/207	15/254
	%	0.00	7.25	5.91
Incisors	N	5/65	26/320	31/385
	%	7.69	8.13	8.05

populations. Larsen (1995) notes that the presence of dental caries in the dentition is clearly related to food composition and its manner of preparation. The gruel-like consistency of soft, boiled foods in many agricultural societies enhances the likelihood that food particles will become caught in the grooves and fissures of molars and premolars during mastication. These grooved areas on the tooth crown are ideal locations for the growth of the bacterial colonies that cause dental caries. Larsen and coworkers (1991) have documented the relationship between dental caries and the increased consumption of maize in the historic period on the Georgia coast. Maize particles remaining in dental fissures provide ideal conditions for the development of dental caries. In general, dental caries rates increase with an increasingly maize-based diet (Larsen 1995, 1997; Larsen et al. 1991).

Of 1,726 deciduous and permanent teeth from Fusihatchee scored for the presence or absence of carious lesions, 15.7 percent were found to be affected. Table 5-3 shows that the prevalence of carious lesions in deciduous dentitions was decidedly lower than in permanent teeth, with rates as low a 0.0 percent for canine teeth and as high as 9.3 percent for molars. Carious lesions were more common in permanent teeth (17.2 percent affected), particularly in permanent molars (32.1 percent affected).

Powell (1988) found that 54.1 percent of individuals and 18.7 percent of teeth were carious at Moundville. These figures are lower than those from the Nodena population and comparable to the Mississippian Lubbub Creek sample. Powell concluded that her original hypothesis, that non-elite individuals from Moundville suffered extreme systemic stress as a result of resource deprivation by the elite, was unsubstantiated by her analysis (Powell 1988).

It should be noted that antemortem tooth loss can introduce complications into calculations of dental caries rates in archaeological populations. True caries rates may be underestimated in samples lacking well-preserved dentitions. Poor preservation in the Fusihatchee sample prevented accurate estimation of antemortem tooth loss, which may have resulted in slightly underestimated rates of dental disease.

Enamel hypoplasia. Enamel hypoplasia is a nonspecific indicator of childhood metabolic stress that occurs when the enamel, the outer covering of the tooth crown, is forming (Larsen 1987). Nutritional or disease stress may disrupt tissue growth in the body; amelogenesis, the process of enamel production, may be halted by a stress episode (or series of episodes), typically producing macroscopic linear bands or pits in the enamel. Goodman and Rose (1990:61) note that "the biological basis and methodology for relating enamel hypoplasias to perturbations during tooth crown development has long been confirmed." Larsen (1987) describes enamel defects as reliable indicators of nonspecific metabolic stress in past populations for a variety of reasons. First, enamel is particularly sensitive to metabolic insult and records such insults as dental defects even in the buffered intrauterine environment (enamel formation in deciduous teeth begins at approximately five months *in utero*). Second, dental enamel is never remodeled; defects serve as permanent records of tissue growth disruption. Finally, because dental tissues are hard and resilient to postmortem degradation, the teeth are often recovered archaeologically and serve as the remaining physical representations of past peoples (Larsen 1987).

Studies of dental enamel hypoplasia have revealed important general trends concerning subsistence shifts to agriculture in prehistoric populations as well as health changes that occurred in Indian populations with European contact. Hutchinson and Larsen (1990) used enamel defects to document a decline in health of native populations from the Georgia coast in the transition from hunting and gathering to agriculture. Health status further declined with additional stressors in the contact period.

Table 5-4 summarizes the prevalence of enamel hypoplasia in deciduous and permanent teeth from Fusihatchee. The highest prevalence of hypoplasia (62.3 percent) was recorded for permanent mandibular canine teeth. Deciduous canine teeth exhibited a much lower prevalence of this condition (0.0 percent). Hypoplastic lesions were present in only 6.3 percent of deciduous central maxillary incisors as compared to 36.5 percent of permanent central maxillary incisor teeth. The overall prevalence of hypoplasia in deciduous maxillary central incisors and mandibular canines was 3.3 percent. Permanent teeth experienced much higher rates of dental defects (50.8 percent). The reason for this is unknown and may be a result of the underenumeration of young juveniles in the sample.

The prevalence of hypoplasia in the permanent dentition of indi-

Table 5-4. Prevalence of Enamel Hypoplasia in Deciduous and Permanent
Teeth

		Deciduous	Permanent	Total
Max I1	N[1]	1/16	31/85	32/101
	%	6.25	36.5	31.7
Man C	N	0/14	66/106	66/120
	%	0.0	62.3	55.0
Total Teeth	N	1/30	97/191	98/221
	%	3.33	50.8	44.3

[1]N signifies number of individuals scored with bilateral presence of hypoplasia.

Table 5-5. Prevalence of Permanent Dentition Hypoplasia in Individuals[1] by
Age

		Subadult[2]	Adult	Total
Max I1	N	7/20	18/42	25/62
	%	35.0	42.86	40.32
Man C	N	8/18	37/53	45/71
	%	44.44	69.81	63.38
Total Teeth	N	10/24	42/66	52/90
	%	41.67	63.64	57.78

[1]Individuals with at least one hypoplastic lesion are scored as affected.
[2]Signifies individuals <16 years of age.

viduals from Fusihatchee is summarized in Table 5-5. Adults experienced higher rates of enamel hypoplasia in their incisors and canines
than did subadults. Mandibular canines were more commonly affected
than were the central maxillary incisors. The prevalence of hypoplasia
in subadult permanent teeth was 41.7 percent, compared to 63.6 percent in those of adult individuals. The prevalence for the combined
subadult/adult sample is 57.8 percent.

Powell's (1988, 1991b) research on diet, health, and status at Moundville provides interesting insights into Mississippian life in a regional
capital with a highly stratified social and political organization. Her
analysis of dental health at Moundville revealed a high general prevalence of hypoplasia (53 percent in 138 adults examined and 59 percent
of 31 subadults examined). However, these figures are lower than those
from other Mississippian populations, including the Dickson Mounds
in Illinois (79 percent) and the late Mississippian Nodena population
in Arkansas (89 percent) (Powell 1988).

DISCUSSION

Creek Ethnohistory

The ethnohistorical record of the changes occurring in Creek societies in the protohistoric and early historic periods is invaluable for interpreting patterns of health and subsistence in the bioarchaeological record. Historian Kathryn Braund (1990) describes the impact of contact on Creek society in the eighteenth century. By the middle 1800s, Creek commerce with Europeans was conducted largely by traders from Augusta, Georgia. The trade good most desired by the European market was the deerskin. Braund (1990:239) states that "the barter of deerskins for European goods was the single most powerful force in Creek history during the eighteenth and early nineteenth centuries." Waselkov (1989) agrees. He details the trade relationship established between the Spanish in *La Florida* and, later, the Dutch, French, and English to the east and north and eastern Muskogeans in the interior Southeast. That relationship extends as far back as the sixteenth century, with exchanges between the Spanish in Florida and the Creeks for deerskins and European goods. In the period from 1565 to 1704, when the Spanish missions of Apalachee were destroyed, trade was conducted either indirectly, through middlemen, or directly, via face-to-face interactions between Europeans and Indians (Waselkov 1989). Waselkov finds evidence for a gradual increase in direct trade through time, and this evidence poses intriguing bioarchaeological questions concerning possible increases in direct pathogen transmission between colonists and native inhabitants. The economic and activity ramifications of the deerskin trade are equally interesting because they heavily impacted subsistence patterns and the lifeways in general of the native peoples of the interior Southeast.

The changes within Creek economic and social life during this time have been explored by Braund (1990) as well, and her research has focused on the changing roles of Creek women in the eighteenth century. Early European accounts of Creek society detail the organization of matrilineal extended family households (Green 1982). During the eighteenth century, however, the prime organizational and economic unit became the more European-style nuclear family. European contact also directly impacted Creek subsistence patterns. According to historic accounts, maize was the major subsistence crop for Creek farmers at this time. Men were responsible for the preparation and planting of communal village maize fields, while women managed the cultivation, collection, preparation, and storage of food. Maize was processed into hominy and meal for consumption. Agricultural products, however, were not the only dietary plant staples. Wild foods also played an important role in the diet (Gremillion 1995), and women were responsible for gathering nuts, wild fruits, berries, and roots for processing as food or medicine (Braund 1990). Maize agriculture and wild food gathering were important economic ventures as well, as the Creeks supplied maize, beans, hickory nut oil, bear oil, and deer oil, as well as fish and venison, to the French traders at Fort Toulouse, ten miles north of modern-day Montgomery (Waselkov 1992).

During winter months, women accompanied their husbands on hunting trips for white-tailed deer. By the early 1700s, the Creeks had become commercial hunters, and their villages and towns were abandoned for the winter season or longer. The European goods the Creeks received in exchange for the deerskins and pelts included thimbles, scissors, rum, axes, knives, cloth, mirrors, and guns. But by the end of the eighteenth century, the deer populations were reduced considerably by overhunting. This, in conjunction with a significant drop in the market price for deerskins, prompted the federal government to assist the Creeks in resolving their economic predicament. The 1790 Treaty of New York between the United States and Creek towns set forth a program of "civilization" to reform the Creek economy. The program included provisioning of agricultural implements and domestic animals to Creeks so that they might become effective herdsmen and full-fledged farmers. This began the crucial transition to an economy based in commercial agriculture and livestock and, for Creek society, a continuing servitude to European forces. In 1813 a Creek civil war began the new century, and Creek Removal by the federal government west of the Mississippi River ensued in 1835. Most of the Creeks settled in the Indian Territory and, to a large extent, resumed traditional Creek lifeways (Braund 1990).

Subsistence in Historic Fusihatchee Town

From the data for moderate prevalence of dental caries in the Fusihatchee skeletal population in conjunction with a high prevalence of enamel hypoplasia, no evidence exists that *directly* implies that the Creek individuals buried at Fusihatchee were malnourished. Ethnohistorical data on the Creek-European trade in the seventeenth and eighteenth centuries documents the exchange of Creek agricultural products for European trade goods. Maize agriculture became more intensive through time (Braund 1990), yet no bioarchaeological evidence was found for a decrease in dietary variation substantial enough to produce obvious skeletal and dental correlates of malnutrition (such as extremely high dental caries rates).

A more detailed recounting of Creek subsistence patterns is provided by Gremillion (1995) in an ethnobotanical analysis of the floral

Table 5-6. Prevalence of Dental Caries: Comparative Data

	% of Carious Individuals	% of Carious Teeth	X Number of Carious Teeth per Individual
Fusihatchee	50.0	15.7	1.44
	(94/188)	(271/1726)	(271/188)
Moundville[1]	54.1	18.7	1.77
	(192/355)	(630/3375)	(630/355)
Santa Catalina de	34.8	8.0	0.81
Guale[2]	(113/324)	(262/3274)	(262/324)
Santa Catalina de	82.1	34.2	5.77
Guale de Santa Maria[3]	(78/95)	(548/1602)	(548/95)

[1] Powell (1988)

[2] Larsen et al. (1991)

[3] Larsen et al. (1991)

remains recovered from Fusihatchee and two other historic assemblages. Gremillion argues that the key element of subsistence in the Southeast in the seventeenth and eighteenth centuries was maize. Because the inhabitants of these historic sites were adapted ecologically to a temperate deciduous forest environment, they also relied on indigenous resources like hickory nuts and acorns. The floral remains from the Fusihatchee site included not only maize cupules and hickory nutshells, but also the remains of Old World crops in the form of peach pits and black-eyed peas. Overall, Gremillion sees commonalties in subsistence in the Southeast from ca. A.D. 1600 to 1800: maize and hickory are ubiquitous taxa, and indigenous grain crops are extremely rare. These findings argue for the continuing importance of mast resources in native subsistence over the last several thousand years.

A comparison to Powell's (1988) data on diet and dental caries at Moundville reveals a prevalence of carious teeth of 3.0 percent higher than that recorded for the Fusihatchee sample (see Table 5-6). Powell notes that the Mississippian diet from A.D. 800–1500 was one of abundant resources. These included a number of wild resources such as fish, migratory waterfowl, white-tailed deer, wild turkey, and raccoon, as well as fruits, berries, nuts such as hickory and acorns, and seed-bearing pioneer plant species.

Cultigens made up the other portion of the Mississippian diet. The inhabitants of Moundville from the Moundville I phase onward practiced full-fledged agriculture (Scarry 1986), and maize dominated the plant food assemblage at Moundville throughout the Moundville and Alabama River phases (Peebles 1987b). Powell (1988) notes that intensive agriculture in the Mississippian period made necessary the adoption of adaptive strategies such as interplanting crops to meet problems that would arise from crop cultivation without artificial fertilization. Additionally, culinary adaptations countered nutritional deficits in cereal-rich diets. Soaking maize kernels in water to which beans or ash had been added increased the content of niacin in the kernels and thus added protection against pellagra. Powell (1988) found that at Moundville, the abundancy of ecological resources precluded large differences in dietary status of individuals of different status segments in the society. Analysis of dental caries prevalence revealed no patterns of evidence that would suggest dietary differences by sex or status.

Dental caries prevalence in the Fusihatchee Town sample closely mirrors the prevalence at Moundville, despite evidence for the increasing intensification of maize agriculture in Creek towns throughout the Lamar region historically. This finding suggests that the inhabitants of Fusihatchee were also balancing their nutritional intake of cereal foods with wild resources such as hickory nuts, berries, and other native plants (as indicated by paleoethnobotanical analysis). They may also have had culinary adaptations that enhanced the nutritional value of a diet rich in maize. Although iron-deficiency anemia was a possible deleterious consequence of the high carbohydrate diet at Moundville, the prevalence of bony pathologies indicative of anemia at Moundville was relatively low (Powell 1991b). It was expected that the Fusihatchee skeletal remains might evidence moderate to high levels of porotic hyperostosis and cribra orbitalia, but unfortunately the fragmentary nature of the remains often prevented scoring for pathological conditions. Few vaults or orbits were well preserved enough to score for these conditions, so no statistically valid estimate exists for their prevalence in the Fusihatchee skeletal series.

Comparison of dental caries prevalence at Fusihatchee Town to contemporaneous populations highlights the sample's similarity to the Mississippian agriculturalists at Moundville. Caries prevalence at Santa Catalina de Guale, an early contact period population (A.D. 1607–1680) on St. Catherine's Island, Georgia, is substantially less than that in the mostly eighteenth-century Fusihatchee sample (see Table 5-6). The temporal differences in the site occupations may account, in part, for differences in prevalence rates by individual as well as by tooth type. Larsen and coworkers (1991) note a general trend toward an increase in dental caries rates from the precontact preagricultural period on the Georgia coast to the late contact period. And they suggest that the increase reflects dietary changes related to increased maize consumption through time. This is potentially the case for the

differences in the early contact Santa Catalina population and the Fusihatchee population.

The results of an analysis of dental caries in the *late* contact-period
population at Santa Catalina de Guale de Santa Maria coincide with
the conclusions of Schoeninger and coworkers' (1990) stable isotope ratio analysis, that a limited dietary repertoire in conjunction with other
stressors brought about by European contact may have contributed to
the extinction of native inhabitants. Larsen and coworkers (1991) recorded high rates of dental caries in this ca. A.D. 1686–1702 population
for individuals, for teeth, and for mean number of carious lesions per
individual. These figures are significantly higher than those for Fusihatchee, despite its conterminous occupation. The data suggest that
the Creeks may have experienced less nutritional stress than their contemporaries on the Georgia coast. Nevertheless, further investigation
of the frequency of infectious diseases, mechanical changes in the long
bones, and stable isotope ratio values associated with agricultural lifestyles would reveal a much more complete picture of diet and health
at Fusihatchee.

Such investigation might be particularly important in light of Hill-
Clark's (1981) research on the biological consequences of the collapse of the settlement and subsistence patterns of stratified societies
in protohistoric Alabama. A series of 200 individuals from five sites
representative of the Mississippian-protohistoric transition period (A.D.
1200–1600) were scored for demographic and pathological data. Hill-
Clark (1981:233) concludes that, from the evidence of a high prevalence
of porotic hyperostosis and dental enamel hypoplasia, the transition
populations were "suffering from extreme nutritional stress." She attributes this stress to a feedback relationship between small, isolated
communities, exhaustion of environmental food resources, inbreeding,
possible prevalence of malaria, and European contact.

*Childhood Stress in the Mississippian and
Historic Periods in Alabama*

The results of the enamel hypoplasia analysis reveal a high prevalence
of hypoplastic lesions by tooth type and by individual in the Fusihatchee dental sample. Powell (1988) also reports a high general prevalence of lesions by individual. In fact, the total prevalence of hypoplasia
by individual in the Moundville sample is only 3.8 percent less than
prevalence in the Fusihatchee sample; the difference is not statistically
significant (Table 5-7). From the temporal, cultural, and ecological differences between the sites, it was expected that the rate of hypoplasia
in the Fusihatchee sample would be significantly higher than Powell's
calculations for Moundville. However, the lack of differentiation between the Moundville and Fusihatchee hypoplastic data necessitates a

Table 5–7. Prevalence of Permanent Dentition Hypoplasia in Individuals by Age[1]: Comparative Data

	Subadults (%)	Adults (%)	Total (%)
Fusihatchee	41.7	63.6	57.8
	(10/24)	(42/66)	(52/90)
Moundville[2]	58.8	53.0	54.0
	(18/31)	(73/138)	(91/169)
Santa Catalina de Guale[3]	81.0	86.0	84.1
	(48/59)	(90/105)	(138/164)

[1]Subadult and adult status were defined differently in all three archaeological samples. Individuals <16 years are defined as subadults in the Fusihatchee sample; adults are 16+ years. Powell (1988) defines subadults as <21 years in the Moundville sample; adults are 21+ years. Subadults in the Santa Catalina de Guale sample are defined as <18 years, and adults are 18+ years.
[2]Powell (1988).
[3]Simpson et al. (1990).

rethinking of the circumstances that affected the appearance of hypo-plastic lesions in individuals at these sites. (It should be noted that prevalence of hypoplasia by age and tooth type in both samples is not directly comparable because of differences in the methods of data collection. The discussion of hypoplasia is based on the similarity of prevalence by *individual*.)

Enamel hypoplasia results from metabolic stress that affects an in-dividual during childhood. Stress during age at weaning, for example, has been documented by a number of researchers. Moggi-Cecchi and coworkers (1994) investigated the age of occurrence of hypoplastic de-fects in an eighteenth-century European skeletal sample and found that the age interval most affected occurred between 2 and 3.5 years. The authors attribute this distribution to weaning stress and the introduc-tion of dietary supplements during weaning. Blakey and coworkers (1994) tested the "weaning hypothesis" in a highly stressed nine-teenth-century African American skeletal population to determine if the age of occurrence of the lesions correlated with the weaning years. They found that weaning stress had only a modest effect on the popu-lation and suggested that other factors, such as differences in suscep-tibility to enamel hypoplasia as well as random factors, affected the frequency of hypoplastic defects in the skeletal sample. In particular, variation in the susceptibility of different portions of the crown to ameloblast disruption may play a key role in producing the "peaks" in age-based stress profiles that have commonly been associated with weaning in the anthropological literature (see Goodman and Armelagos 1985).

Alternately, Goodman (1991) has argued that the presence of hypoplastic defects in teeth may be representative of relative good, rather than bad, health because hypoplasia presence indicates that the individual *survived* the metabolic insult resulting in the defect. This interpretation is plausible in the instance when hypoplastic defects are accompanied by demographic data that show relatively low rates of mortality or high rates of fertility. Otherwise, high rates of enamel defects coupled with high rates of childhood mortality likely indicate a (relatively) less healthy population. Conclusions based on dental health analyses coupled with the demographic profiles of both the Fusihatchee and Moundville sites are problematic. Both samples show an underenumeration of young juveniles and are unreliable for estimates of childhood mortality.

Compared to other contact-period rates of hypoplasia prevalence, the Fusihatchee material shows low to moderate prevalence. For example, comparison with the missionized Santa Catalina de Guale sample from the Georgia coast reveals large differences in frequency of affected individuals (Table 5-7); dental caries prevalence is approximately 25 percent higher in the Santa Catalina sample. One might expect the Fusihatchee and Santa Catalina populations to differ in health status because of the harsh conditions of European missionization versus the more isolated, inland location of Fusihatchee. Because Fusihatchee deerskin traders often traded with Indian middlemen as opposed to Europeans, lower rates of exposure to European diseases might be expected. French Fort Toulouse near the Fusihatchee Town site was a major trading center for the Creeks in the early eighteenth century, however. Direct contact appears, therefore, to have increased through time in Creek Alabama (Waselkov 1989) and may have altered the possibilities for disease transmission.

Relationship Between Dental Pathologies

A last point to consider in evaluations of enamel hypoplasia and dental health is the relationship between enamel defects and dental caries. Pascoe and Seow (1994) have studied that relationship in the deciduous dentitions of living Australian Aboriginal children. The results of their study indicate that dental caries occurred primarily in teeth with hypoplasia; a significant association was found between hypoplastic lesions and dental decay. The authors hypothesize that the defective enamel surface predisposes a tooth to carious attack in individuals with a diet high in refined carbohydrates (who also consume nonfluoridated drinking water); in short, food particles can easily become caught in a pit or groove in the enamel, eventually leading to a carious lesion at the site of the defect (Pascoe and Seow 1994). Duray (1990) found a similar correlation between dental caries and enamel hypocalcification in the prehistoric Libben series but suggests that the hypermineralization of linear defects may actually prevent caries. The implication of the potential relationship between dental defects and dental caries may become important in altering bioarchaeological interpretation of subsistence strategies and health levels in past populations. Dental caries in the Fusihatchee population are generally occlusal and not associated with hypoplastic lesions; thus, the caries-hypoplasia relationship does not appear to be relevant for the interpretation of the dental data presented here.

CONCLUSIONS

The principal findings that emerge from the dental analysis of the Fusihatchee Town population include the following: (1) the archaeological populations from Fusihatchee and Moundville exhibit similar prevalence of dental caries, and (2) both populations exhibit similar prevalence of dental enamel hypoplasia. These findings do not support the original expectation that both nutritional and health stress increased in the post-Moundville contact period. No direct evidence was found for an increase in nutritional stress at Fusihatchee; in fact, the prevalence of dental caries is similar to that of the Moundville population, suggesting a carryover from the decline in maize consumption at Moundville in late prehistory (Schoeninger et al. 1996).

The results of the analysis also lend some support to Waselkov and coworkers' (1987) proposition that cultural reorganization after the Mississippian decline in Alabama did occur in a near absence of "a direct European presence." Indirect presence may account for the lower rates of enamel hypoplasia in the Fusihatchee sample as compared to those of populations more deeply entrenched in a relationship of direct contact with Europeans (mission populations, for example). Historical and archaeological documentation of indirect Creek-European trade via Apalachee middlemen in the seventeenth and eighteenth centuries suggests a less intensive mode of contact at Fusihatchee. This is not to say that Fusihatchee Town residents were healthy in life. The general prevalence of hypoplasia was high, indicating a concomitantly high disease or dietary stress level.

From the results of the comparative dental analysis of skeletal samples from Fusihatchee Town and Moundville, several conclusions can be drawn about the health changes in the Native American population at Fusihatchee following the collapse of complex chiefdoms in Alabama. First, the diverse resource base, although centered on maize agriculture, included a significant dietary component from nonagricultural resources that may have helped to buffer the population against nutritional stress. The similarity in dental caries prevalence to that observed at Moundville may also indicate a carryover of the trend toward a decline in maize consumption in late prehistory. Second, similar enamel hypoplasia rates in both populations indicate similar levels of childhood stress, rather than increased health stress in the contact period. The Fusihatchee remains suggest a kind of continuity in health stress from the Mississippian to contact periods. Finally, non-missionized Indian townspeople actively involved in the deerskin trade with Europeans experienced generally lower levels of health stress than their missionized counterparts in Florida and along the Georgia coast.

Further research on the health status of protohistoric and historic populations in Alabama will provide a larger comparative base for interpreting the results of the Fusihatchee dental analysis. That area of research, however, remains largely unexplored, and it is the hope of the author that future endeavors in historic Creek archaeology will include bioarchaeological analyses.

ACKNOWLEDGMENTS

Gregory A. Waselkov of the University of South Alabama, Craig Sheldon of Auburn University at Montgomery, and John Cottier of Auburn University at Auburn are gratefully acknowledged for their support in conducting the Fusihatchee skeletal inventory and dental analysis. Clark Spencer Larsen of the University of North Carolina at Chapel Hill and Patricia M. Lambert of Utah State University were also invaluable for their knowledge and expertise in skeletal analysis. Thanks are also extended to Mintcy Dana Maxham and Lewis Maxham for their aid in transporting the remains back to Alabama. This research was funded by the University of South Alabama Center for Archaeological Studies and NSF grants BNS-8718934 and BNS-8907700.

6 Agricultural Melodies and Alternative Harmonies in Florida and Georgia

Dale L. Hutchinson
Clark Spencer Larsen
Lynette Norr
Margaret J. Schoeninger

Late prehistoric cultural development in eastern North America is often characterized by the emergence of nonegalitarian societies organized into hierarchical political formations and associated with increased reliance on horticultural products, specifically maize (Griffin 1985; Peebles and Kus 1977; B. D. Smith 1987, 1990, 1992). Archaeological and bioarchaeological evidence for the most part substantiate an increased reliance on maize that began between A.D. 800 and 1000 (Bender et al. 1981; Dunn 1981; Moore 1985; van der Merwe and Vogel 1978; Vogel and van der Merwe 1977; Watson 1989; Yarnell and Black 1985). In addition to the increased recovery of maize at archaeological sites, life during this "age of agriculture" is often marked by Mississippian settlements composed of large mound centers with plazas and adjacent residential areas, such as at Moundville (Peebles 1978, 1983a; Powell 1988; Scarry 1993a; Steponaitis 1983), Etowah (Blakely 1977; Moorehead 1979) and Cahokia (Johannessen 1984, 1993; Johannessen and Whalley 1988).

Just as there was deviation from an idealized modal Mississippian center of occupation, however, there was variability in subsistence production strategies and use of maize (Hally and Rudolph 1986; Scarry 1993a, 1993b). For instance, some have suggested that coastal zones in the Southeast experienced differences in both the timing and influence of maize horticulture. Reitz (1988) has argued that there is little archaeological evidence supporting horticulture before European contact along the Georgia and South Carolina coasts. Furthermore, the available evidence suggests that the use of maize in Florida was different from much of the prehistoric Mississippian Southeast and that maize was not much utilized in central or southern Florida prior to European influence (Hutchinson and Norr 1994; Newsom 1987; Newsom and Quitmyer 1992). In order to examine the patterns and anomalies of prehistoric and protohistoric diet of Native Americans in Georgia and Florida, we examined the stable isotope ratios of carbon and nitrogen obtained from populations inhabiting this broad region between 1100 B.C. and A.D. 1700.

We have previously summarized the geological, zoological, botanical, and archaeological evidence for environmental context and subsistence in this broad region during the time periods encompassed by this study (Hutchinson, Larsen, Schoeninger, Norr 1998) and will summarize that discussion below. The study region in Georgia and Florida is broadly subtropical with varying ecological zones that are undoubtedly important in dietary strategies. The broad ecological zones consist of coastal marsh and barrier islands, interior lowlands, and interior uplands. The coastal marshes and barrier islands that extend along the Georgia and Florida Atlantic coast support a variety of plants and animals, including oak and pine forests, edible wild plants, white-tailed deer, small mammals, birds, and marine fish, and shellfish. Botanical and faunal evidence from archaeological contexts in these localities suggests that maritime resources were heavily utilized (Hutchinson, Larsen, Schoeninger, Norr 1998).

The northern portion of Florida is characterized by upland and flatland pine forests and hardwood hammocks broken by rivers, lakes, and swamps (Myers and Ewel 1991). At sites in the panhandle region of Florida and in the central Gulf coast region, freshwater fish such as gar, catfish, and sunfish are found in archaeological contexts as well as saltwater fish such as catfish, sheepshead, drum, and mullet. Mammals found include white-tailed deer and squirrel. Plant remains include hickory nuts, acorns, persimmon, maypop, and wild cherry. Although maize is found in the northwestern corner of the Florida panhandle after A.D. 1000, it is absent from archaeological contexts farther south in the central Gulf coast region (Hutchinson and Norr 1994).

Missionization brought about several changes for native populations in the region, and native populations experienced dramatic reorganization of their traditional social and political organization, settlement behaviors, and diet. Through the missions, the Spanish encouraged devotion to agricultural production of native maize and introduced Old World domesticates such as wheat, peach, and pea. Although reliance on previously utilized wild fauna and flora appears to have continued in some of the missions in *La Florida* (Newsom and

Quitmyer 1992), there was certainly a trend toward more reliance on maize.

MATERIALS AND METHODS

Information on the diet of humans can be extracted by comparing isotopic analysis of human bones with isotopic analyses of the tissues of plants and animals that they have consumed (Ambrose and Norr 1993; Schoeninger and Moore 1992). The foods have distinct ratios of the stable isotopes of carbon $(^{13}C/^{12}C)$ and nitrogen $(^{15}N/^{14}N)$. When eaten, the isotopic composition of the diet is incorporated into body tissues such as bone collagen (DeNiro and Epstein 1978, 1981). In cases where collagen is preserved in adequate quantities, the biogenic isotope signal is retained (Ambrose 1990; DeNiro 1985; Schoeninger and DeNiro 1981). Isotope ratios are expressed using the delta symbol (δ) as parts per thousand (‰) difference from a reference standard, Pee Dee Belemnite (PDB) for carbon and atmospheric nitrogen (AIR) for nitrogen. The δ values for carbon are generally negative and those for nitrogen are usually positive. The delta values of a sample are calculated relative to a standard using the following equations:

$$\delta^{13}C = \frac{(^{13}C/^{12}C)_{sample} - (^{13}C/^{12}C)_{PDB}}{(^{13}C/^{12}C)_{PDB}} \times 1000‰$$

$$\delta^{15}N = \frac{(^{15}N/^{14}N)_{sample} - (^{15}N/^{14}N)_{AIR}}{(^{15}N/^{14}N)_{AIR}} \times 1000‰$$

Carbon isotopic variation is used to differentiate C_3, C_4, and CAM photosynthetic pathway plant foods, animals feeding on those plants, and animals in terrestrial versus marine ecosystems (Bender 1968; DeNiro and Epstein 1978; Schoeninger and DeNiro 1984; Smith and Epstein 1971; Tieszen 1991). C_3 plants have $\delta^{13}C$ values averaging near −26‰ and include most temperate grasses, trees, fruits, and tubers. C_4 plants have less negative $\delta^{13}C$ values averaging near −12‰ and include tropical grasses native to the New World such as corn, some amaranths, chenopods, and setarias. CAM (Crassulacean Acid Metabolism) plants have $\delta^{13}C$ values that occur between the entire range of C_3 and C_4 plants and include succulents, cacti, and bromeliads (O'Leary 1988). Nitrogen isotopic variation distinguishes between most terrestrial and marine organisms (Schoeninger and DeNiro 1984; Schoeninger et al.

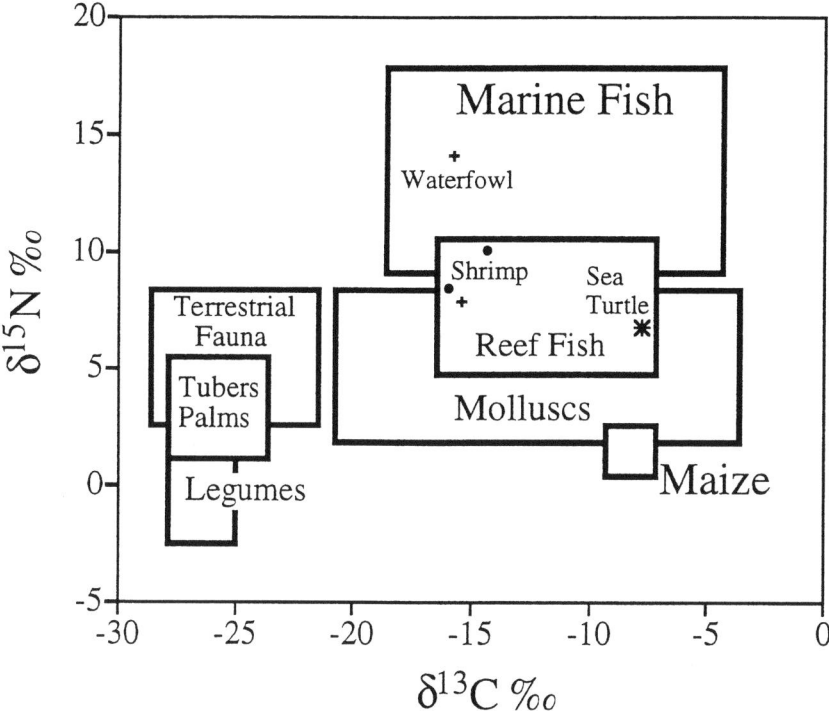

Figure 6-1. Isotopic Composition of Preindustrial Food Resources in the Circum-Caribbean Region (1.5 percent was added to the $\delta^{13}C$ value of modern foods to compensate for ^{12}C enrichment of the atmosphere from the burning of fossil fuels, as per Tieszen 1991). Figure is based on data from Keegan and DeNiro 1988; Norr 1990; Schoeninger and DeNiro 1984; Schoeninger et al. 1990; Hutchinson and Norr 1998; Norr and Cooke unpublished data. (Reprinted by permission of *American Antiquity* 63, no. 3.)

1983). Animals generally exhibit a trophic effect with higher $\delta^{15}N$ values for carnivores than for herbivores (Schoeninger and DeNiro 1984; Wada 1980). In most cases where legumes utilize atmospheric nitrogen they show values close to zero (Shearer and Kohl 1994). The general signatures of some of the foods commonly eaten by humans are displayed in Figure 6-1. It is necessary to obtain isotopic information from modern plants and animals living in the same climatic zone as the human samples to which they are being compared in order to establish an interpretive baseline.

Now extensive stable isotope dietary data exist for prehistoric humans from eastern North America (Ambrose 1987; Buikstra 1992; Buikstra and Milner 1991; Buikstra et al. 1988; Katzenberg et al. 1995; Little and Schoeninger 1995) and more specifically for coastal Georgia and Florida (Hutchinson and Norr 1994, 1998; Larsen, Schoeninger, et

al. 1992; Schoeninger et al. 1990; Tuross et al. 1994). The most comprehensive of these studies by Larsen and coworkers for the Georgia
coast documented stability and change for Georgia coastal populations
during a 4000-year period that encompasses the transition to agriculture and the arrival of Europeans. In their analyses, Larsen, Schoeninger and coworkers (1992; Schoeninger et al. 1990) demonstrated a trend
toward increased consumption of maize that began approximately A.D.
1000 and was accentuated during the mission period (A.D. 1600–1700).
Associated with a diet increasingly focused on maize was a concomitant decrease in the use of maritime resources. Hutchinson and Norr
(1994, 1998) examined the role of maize in the diet of a protohistoric
population from the central Gulf coast of Florida composed of late prehistoric and early historic individuals. Their analysis indicated that the
individuals interred at Tatham Mound had a diet consisting of limited
maize and local lacustrine/riverine resources. There was little change
in dietary focus between A.D. 1200 and 1550.

Several questions remained, however, regarding the broader regional patterns (Florida and Georgia) of diet and the effects of European
contact, particularly in the intermediate area of northern Florida. This
area is especially interesting because of the abundant archaeological
data that indicate Mississippian influence and the well-documented
mission activity that occurred during the seventeenth century. Consequently, in this study we added stable isotope dietary data from the
northern Florida populations and further organized the samples into
three temporal categories generally corresponding with prevailing subsistence trends as indicated by our previous studies. The data come
from the analysis of stable carbon and nitrogen isotope ratios from human skeletal remains of 184 individuals from populations dwelling in
a range of coastal and interior environments between 400 B.C. and A.D.
1700 (Figure 6-2; Table 6-1).

The addition of samples from northern and central Florida to our
previous data provides further documentation of the precontact and
contact period dietary variation between coastal and inland areas as
well as between Florida and Georgia. Furthermore, it extends the temporal span of the contact period from initial contact through the late
mission period. The addition of the northern Florida mission data is
particularly important. Although some recent documentation for the
early contact mission Santa Catalina de Guale on St. Catherines Island
in Georgia has been translated (Worth 1995), the chain of missions that
extended east to west across northern Florida is generally more extensively documented, facilitating more extensive hypothesis formulation
and testing (e.g., Bushnell 1994; Hann 1990; McEwan 1993).

We concentrated on the following issues: (1) variation in the subsistence regime prior to horticulture in Georgia and Florida—the effect
of coastal versus inland habitation; (2) variation exhibited in the chro-

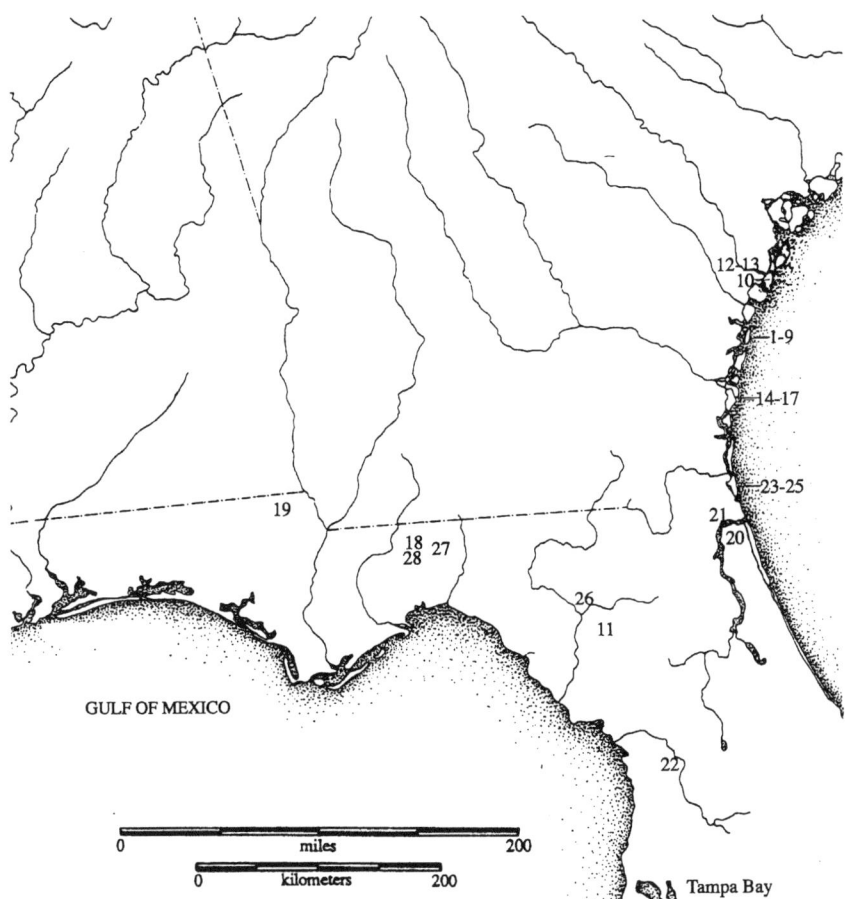

Figure 6-2. Locations of Sites Mentioned: 1 = McLeod Mound; 2 = Seaside Mound I; 3 = Seaside Mound II; 4 = Cunningham Mound C; 5 = Cunningham Mound D; 6 = Johns Mound; 7 = Marys Mound; 8 = Southend Mound I; 9 = Santa Catalina de Guale; 10 = Deptford Site; 11 = Henderson Mound; 12 = Irene Burial Mound; 13 = Irene Mortuary; 14 = Martinez B; 15 = Indian Field; 16 = Taylor Mound; 17 = Couper Field; 18 = Lake Jackson; 19 = Waddells Mill Pond; 20 = Browne Mound; 21 = Holy Spirit; 22 = Tatham Mound; 23 = Santa Maria de Yamassee; 24 = Ossuary at Santa Catalina de Santa Maria; 25 = Santa Catalina de Amelia; 26 = San Martin de Timucua; 27 = San Pedro y San Pablo de Patale; 28 = San Luis. (Map adapted from C. Hudson, M. T. Smith, C. B. DePratter, and E. Kelley, The Tristán de Luna Expedition: 1559–1561. *Southeastern Archaeology* 8 (1989): 31–45. Reprinted by permission of *American Antiquity* 63, no. 3.)

nology of maize adoption; (3) how the use of local, wild dietary resources changed with the adoption of maize; (4) whether changes in the use of local resources after European contact were of the same pattern and magnitude as those that occurred with the introduction of

Table 6-1. Human Isotope Samples by Geographic Location and Time Period

SITE	LOCATION	N	REFERENCES
Georgia Early Prehistoric: 400 B.C.–A.D. 1000			
McLeod Mound	Coastal Georgia	4	Thomas and Larsen 1979a; Larsen 1982
Seaside Mound I	Coastal Georgia	1	Thomas and Larsen 1979a; Larsen 1982
Seaside Mound II	Coastal Georgia	3	Thomas and Larsen 1979a; Larsen 1982
Cunningham Mound C	Coastal Georgia	2	Thomas and Larsen 1979a; Larsen 1982
Cunningham Mound D	Coastal Georgia	1	Thomas and Larsen 1979a; Larsen 1982
Deptford Site	Inland Georgia	11	Thomas and Larsen 1979a; Larsen 1982
Florida Early Prehistoric: A.D. 600–1200			
Henderson Mound	Inland Florida	4	Loucks 1976
Georgia Late Prehistoric: A.D. 1000–1450			
Johns Mound	Coastal Georgia	10	Larsen and Thomas 1982; Larsen 1982
Mary's Mound	Coastal Georgia	2	Larsen and Thomas 1982; Larsen 1982
Southend Mound I	Coastal Georgia	5	Larsen and Thomas 1986
Irene Burial Mound	Inland Georgia	9	Caldwell and McCann 1941; Hulse 1941; Larsen 1982; Anderson 1994
Irene Mortuary	Inland Georgia	12	Caldwell and McCann 1941; Hulse 1941; Larsen 1982; Anderson 1994
Martinez B	Coastal Georgia	2	Martinez 1975
Indian Field	Coastal Georgia	2	Wallace 1975; Zahler 1976
Taylor Mound	Coastal Georgia	9	Wallace 1975; Zahler 1976
Couper Field	Coastal Georgia	7	Wallace 1975; Zahler 1976
Florida Late Prehistoric and Protohistoric: A.D. 1200–1600			
Lake Jackson	Inland Florida	4	Jones 1982
Waddells Mill Pond	Inland Florida	1	Gardner 1966
Browne Mound	Coastal Florida	5	Sears 1959

Table 6–1. continued

Holy Spirit	Coastal Florida	4	Larsen 1996
Tatham Mound	Inland Florida	20	Hutchinson 1991; Hutchinson and Norr 1994; Mitchem 1989

Georgia Early Mission: A.D. 1600–1680

Santa Catalina de Guale	Coastal Georgia	22	Thomas 1987; Larsen 1990b; Larsen, Schoeninger, Hutchinson, et al. 1990

Florida Early Mission: A.D. 1600–1680

Santa Maria de Yamassee	Coastal Florida	7	Larsen 1993; Saunders 1988
Ossuary at Santa Catalina de Santa Maria	Coastal Florida	8	Larsen 1993; Simmons et al. 1989
San Martin de Timucua (Fig Springs)	Inland Florida	2	Hann 1990; Hoshower 1992; Hoshower and Milanich 1993; Weisman 1992, 1993
San Pedro y San Pablo de Patale	Inland Florida	5	Hann 1990; Jones et al. 1991; Marrinan 1993

Florida Late Mission: A.D. 1680–1700

San Luis	Inland Florida	1	Shapiro and McEwan 1992; McEwan 1993
Santa Catalina de Amelia	Coastal Florida	21	Larsen 1993; Saunders 1988

horticultural products; (5) broad differences brought about by dependence on local resources, such as differences between coastal and inland dietary patterns; and (6) broad differences in dietary focus between Florida and Georgia.

For this study, we used methods of isotope analysis that have been published previously (Hutchinson and Norr 1994; Schoeninger et al. 1990). Human bone samples were primarily taken from long bones and ribs, were cleaned of soil and other matrix, and the organic portion known as "collagen" was isolated. The collagen was then analyzed in three laboratories by comparable methods. Except for one individual from St. Catherines Island (MS2876), all are adults. Table 6-2 presents the data for all sites and time periods by individual. All samples were assessed for quality by examination of percent collagen weight yield and carbon to nitrogen ratios. We established the baseline for dietary

Table 6–2. Stable Isotope Results by Individual

LAB NO.	SITE	BURIAL	SEX	$\delta^{13}C$	$\delta^{15}N$
UCT389	McLeod Mound	13	F	−17.1	13.1
UCT391	McLeod Mound	15	F	−18.6	12.9
UCT392	McLeod Mound	16	F	−13.8	12.6
UCT393	McLeod Mound	17	F	−13.6	12.4
UCT385	Seaside I	14	M	−15.0	
UCT386	Seaside II	11	M	−13.8	10.6
UCT387	Seaside II	13	F	−15.7	
UCT388	Seaside II	14	F	−13.4	13.2
UCT394	Cunning. Mound C	1	F	−16.0	14.4
UCT395	Cunning. Mound C	3	F	−14.8	
UCT396	Cunning. Mound D	2	M	−13.9	12.9
UCT335	Deptford	4	F	−14.5	11.3
UCT384	Deptford	4	F	−13.4	11.3
UCT382	Deptford	8	F	−18.6	10.7
UCT337	Deptford	13	F	−17.5	9.6
UCT338	Deptford	16	F	−17.7	
UCT339	Deptford	17	F	−16.7	11.6
UCT340	Deptford	18	M	−15.6	12.9
UCT341	Deptford	22	F	−16.0	11.8
UCT342	Deptford	28	M	−16.8	12.0
UCT343	Deptford	29	M	−17.1	9.6
UCT344	Deptford	40	M	−12.6	10.4
UCT372	Johns Mound	1	M	−14.2	11.6
UCT379	Johns Mound	14	M	−13.4	13.1
UCT377	Johns Mound	16	F	−14.6	13.3
UCT376	Johns Mound	18	F	−13.9	13.6
UCT374	Johns Mound	26	I	−13.7	12.3
UCT370	Johns Mound	36	I	−14.1	13.0
UCT375	Johns Mound	37	F	−14.4	12.7
UCT378	Johns Mound	47	M	−14.3	13.5
UCT373	Johns Mound	—	M	−14.2	12.9
UCT371	Johns Mound	11A	M	−14.2	13.3
UCT380	Marys Mound	1	F	−14.3	11.8
UCT381	Marys Mound	5	F	−14.7	12.9
UCT349	Irene Bu. Mound	2	F	−14.0	9.6
UCT350	Irene Bu. Mound	3	M	−13.3	10.4
UCT351	Irene Bu. Mound	4	M	−10.0	10.6
UCT353	Irene Bu. Mound	5	M	−12.4	10.5
UCT352	Irene Bu. Mound	7	F	−10.8	9.5
UCT355	Irene Bu. Mound	12	F	−16.4	10.1
UCT356	Irene Bu. Mound	14	F	−13.9	11.2

Table 6–2. continued

UCT357	Irene Bu. Mound	16	M	−14.4	10.8
UCT358	Irene Bu. Mound	72	F	−11.5	13.3
UCT359	Irene Mortuary	8	M	−17.4	10.7
UCT354	Irene Mortuary	9	F	−16.4	
UCT360	Irene Mortuary	64	M	−16.8	9.2
UCT361	Irene Mortuary	69	M	−17.9	8.7
UCT362	Irene Mortuary	70	M	−17.0	10.4
UCT363	Irene Mortuary	74	F	−14.5	9.7
UCT364	Irene Mortuary	75	M	−13.7	10.2
UCT365	Irene Mortuary	107	M	−17.7	9.9
UCT366	Irene Mortuary	108	F	−17.0	9.6
UCT367	Irene Mortuary	109	M	−17.9	10.2
UCT368	Irene Mortuary	110	F	−15.6	10.0
UCT369	Irene Mortuary	111	F	−17.2	9.6
MS4843	Southend Md I	5	M	−13.3	13.1
MS4844	Southend Md I	6	F	−	12.5
MS4847	Southend Md I	16	F	−	10.4
MS4850	Southend Md I	24	F	−13.2	12.8
MS4851	Southend Md I	27	F	−12.4	11.7
$386	Couper Field	2	F	−13.8	12.8
$382	Couper Field	5	M	−14.0	12.8
$387	Couper Field	7	F	−14.2	12.1
$383	Couper Field	8	M	−12.4	11.8
$384	Couper Field	11	M	−13.9	11.4
$388	Couper Field	13	F	−14.5	11.7
$385	Couper Field	15	M	−13.6	13.5
$371	Indian Field	4	M	−14.8	14.8
$372	Indian Field	5	F	−14.8	13.2
$369	Martinez B	2	M	−13.4	14.1
$370	Martinez B	3	M	−12.7	13.6
$376	Taylor Mound	2	F	−13.0	12.7
$373	Taylor Mound	3	M	−12.5	13.6
$377	Taylor Mound	4	F	−13.7	12.1
$378	Taylor Mound	5	F	−13.9	12.7
$374	Taylor Mound	6	M	−9.9	12.2
$375	Taylor Mound	8	M	−10.2	12.8
$379	Taylor Mound	9	F	−13.3	11.5
$380	Taylor Mound	11	F	−11.1	11.0
$381	Taylor Mound	379	F	−11.1	12.5
MS4610	Browne Mound	7	F	−12.4	14.0
MS4604	Browne Mound	11	F	−17.1	13.2

Table 6-2 continued on next page

Table 6–2. continued

LAB NO.	SITE	BURIAL	SEX	$\delta^{13}C$	$\delta^{15}N$
MS4608	Browne Mound	18	M	−12.3	14.2
MS4603	Browne Mound	19	M	−17.4	9.2
MS4607	Browne Mound	46	M	−13.4	13.2
MS4617	Holy Spirit	7	F	−17.3	12.2
MS4619	Holy Spirit	8	M	−18.1	
MS4620	Holy Spirit	9	M	−19.4	12.8
MS4622	Holy Spirit	11	F	−17.1	11.8
MS4615	Henderson Mound	14	I	−17.9	9.0
MS4613	Henderson Mound	27	I	−16.1	11.2
MS4612	Henderson Mound	32	I	−13.2	9.1
MS4614	Henderson Mound	34	I	−16.3	11.9
DH39	Waddell's Mill Pond	65	I	−12.8	10.4
MS4599	Lake Jackson	6	M	−14.6	9.1
MS4600	Lake Jackson	7	F	−13.7	13.0
MS4601	Lake Jackson	10	F	−14.0	8.8
MS4602	Lake Jackson	16	F	−13.6	9.3
DH10	Tatham Mound	113	F	−17.5	10.9
DH7	Tatham Mound	127	M	−20.3	11.9
DH23	Tatham Mound	1	F	−18.8	11.8
DH48	Tatham Mound	2	F	−13.8	10.1
DH24	Tatham Mound	9	M	−18.7	12.0
DH8	Tatham Mound	14	F	−15.6	10.9
DH4	Tatham Mound	16	M	−13.9	11.4
DH11	Tatham Mound	17	M	−15.8	11.5
DH13	Tatham Mound	24	I	−18.4	12.0
DH9	Tatham Mound	30	M	−17.7	11.7
DH16	Tatham Mound	33	I	−16.9	10.8
DH1	Tatham Mound	42	I	−18.1	12.0
DH17	Tatham Mound	48	I	−18.6	12.0
DH14	Tatham Mound	51	M	−18.5	12.6
DH15	Tatham Mound	55	I	−19.1	11.9
DH6	Tatham Mound	56	I	−19.7	11.7
DH30	Tatham Mound	66	F	−17.8	10.3
DH42	Tatham Mound	77	F	−15.0	10.4
DH29	Tatham Mound	86	F	−17.3	11.7
DH12	Tatham Mound	120	I	−18.6	11.6
MS2835	Santa Cat. SC	9	F	−9.6	7.4
MS2836	Santa Cat. SC	18	M	−11.7	9.6
MS2838	Santa Cat. SC	22	F	−12.4	9.6
MS2839	Santa Cat. SC	39	M	−11.6	10.4
MS2840	Santa Cat. SC	41	M	−11.0	9.8

Table 6–2. continued

MS2841	Santa Cat. SC	46	M	−10.4	8.5
MS2844	Santa Cat. SC	58	F	−12.0	9.5
MS2832	Santa Cat. SC	60	F	−14.3	9.5
MS2848	Santa Cat. SC	64	F	−11.8	9.9
MS2849	Santa Cat. SC	74	M	−9.7	7.5
MS2850	Santa Cat. SC	88	F	−11.0	9.7
MS2851	Santa Cat. SC	98	F	−11.2	8.9
MS2857	Santa Cat. SC	99	F	−12.1	9.0
MS2861	Santa Cat. SC	107	M	−10.8	10.8
MS2865	Santa Cat. SC	123	F	−11.2	10.2
MS2862	Santa Cat. SC	160	I	−12.9	9.9
MS2869	Santa Cat. SC	169	M	−11.6	9.3
MS2871	Santa Cat. SC	219	I	−11.0	8.9
MS2876	Santa Cat. SC	235	I	−10.6	10
MS2879	Santa Cat. SC	276	F	−11.3	9.4
MS2877	Santa Cat. SC	294	M	−11.4	9.8
MS2859	Santa Cat. SC	iso	I	−12.6	9.6
MS3280	Ossuary Am.	1	M	−12.1	9.8
MS3281	Ossuary Am.	2	M	−12.1	10.6
MS3282	Ossuary Am.	3	M	−11.5	10.0
MS3283	Ossuary Am.	4	M	−13.4	10.1
MS3284	Ossuary Am.	5	F	−12.8	10.2
MS3285	Ossuary Am.	6	F	−11.3	10.8
MS3286	Ossuary Am.	7	F	−12.4	9.4
MS3287	Ossuary Am.	8	F	−12.0	10.8
MS4575	Santa Maria Y	15	M	−12.0	14.5
MS4585	Santa Maria Y	16	F	−12.0	12.2
MS4586	Santa Maria Y	42	F	−11.6	11.9
MS4587	Santa Maria Y	51	M	−12.8	11.2
MS4588	Santa Maria Y	67	F	−12.0	9.5
MS4589	Santa Maria Y	74	M	−13.6	7.3
MS4590	Santa Maria Y	83	F	−12.5	9.5
MS4591	Fig Springs	91	M	−12.7	7.9
MS4595	Fig Springs	92	M	−12.1	9.4
MS4581	Patale	14	M	−12.2	9.0
MS4582	Patale	34	F	−14.2	5.8
MS4578	Patale	41	F	−10.2	8.7
MS4577	Patale	46	M	−10.0	9.6
MS4584	Patale	61	F	−11.0	6.4
MS4611	San Luis	3	M	−16.5	12.3
MS3248	Santa Cat. Am	1	F	−11.1	10.9

Table 6-2 continued on next page

Table 6–2. continued

LAB NO.	SITE	BURIAL	SEX	$\delta^{13}C$	$\delta^{15}N$
MS3249	Santa Cat. Am	6	M	−10.2	11.0
MS3250	Santa Cat. Am	7	F	−11.3	10.1
MS2832	Santa Cat. Am	11	M	−12.4	9.8
MS3251	Santa Cat. Am	15	M	−11.3	10.1
MS2834	Santa Cat. Am	19	F	−12.1	8.8
MS3252	Santa Cat. Am	20	F	−11.8	10.5
MS3254	Santa Cat. Am	30	F	−11.1	9.6
MS3255	Santa Cat. Am	34	M	−10.9	9.8
MS3256	Santa Cat. Am	36	F	−11.3	9.4
MS3257	Santa Cat. Am	45	M	−10.0	8.6
MS3258	Santa Cat. Am	50	F	−12.2	10.3
MS3271	Santa Cat. Am	59	M	−11.4	10.3
MS3272	Santa Cat. Am	60	F	−12.2	9.6
MS3273	Santa Cat. Am	65	M	−10.4	10.2
MS3274	Santa Cat. Am	66	F	−12.5	8.3
MS3275	Santa Cat. Am	73	M	−10.5	8.8
MS3276	Santa Cat. Am	78	M	−12.5	11.6
MS3277	Santa Cat. Am	88	F	−12.6	10.1
MS3278	Santa Cat. Am	91	F	−12.1	9.7
MS3279	Santa Cat. Am	94	M	−12.5	10.9

reconstruction by stable carbon and nitrogen signatures of local flora and fauna collected at or near the habitation areas of the Florida and Georgia populations (Figure 6-2). Modern samples were processed using the same methods as for prehistoric samples with the exception of the collagen extraction stages.

Results

Early Prehistoric Period (1100 B.C.–A.D. 1000)

Represented by 2,000 years, this early time span (Refuge, Deptford, and Wilmington periods) may show more dietary diversity than the later periods, which have much shorter time spans. Nonetheless, there is some consistency in the early data. Local ecological circumstances undoubtedly influenced dietary selection during this period as evidenced by the stable isotope values for coastal dwelling populations as compared to those dwelling inland (Figure 6-3). The Deptford site, for instance, reflects the dietary inclusion of terrestrial resources that is not exhibited by the more coastal dwelling groups (McLeod Mound, Seaside I and II, Cunningham Mounds C and D). Florida isotopic sig-

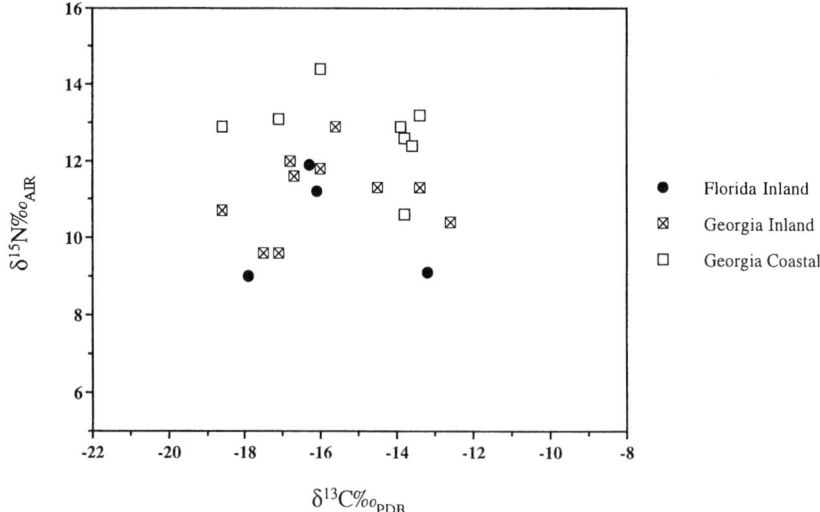

Figure 6-3. Dietary Signatures from Early Prehistoric Georgia and Florida Populations. In this and all other plots filled and solid symbols indicate inland populations, and open symbols indicate coastal populations. (Reprinted by permission of *American Antiquity* 63, no. 3.)

Table 6-3. Summary of Stable Isotope Results for Early Prehistoric Georgia and Florida Populations by Total Sample and by Sex

	N	$\delta^{13}C$	S.D.	$\delta^{15}N$	S.D.
COASTAL GEORGIA					
FEMALES	8	−15.4	1.8	13.1	.7
MALES	3	−14.2	.7	11.8	1.6
ALL	11	−15.1	1.7	12.8	1.1
INLAND GEORGIA					
FEMALES	7	−16.3	1.9	11.1	.8
MALES	4	−15.5	2.1	11.2	1.5
ALL	11	−16.0	1.9	11.1	1.1
INLAND FLORIDA					
ALL	4	−15.9	2.0	10.3	1.5

natures from individuals interred at the noncoastal Henderson Mound (A.D. 600–1200) located at the mouth of the St. Johns River on the Atlantic coast indicate little consumption of maize and a mixed dietary regime of terrestrial and marine animals combined with C_3 plants. Table 6-3 presents the summary data by total sample and by sex for each of the sample classes.

Late Prehistoric Period (A.D. 1000–1600)

Following A.D. 1000, the isotope data indicate a general trend in Georgia toward increased consumption of maize (Figure 6-4). The period between A.D. 1000 and 1150 (St. Catherines period—Johns and Marys Mounds) marks the beginning of a general trend toward increased consumption of C_4 plants, presumably maize, with a continued reliance on marine resources. This trend continues until the period of European missionization, although there appears to be less reliance on marine resources for individuals interred at the mainland Irene Mound (A.D. 1150–1300), and particularly at the Irene mortuary (A.D. 1300–1550). Individuals interred on St. Simons Island (Martinez B, Indian Field, Taylor Mound, Couper Field) contemporary with those from the Irene Mound mortuary illustrate the differences in dietary focus, with the St. Simons individuals consuming a diet more focused on marine resources and other resources distinct from terrestrial C_3 plants. In contrast, those interred at Irene Mound appear to have consumed far more terrestrial food resources and less marine resources, indicating a strong preference for local subsistence resources. Summary data for the total sample and by sex are shown in Table 6-4. There are significant differences (t-test; $p \leq .05$) for males and females as indicated by the $\delta^{15}N$ values (males = 12.3; females = 13.0).

The Florida data suggest that during the period designated as "agricultural" in Georgia, there was little use of maize except for the extreme northern part of the state. In fact, prior to contact there was little maize in the diet (Figure 6-5). Only at the larger mound complex site of Lake Jackson and at Waddells Mill Pond does maize appear to have increased in dietary importance between A.D. 1100 and 1400. Maize is certainly more important at Lake Jackson than at Tatham Mound in central Florida, during both the precontact (A.D. 1200–1450) and early contact periods (A.D. 1525–1550). This pattern of maize use is consistent with the ethnohistoric accounts of the Spanish exploratory expeditions of Narváez and De Soto that report limited observations of maize fields and availability of maize in central Florida between A.D. 1525 and 1550 (Smith 1968). Individuals interred at two late prehistoric Atlantic coastal mortuary sites, Holy Spirit and Browne Mound, indicate the use of maritime resources with little consumption of maize. Examination of the data by sex for each of the sample classes (Table 6-5) showed significant differences in diet (t-test; $p \leq .01$) of the inland central Florida individuals as indicated by the $\delta^{15}N$ values (males = 11.9; females = 10.9).

Mission Period (A.D. 1600–1700)

Between A.D. 1600 and 1700, the time of the missions in *La Florida*, the stable isotope evidence indicates that the native populations were

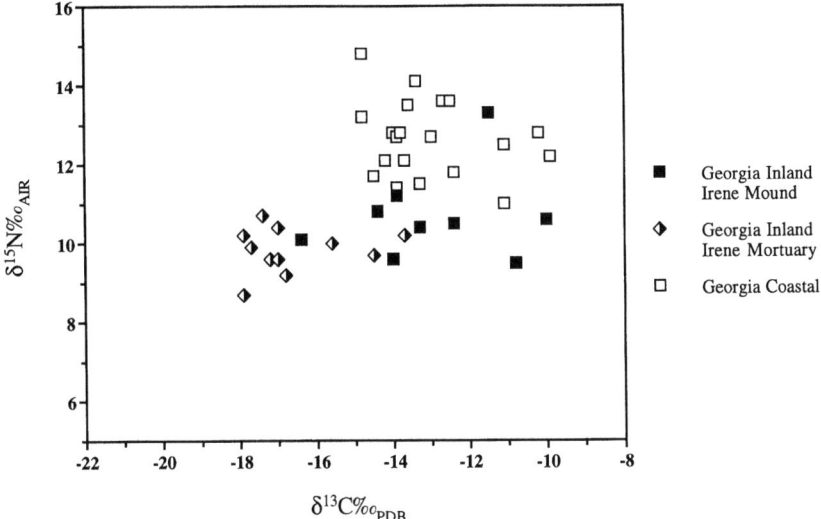

Figure 6-4. Dietary Signatures from Late Prehistoric Georgia Populations. (Reprinted by permission of *American Antiquity* 63, no. 3.)

Table 6–4. Summary of Stable Isotope Results for Late Prehistoric Georgia Populations by Total Sample and by Sex

	N	δ^{13}C	S.D.	δ^{15}N	S.D.
COASTAL GEORGIA					
FEMALES	19	−13.6	1.1	12.3*	.8
MALES	16	−13.2	1.4	13.0*	.9
ALL	37	−13.4	1.2	12.6	.9
INLAND GEORGIA					
FEMALES	10	−14.7	2.2	10.3	1.2
MALES	11	−15.3	2.7	10.1	.7
ALL	21	−15.0	2.4	10.2	.9

*Significant difference in *t*-test at $p \leq 0.05$ level.

relying increasingly on a C_4 plant, undoubtedly maize (Figure 6-6). All evidence—ethnohistoric, biological, and archaeological—supports an increase in the maize production and consumption as part of the Spanish colonial effort. Although increased reliance on maize may have resulted in a decreased reliance on marine resources, as suggested by the stable isotope data, recent examination of strontium and barium trace elements by Ezzo and coworkers (1995) may indicate that the decrease in marine resources was minor. Table 6-6 presents the summary data by total sample and by sex for each of the sample classes.

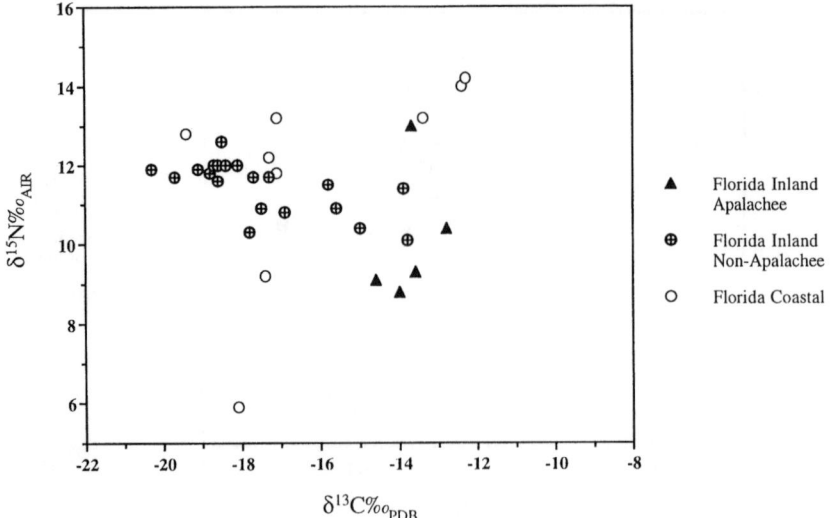

Figure 6-5. Dietary Signatures from Late Prehistoric Florida Populations. (Reprinted by permission of *American Antiquity* 63, no. 3.)

Table 6-5. Summary of Stable Isotope Results for Late Prehistoric Florida Populations by Total Sample and by Sex

	N	$\delta^{13}C$	S.D.	$\delta^{15}N$	S.D.
NORTHERN COASTAL FLORIDA					
FEMALES	4	−16.0	2.4	12.8	1.0
MALES	5	−16.1	3.1	12.4	2.2
ALL	9	−16.1	2.6	12.6	1.6
NORTHERN INLAND FLORIDA					
FEMALES	3	−13.8	.2	10.4	2.3
MALES	1**	−14.6	**	9.1	**
ALL	5	−13.7	.7	10.1	1.7
CENTRAL INLAND FLORIDA					
FEMALES	7	−16.5	1.8	10.9*	.7
MALES	6	−17.5	2.3	11.9*	.4
ALL	20	−17.5	1.8	11.5	.7

*Significant difference in *t*-test at $p \leq 0.01$ level

**Small sample size

DISCUSSION

Our data indicate clear differences among the broad regional patterns of maize consumption, in part due to consumption of local resources. In particular, consumption of local resources contributes to the isotope

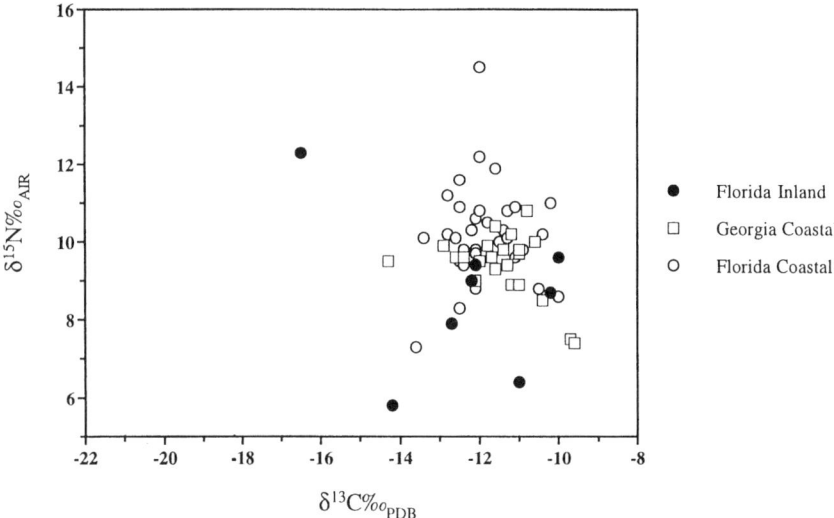

Figure 6-6. Dietary Signatures from Mission Period Georgia and Florida Populations. Reprinted by permission of *American Antiquity* 63, no. 3.)

Table 6–6. Summary of Stable Isotope Results for Mission Period Georgia and Florida Populations by Total Sample and by Sex

	N	$\delta^{13}C$	S.D.	$\delta^{15}N$	S.D.
COASTAL FLORIDA					
FEMALES	19	−11.9	.5	10.1	1.0
MALES	17	−11.7	1.1	10.3	1.5
ALL	36	−11.8	.8	10.2	1.2
COASTAL GEORGIA					
FEMALES	10	−11.7	1.2	9.3	.8
MALES	8	−11.0	.7	9.5	1.1
ALL	22	−11.5	1.0	9.4	.8
INLAND FLORIDA					
FEMALES	3	−11.8	2.1	7.0	1.5
MALES	5	−12.7	2.4	9.6	1.6
ALL	8	−12.4	2.2	8.6	2.0

patterns that serve to differentiate coastal from inland populations. When Florida and Georgia are compared, it is clear that marine resources were an important part of the diet on the Georgia islands (Figure 6-7). The stable isotope data from Georgia indicate that foraging gave way to horticulture after A.D. 1000. There is a steady increase in

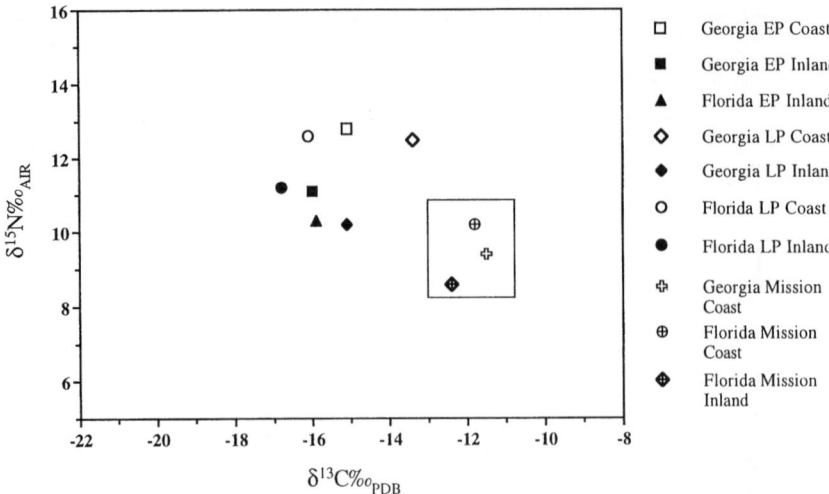

Figure 6-7. Mean Dietary Signatures from the Total Sample of Georgia and Florida Populations. Box indicates Mission Period populations. (Reprinted by permission of *American Antiquity* 63, no. 3.)

maize reliance through time that continues into the contact period. It is also clear, however, that local dietary variation continued until the arrival of the Spaniards. Island dwellers differ significantly in nitrogen signatures from mainland dwellers, such as at the Irene site ten miles up the Savannah River. Irene is also interesting as it appears that maize consumption declines between the Savannah and Irene components, possibly a sign of the collapse of the Savannah-period chiefdom (Anderson 1994).

The Florida dietary signatures, with the exception of Lake Jackson, show little evidence of maize consumption prior to the mission period. A combination of cultural and climatic differences in Florida probably contributed to departures from the expected Mississippian pattern. Because of the absence of the large mound centers with plazas, many have suggested that Florida, with the exception of northern Florida, had only marginal connections with Mississippian societies (Milanich 1994; Willey 1982). Furthermore, although stratified societies were present, some such as the Calusa appear to have focused on subsistence regimes that did not include maize (Goggin and Sturtevant 1964; Hutchinson and Norr 1991; Marquardt 1992; Widmer 1988). Dietary reconstruction for 24 individuals from prehistoric sites along the Florida Gulf coast corroborates the absence of maize in archaeological contexts in south Florida. Although the $\delta^{13}C$ values from collagen are consistent with maize consumption, the $\delta^{13}C$ values from apatite are not consistent with maize consumption. Our conclusions (Norr and Hutchinson

1998) are that the prehistoric Calusa focused their diet on maritime resources. This interpretation is also supported by the archaeological recovery of pinfish, mullet, catfish, sheepshead, sea trout, shark, and sea turtle (Walker 1992). As well, the climatic and biogeographical conditions in Florida are far different from most of the eastern United States (Myers and Ewel 1991).

There is a general convergence of diet in the mission period. We see a shift from a heterogeneous diet with distinctions occurring between Florida and Georgia and between coastal and noncoastal to a largely homogeneous diet in the mission period, due in no small part to the impact of Europeans on native subsistence patterns. Although there are still some distinctions between coastal mission sites and those located inland, there is a general trend toward increased maize consumption and decreased consumption of marine foods, in accord with the archaeological and ethnohistoric data.

Our data suggest that the process of agricultural transition was not homogeneous in either geographic or chronological location. The adoption of maize appears to have occurred later in most Florida populations. With the advent of European colonization, the Spaniards introduced more homogeneity in subsistence patterns, particularly with regard to an increased emphasis on horticulture and a decreased emphasis on foraging.

ACKNOWLEDGMENTS

We thank Douglas H. Ubelaker and Jerald T. Milanich for permission to sample the skeletal series reported here and currently housed in the National Museum of Natural History and the Florida Museum of Natural History. For assistance in field excavations, we thank David Hurst Thomas, Kenneth W. Hardin, Jerald T. Milanich, Jeffrey M. Mitchem, Rebecca Saunders, and many field workers too numerous to name. Funding for excavations on St. Catherines Island came from the Edward John Noble and St. Catherines Island Foundations. Funding for excavations on Amelia Island was contributed by Dr. and Mrs. George H. Dorion. Funding for excavations at Tatham Mound was contributed by Piers Anthony. The analysis was funded by the University of Florida, the University of Illinois, East Carolina University, the Margaret Cullinan Wray Research Fund (to DLH and LN), and the National Science Foundation (grant awards SBR-9305391, BNS-8406773, and BNS-8703848 to CSL and MJS). For editing and comments we thank Lorraine V. Aragon, Lori Higginbotham, Bree Tucker, and M. Anne Katzenberg.

7 Inferring Iron-Deficiency Anemia from Human Skeletal Remains: The Case of the Georgia Bight

Clark Spencer Larsen
Leslie E. Sering

A nemia is a condition present when an individual's hemoglobin or red blood cell amount—as measured by count or volume—is below normal. This is problematic because the body is less able to transport oxygen to the tissues. There are various types of anemias, but most fall into one of two groups: genetic hemolytic (abnormal hemoglobin) and acquired. A distinctive pattern of skeletal pathology associated with anemia has been observed with frequency in archaeological human remains worldwide (reviewed in Stuart-Macadam 1992; Larsen 1997). This chapter documents and interprets skeletal pathology in precontact and contact-era Native American remains from the Georgia Bight, a region in the northern periphery of New Spain called the Spanish borderlands. This region has provided an abundance of data on the history of health and the human condition (Larsen, Ruff et al. 1992; Larsen et al. n.d.). In particular, we explore how the bioarchaeological record informs our understanding of two major events and their impact on iron status and quality of life: (1) the adoption of maize agriculture in the last few centuries prior to European contact; and (2) the arrival of Europeans, establishment of mission centers, and intensification of agricultural production in native populations.

THE ENVIRONMENTAL AND BIOCULTURAL CONTEXT

The Georgia Bight is a large embayment extending north to south from Cape Hatteras, North Carolina, to Cape Canaveral, Florida (Reitz 1988).

The dominant feature of this embayment is a chain of offshore barrier islands sharing similar depositional and ecological histories that began during the late Pleistocene. These islands are separated from the mainland by a series of marsh islands and tidal rivers and creeks. The topography of the region is characterized by very low relief. Its subtropical flora and fauna are diverse. Primary plant communities include maritime oak and pine forests. The inshore zone contains a very rich and variable estuarine/marine fauna, including various fishes and invertebrates (shellfish). These marine resources were a dominant food for native populations throughout much of prehistory and into the historic period (Reitz 1988; Larsen, Schoeninger et al. 1992). The abundance of remains of terrestrial plants (e.g., acorns from live oaks) and animals (e.g., deer) found in archaeological sites attests to the importance of these foods in native foodways (Reitz 1988).

There is an abundant archaeological record of human occupation of the Georgia Bight. We divide this record into four periods or population groupings, including the precontact preagricultural, precontact agricultural, early contact, and late contact groups. In addition to archaeological information, a wealth of historical written sources reveals important information on human adaptation, lifestyle, and health during the contact period.

THE POPULATION GROUPS

This study uses a large sample of human skeletons from prehistoric and historic mortuary sites in present-day Georgia and Florida in assessing anemia. A summary of the mortuary sites is presented in Table 7-1.

Precontact Preagricultural Group (pre-A.D. 1150)

The first occupation of islands and the adjacent mainland occurred by at least 4,000 years ago by primarily foraging groups who acquired resources from hunting, gathering, and fishing (Thomas and Larsen 1979a; Larsen 1982). Foods of these foragers included the aforementioned nondomesticated terrestrial plants and animals and marine animals. Dietary reconstruction using stable isotopic (carbon and nitrogen) and elemental (barium and strontium) analysis of human bone (collagen) shows a heavy reliance on marine foods (Larsen, Schoeninger, et al. 1992; Ezzo et al. 1995; Hutchinson, Larsen, Schoeninger, and Norr 1998). Pattern of settlement and the size and density of habitation sites indicate that populations were small, dispersed, and probably transitory, at least on a seasonal basis (Larsen 1982; Crook 1984; De-Pratter 1976, 1978, n.d.).

The precontact preagricultural occupation spans the Woodland period of the southeastern United States, known locally as the Refuge (1100–400 B.C.), Deptford (400 B.C.–A.D. 500), Wilmington (A.D. 500–

Table 7-1. Skeletal Samples and Mortuary Localities, Georgia Bight

Site	N[a]	Reference
Precontact Preagricultural (pre-A.D. 1150)		
Cunningham Mound C	2	Thomas and Larsen 1979a
Cunningham Mound D	2	Thomas and Larsen 1979a
McLeod Mound	5	Thomas and Larsen 1979a
Seaside Mound I	5	Thomas and Larsen 1979a
Seaside Mound II	4	Thomas and Larsen 1979a
Evelyn Plantation	1	Larsen 1982
Airport	18	Larsen 1982
Deptford (nonmound)	17	Larsen 1982; DePratter 1991
Cannons Point	5	Larsen 1982
Cedar Grove, Mound B	1	Larsen 1982; DePratter 1991
Sea Island Mound	11	Larsen 1982
Johns Mound	26	Larsen and Thomas 1982
Marys Mound	4	Larsen and Thomas 1982
Charlie King Mound	1	Larsen 1982
Cedar Grove Mound C	4	Larsen 1982; DePratter, 1991
South End Mound II	10	Larsen and Thomas 1986
Precontact Agricultural (A.D. 1150–1500)		
North End Mound	1	Moore 1897
Low Mound, Shell Bluff	1	Moore 1897
Townsend Mound	1	Moore 1897; Cook 1970
Deptford Mound	2	Larsen 1982; DePratter 1991
Norman Mound	16	Larson 1957; Larsen 1982
Kent Mound	19	Cook 1978; Larsen 1982
Lewis Creek, Mound III	1	Cook 1966; Larsen 1982
Lewis Creek, misc.	3	Cook 1966; Larsen 1982
Lewis Creek, Mound E	1	Cook 1966; Neighbors and Rathbun 1973; Sexton and Rathbun 1977
Seven Mile Bend	10	Larsen 1982, unpublished
Oatland Mound	2	Cook and Pearson 1973; Larsen 1982
Irene Mound	187	Hulse 1941; Larsen 1982
Grove's Creek	1	Larsen, unpublished
South End Mound I	13	Moore 1897; Larsen, unpublished
Little Pine Island	9	Larsen, unpublished
Red Bird Creek Mound	1	Pearson 1984; Larsen, unpublished

Table 7–1. continued

Couper Field	23	Wallace 1975; Zahler 1976; Larsen, unpublished
Taylor Mound	16	Wallace 1975; Zahler 1976; Cook and Pearson 1973; Larsen, unpublished
Indian Field	8	Wallace 1975; Zahler 1976; Larsen, unpublished
Taylor Mound/ Martinez B	1	Martinez 1975; Larsen, unpublished
Early Contact (A.D. 1550–1680)		
Santa Catalina de Guale	32	Larsen 1990a, 1993
Santa Maria de los Yamassee	48	Larsen 1993
Late Contact (A.D. 1686–1702)		
Santa Catalina de Santa Maria	91	Larsen 1993, unpublished

[a]N = number of individuals with at least one eye orbit and/or vault element complete enough for observation.

1000), and St. Catherines (A.D. 100–1150) periods (DePratter 1979). Human remains are available from all periods, but most postdate A.D. 700. The precontact preagricultural group is represented by a composite of human remains drawn from 16 mortuary sites on the islands and the mainland Georgia coast.

Precontact Agricultural Group (A.D. 1150–1550)

The populations from this group are from the Mississippian period occupation of the region, known locally as the Savannah (A.D. 1150–1300) and Irene (A.D. 1300–1550) periods (DePratter 1979). Analysis of food remains from late prehistoric sites indicates a continued reliance on wild plants and animals, the latter drawn especially from marine/ estuarine settings (Reitz 1988). Little ethnobotanical evidence of maize has been recovered from Georgia coastal archaeological sites, suggesting a minor role of this domesticate in native foodways (see Larsen 1982; Reitz 1988). This reconstruction of diet is based, however, on incomplete evidence, since carbon and nitrogen stable isotope analysis reveals a significant use of C_4 terrestrial resources, namely maize, beginning in the twelfth century A.D. (Larsen, Schoeninger et al. 1992). In the last prehistoric period, the Irene period, isotopic analysis indicates a clear decline in use of maize at the primary Mississippian center located at the Irene site, which may have been due to environmental stress (e.g., drought) or social disruption or some combination of these two factors (Larsen, Schoeninger et al. 1992; Anderson 1994).

Settlement systems in the Mississippian populations occupying the Georgia coastal region are different from earlier times. After the twelfth century, there is an increase in the number of habitation sites and spatial extent of some habitation sites (e.g., Crook 1984, 1986; Pearson 1979). We believe that this shift reflects population increase and sedentism such as that seen throughout the Eastern Woodlands of North America. Increasing sedentism appears to be linked with maize production. Moreover, analysis of site structure and mortuary archaeology indicates that these population changes are linked with the appearance of complex chiefdoms and elaboration of social order and structure (Anderson 1994; Crook 1984, 1986).

The human skeletal remains representing this period are a composite of some 18 mortuary sites dating to the last several centuries of prehistory. Most of the remains are from the Irene site on the north coastal zone (Caldwell and McCann 1941).

Early Contact Group (A.D. 1550–1680)

Interaction between native populations and Europeans in the Georgia Bight came in two primary stages, involving an initial series of explorations and attempts at colonization during the first half of the sixteenth century by two major European powers, France and Spain (Jones 1978; Worth 1995). The exploratory period ended after the expulsion of France from the region by Spain in 1565 and subsequent establishment of the first permanent European colony north of Mexico at St. Augustine, Florida, by Pedro Menéndez de Avilés (Jones 1978). After the founding of this settlement, a series of Roman Catholic missions were established north of St. Augustine on the Atlantic coastline in the present-day states of Florida and Georgia. The northernmost mission was established on St. Catherines Island among the Guale Indians and named Santa Catalina de Guale (Thomas 1987).

Santa Catalina de Guale served as a mission from the 1570s to 1680, when abandonment was forced as the English began to encroach on and claim the Georgia coast. Ethnobotanical evidence from archaeological sites, coupled with isotopic (carbon and nitrogen) and elemental (barium and strontium) data, indicates a marked reorientation of diet, involving mainly an increase in consumption of maize by native populations (Larsen, Schoeninger et al. 1992; Ezzo et al. 1995). Analysis of historical records and archaeological settlement data reveals that populations became increasingly sedentary during this period. Most of the increased sedentism involved relocation and nucleation of native groups around the mission in an associated village located on the western side of St. Catherines Island.

In addition to the Guale, missions were established among other native groups throughout Spanish Florida in the late sixteenth and early seventeenth centuries. Throughout this period, extensive population movement occurred involving the relocation of refugee groups from the north to the south. The Yamassee—a group closely related to the Guale—were especially prominent in this regard. They migrated from coastal South Carolina, establishing at least one settlement with a mission on Amelia Island, Florida, during the first half of the seventeenth century. The mission, Santa Maria de los Yamassee, was abandoned in 1683 (Larsen 1993; Worth 1995). Analysis of stable isotopes from skeletal remains recovered from Santa Maria de los Yamassee indicates a reliance on maize agriculture at a level similar to that of Guale living at Santa Catalina (Hutchinson et al., this volume). The early contact group is represented by crania from Santa Catalina de Guale on St. Catherines Island, Georgia, and Santa Maria de los Yamassee on Amelia Island, Florida.

Late Contact Group (A.D. 1686–1702)

The late seventeenth century was a period of increased turmoil for the native populations and Spaniards living in the Georgia Bight. Following attacks on St. Catherines Island by British and British-ally Indians, the native population fled and subsequently resettled on Amelia Island several years after the departure of the Yamassee group. The Guale and Spaniards from St. Catherines Island reestablished the new mission on Amelia Island, calling it Santa Catalina de Guale de Santa Maria (hereafter referred to as Santa Catalina de Santa Maria). Historical, ethnobotanical, and other analyses indicate the same basic continuation of subsistence practices and settlement pattern as during the early contact period. Indeed, the population was heavily focused on maize agriculture, and it was concentrated at the mission. Because of Britain's interest in the region the mission was abandoned in 1702, marking the terminal date of native occupation of this region of the Georgia Bight. Human remains recovered from Santa Catalina de Santa Maria comprise the late contact group in this study.

THE BIOCULTURAL CONTEXT FOR ANEMIA IN ARCHAEOLOGICAL SETTINGS

The skeletal changes associated with anemia are part of a generalized syndrome called *porotic hyperostosis,* a term first introduced by Angel (1966) and used to describe a pathological condition involving the diploë and outer table of compact bone, especially in the squamous portions of the frontal, occipital, and parietals. Similar lesions found in the roof areas of the eye orbits, called cribra orbitalia, are also frequently encountered in archaeological human remains. The skeletal changes result from the hypertrophy of the erythropoietic tissues in the diploic space in response to the anemia. The increase in activity results in the replacement of the outer table of compact bone with ex-

posed diploic bone, giving the appearance of sieve-like porosity, sometimes with raised and hypervascularized areas of skeletal tissue (Larsen
1997).

There is a wide degree of variation in frequency of orbital versus
nonorbital lesions in human populations from archaeological settings.
For example, in prehistoric Ecuador, most lesions are found on the cranial vault (Ubelaker 1992), whereas in Australian samples, lesions are
primarily orbital (Webb 1995). Some argue that the etiologies of porotic
hyperostosis and cribra orbitalia are different or represent different
levels of progression of anemia (Carlson et al. 1974; Lallo et al. 1977).
The preponderance of clinical and paleopathological evidence indicates, rather, a common etiology for orbital and vault lesions (Stuart-
Macadam 1989; Walker 1985; Larsen 1997).

Although porotic hyperostosis and cribra orbitalia have been found
in individuals of all ages, the active, unhealed form is predominantly
found in juvenile remains (less than five years of age), regardless of geographic or cultural circumstances (Lallo et al. 1977; Larsen, Ruff et al.
1992; Mensforth et al. 1978; Mittler and Van Gerven 1994; and others).
In adults, the lesions tend to be remodeled and well healed. After ob-
serving the differences between juveniles and adults, Stuart-Macadam
(1985) contends that porotic hyperostosis is derived from anemia occurring during early childhood. This appears to be the case because
the blood-forming spaces in young children are completely filled with
red marrow—expansion arising from marrow production thus places
increased stress on the bone tissue. In adults, by contrast, an increase
in red blood cell production does not involve the use of all available
marrow space. Therefore, the adult component of the population, although it may be experiencing anemia, does not express a record of
active iron deficiency in its skeletal tissues.

Other pathological conditions, including scurvy, rickets, and infection, produce skeletal changes similar to those of anemia (Henschen
1961; Ortner 1992; Schultz 1993). These conditions can be distinguished on the basis of histological and morphological differences
(Schultz 1993; and see Ortner 1992).

METHODS OF STUDY

All crania with cranial flat and orbital surfaces intact enough for observation were included in the present study. Porotic hyperostosis for
flat cranial surfaces (frontal, parietals, occipital) and cribra orbitalia for
orbital surfaces were recorded. Lesions ranged from clearly discernible,
usually healed, porosity (Figure 7-1) to extreme diploic expansion and
hypervascularization (Figure 7-2). In view of this variation, we also collected data in regard to severity of expression, distinguishing between
presence of cribrotic or porotic lesions of minor to moderate severity

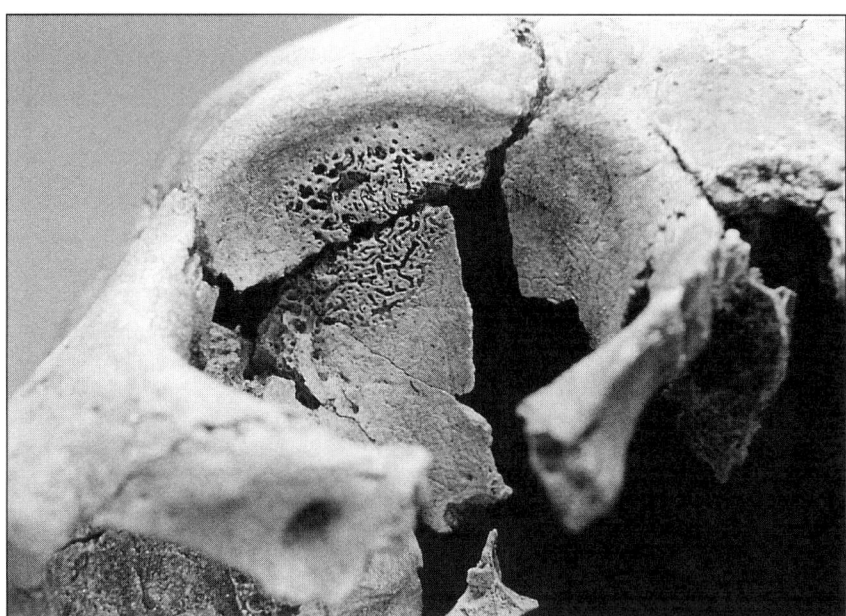

Figure 7-1. Mild Expressions of Cribra Orbitalia (above) and Porotic Hyperostosis (below) in Two Adults, Amelia Island, Florida. (Photographs by Mark C. Griffin)

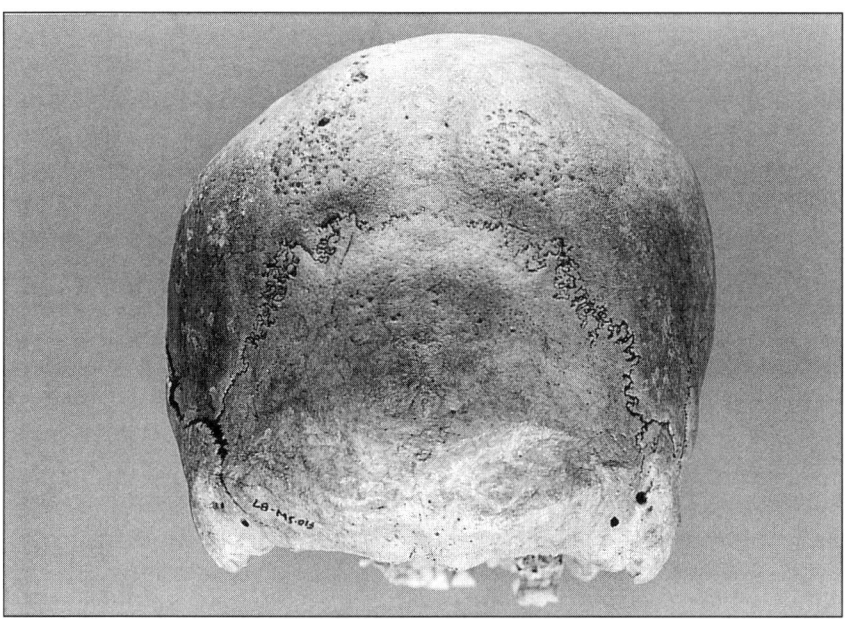

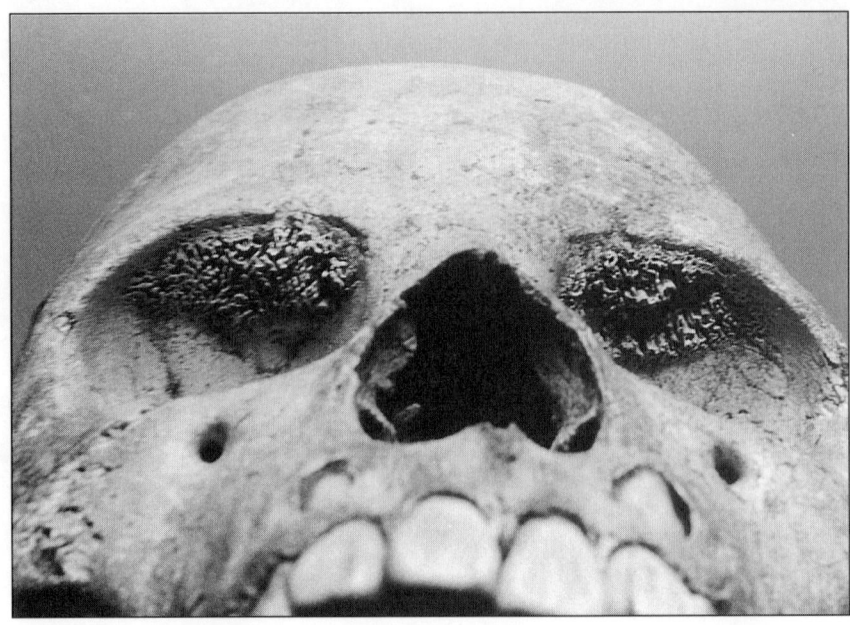

Figure 7-2. Severe Expressions of Cribra Orbitalia (above) and Porotic Hyperostosis (below) in Two Juveniles, Amelia Island, Florida. (Photographs by Mark C. Griffin)

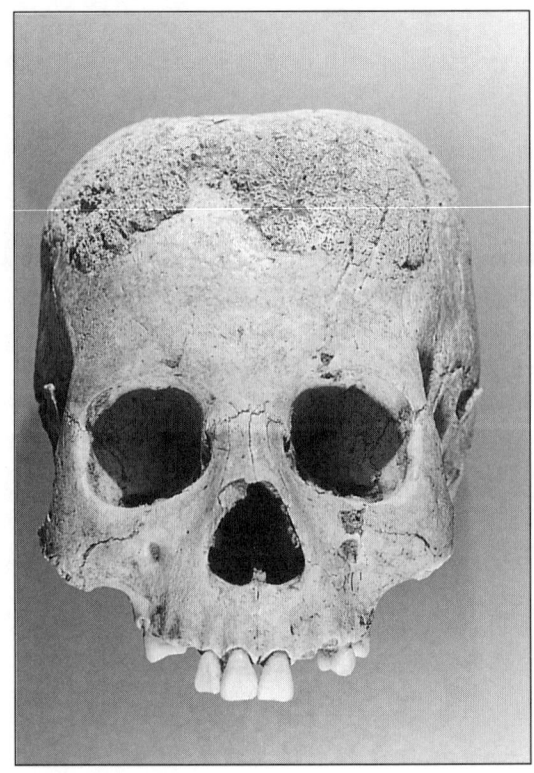

from gross lesions with excessive expansion and large areas of diploic exposure. Minor lesions are those with fine porosity, usually well healed; moderate lesions have a mix of fine porosity with at least some perforations that appear to be active at the time of death; and gross lesions are expressed as extreme porosity with pronounced elevation from the normal bone surface.

The present investigation distinguishes pathology by age and sex in order to identify diachronic changes in and differences between these subgroups. Age and sex were determined by use of a standard osteological protocol (Bass 1995). Age is expressed with regard to either juvenile (individuals less than 10 years of age at death) or adult (greater than or equal to 16 years). Individuals between ages 10 and 16 contain virtually no evidence of porotic hyperostosis or cribra orbitalia and are not considered in the analysis.

GROUP COMPARISONS

Comparisons of cribra orbitalia and porotic hyperostosis prevalence for each of the four groups are presented in Table 7-2. Temporal comparisons reveal a clear dichotomy between the precontact and contact groups. The precontact preagriculturalists and agriculturalists have a relatively low prevalence of cribrotic and porotic lesions, well under 10 percent for most subsamples in either group. In the precontact preagriculturalists, no individuals have porotic hyperostosis. In contrast to the precontact groups, the early and late contact samples express considerably elevated prevalences of cribra orbitalia and porotic hyperostosis, with some evidence for increase from the early to late contact periods. For all individuals combined, both groups show more than 20 percent prevalence of cribra orbitalia and porotic hyperostosis. Severity of lesions increases over the temporal span, indicating the presence of some expression of severe forms of porotic hyperostosis and cribra orbitalia in the late contact group.

Examination of subgroups within each of the periods reveals important distinctions between them. Most obvious is the very high prevalence of cribrotic and porotic lesions in the contact-period juveniles, equal to or exceeding 50 percent in the late contact group and contrasting with the precontact juveniles (no porotic hyperostosis in precontact preagricultural juveniles). In the adults, there are no statistically significant differences between males and females (chi-square: $p > 0.05$).

INTERPRETING LESION PATTERN AND PREVALENCE

Two principal findings emerge from this study. First, there is an appreciable increase in prevalence and severity of cribra orbitalia and porotic

Table 7–2. Cribra Orbitalia and Porotic Hyperostosis Prevalence and
Severity, Georgia Bight

	PP[a]		PA		EC		LC		Significant
	%	n[b]	%	n	%	n	%	n	change[c]
Cribra orbitalia									
Total[d]	5.7	104	3.1	287	11.8	68	22.9	70	none
Juveniles[e]	38.5	13	6.1	33	33.3	12	73.3	15	PP/PA, PA/EC
Males	0.0	29	2.4	84	9.5	21	10.3	29	none
Females	0.0	39	2.4	123	0.0	22	4.2	24	none
Severity[f]	1.06	104	1.03	287	1.12	68	1.23	70	none
Porotic hyperostosis									
Total	0.0	113	3.3	308	18.8	80	21.1	90	none
Juveniles	0.0	13	0.0	33	21.4	14	50.0	18	EC/LC
Males	0.0	35	5.7	88	23.8	21	11.4	35	none
Females	0.0	42	0.7	137	7.7	26	11.4	35	PA/EC
Severity	1.00	113	1.03	308	1.09	80	1.21	90	none

[a]PP = precontact preagricultural; PA = precontact agricultural; EC = early contact;
LC = late contact.
[b]Percent of orbits/vaults affected; n = total number of orbits/vaults examined (pathological + nonpathological).
[c]Statistically significant change (chi-square: $p<0.05$, two-tailed).
[d]Total = juveniles, unsexed adults, adult females, adult males.
[e]Juveniles = <10 years.
[f]Mean of severity determined from the following scores: 1 = absent on at least one
observable orbit or parietal; 2 = presence of lesion; 3 = gross lesions with excessive
expansion and large areas of diploë exposed. All individuals combined.

hyperostosis in Georgia Bight native populations, especially in relation
to the increase in the contact period relative to the precontact period.
Second, the increase is more pronounced for the juvenile component
of the population. The following discussion presents potential causes
of anemia, including the role of genetics, diet, and nondietary environmental factors.

Genetic Factors

Angel (1966) argued that porotic hyperostosis in prehistoric populations resulted from hemolytic genetic anemias (sickle cell anemia,
thalassemia), particularly in reference to his long-term study of archaeological skeletons from the eastern Mediterranean, principally in
Greece, Cyprus, and western Turkey. In present-day populations, ma-

laria is endemic in the region. The very high frequency of abnormal hemoglobins for this and other regions having endemic malaria led Haldane (1949) to hypothesize that individuals who are heterozygous carriers have a selective advantage over individuals with normal hemoglobin. Indeed, there are distinctive geographic correlations of endemic malaria and abnormal hemoglobins throughout the Old World (Livingstone 1973).

For Old World populations, an explanation of high prevalence of porotic hyperostosis in relation to abnormal hemoglobins is difficult to prove since all manner of anemias, genetic and acquired, leave a similar skeletal signature (Ortner and Putschar 1985). Identification of the thalassemia mutation via analysis of DNA from a child's skeleton from Israel lends support for Angel's hypothesis (Filon et al. 1995). It is highly unlikely, however, that some underlying genetic condition is the cause of anemia in Georgia Bight groups. Native populations living in the Americas were not exposed to malaria prior to European contact (Dunn 1965), thus hemolytic genetic anemias were not present in the New World prior to or well after the arrival of Europeans. As noted by Livingstone (1973:42), native populations in the Americas are "dismally homozygous for normal (hemoglobin) alleles."

Dietary Factors

The bioavailability of iron from dietary sources is related to several factors, mostly associated with the efficiency by which it is absorbed by the body (Baynes and Bothwell 1990; Hallberg 1981). This efficiency is dependent on the source of the iron, whether derived from heme or nonheme sources. Heme sources, derived primarily from meat, fish, and poultry, are efficiently absorbed by the gut. Moreover, iron in meat does not require processing in the stomach, and the amino acids from digestion of meat enhance iron absorption (Wadsworth 1992). Nonheme sources of iron, forming most of iron acquired by the body, are found in plants and are the least efficiently absorbed. A number of plant substances actually inhibit iron absorption, such as phytates found in maize. Some foods consumed in combination enhance iron absorption. Layrisse and coworkers (1968) demonstrated via experimental evidence that absorption of (nonheme) iron in maize is considerably enhanced—by as much as 300 percent—when consumed with fish.

Because diets severely deficient in iron or inhibiting iron bioavailability are known to cause iron-deficiency anemia, many researchers conclude that diet is the leading cause of the illness. Considering a body of evidence showing iron loss through a variety of secretions (urine, stools, sweat, and so forth), however, some workers suggest that iron deficiency via dietary causes alone is unusual (Daly 1989; Kent

1992). Most water and foods contain small but sufficient amounts of iron (Wadsworth 1992). Thus, even the most minimalist diets contain enough iron to meet physiological needs of the body.

Unlike some other eastern or southwestern North American settings that show increases in porotic hyperostosis with the adoption and intensification of maize agriculture (various authors in Cohen and Armelagos 1984; see Larsen 1995, 1997), the late prehistoric Georgia Bight shows no appreciable increase. This observation, combined with the clinical evidence underplaying the role of diet in anemia, suggests that diet is probably not an important cause of iron deficiency in this setting. Indeed, the strong dependence on marine resources in the agricultural period before contact may have served to increase the bioavailability of iron in these maize consumers, thus resulting in low prevalence of porotic hyperostosis in the precontact agriculturalists (and see Rathbun et al. 1980).

Nondietary Environmental Factors

Iron-deficiency anemia may also be caused by a variety of nondietary factors. Children with low birth weights are predisposed to iron-deficiency anemia; and blood loss, hemorrhage, chronic diarrhea, and dysentery have also been implicated as causes of the disease (Kent 1986). Children are especially vulnerable to iron-deficiency anemia because of rapid growth of the red cell mass. In adults, gastrointestinal bleeding causes iron-deficiency anemia (Farley and Foland 1990). A newly recognized cause of iron-deficiency anemia is found in endurance athletes, especially marathon runners (Newhouse and Clement 1988; Farley and Foland 1990). In these individuals, blood loss from ischemia of the gastrointestinal mucosa results from the shunting of blood to muscles in strenuous activities.

Parasitic infections can also cause severe anemia. In some regions of the world, parasitism is highly endemic. Schistosomiasis ("snail fever") triggers an immunological response after the eggs of worms (Schistosoma) inhabiting blood vessels become lodged in body organs, such as the liver, intestinal walls, and urogenital tract. The disease has a tropical worldwide distribution (Farley 1993). Similarly, hookworms are geographically widespread but are mostly limited to tropical and subtropical settings. Hookworm disease is caused by the ingestion or inhalation of infective larvae (Ancylostoma duodenale, Necator americanus). The worm extracts blood by grasping the host's intestinal wall with its sharp teeth (Despommier et al. 1995; Hotez and Pritchard 1995). One or several hookworms are inconsequential for the host. When several hundred or more worms are simultaneously feeding, however, enormous amounts of blood are potentially lost—upwards of

0.21 ml of blood per hookworm per day—thus linking the organism to iron-deficiency anemia (Layrisse and Roche 1964; Woodruff 1982).

The striking increase in prevalence of porotic hyperostosis in contact-era coastal Georgia and Florida populations may be related to conditions not unlike those described by various workers where parasitism was endemic because of widespread contamination of water sources in some regions of the world, for example in Nubia (Carlson et al. 1974; Mittler and Van Gerven 1994), Australia (Webb 1995), southern coastal California (Lambert and Walker 1991; Walker 1986), the American Southwest (Kent 1986), and Ecuador (Ubelaker 1992). In these settings, it is possible to identify sources of water contamination by parasites, especially where drinking water is obtained. Lambert and Walker (1991; Walker 1986) observe that increased prevalence of iron-deficiency anemia in populations living on islands in the Santa Barbara Channel Island region of California coincided with a period of increasing sedentism and population size and a shift from dietary focus on terrestrial to marine-based diets, especially fish. In the latest prehistoric period in the California sequence, groups became concentrated around a limited number of water sources on the islands. As a result, diarrhea-causing enteric bacteria and parasites may have contaminated these water sources, thus leading to iron-deficiency anemia. Ethnographic evidence indicates that island populations had a preference for eating raw fish (Walker 1986), thus further exposing them to parasitic infections and other factors that would deplete iron stores.

The California setting serves as an important model for what may have occurred after the establishment of missions and population relocation among Guale and Yamassee Indians in the sixteenth and seventeenth centuries in the Georgia Bight. In the mission settings of St. Catherines and Amelia Islands, the increased concentration of population in crowded mission villages would have contributed to reduced sanitary conditions. Unlike their prehistoric forebears, mission Indians constructed wells by digging shallow holes into a high water table. This practice was introduced to native populations by the Spaniards. Archaeological documentation of a well at Santa Catalina de Guale on St. Catherines Island indicates that it was quite shallow (Thomas 1987). These wells are easily contaminated and serve as potential breeding grounds for parasites and, hence, increased iron-deficiency anemia in the humans drinking the water. Moreover, a freshwater stream located near the St. Catherines Island mission appears to have been dammed and utilized as a primary water source (Royce Hayes, personal communication 1985). We have observed a profusion of early contact-period trash middens in and surrounding the dammed area. The unsanitary nature of this setting during the occupation of the mission may have also contributed to parasitism and other factors leading to iron-deficiency anemia.

The presence of anemia-related pathology in primarily young juveniles is consistent with the general findings of greater prevalence of pathology in juveniles from other settings (see Stuart-Macadam 1985). More important, the high prevalence in juveniles serves as a barometer for measuring iron status in the population as a whole. Histological analysis of a small sample of juvenile and adult crania dating to the contact period with porotic hyperostosis and cribra orbitalia indicates that at least some instances of pathology are related to infection and other causes not related to iron-deficiency anemia (Schultz and Larsen 1997). Nevertheless, the overall pattern of bony response indicates that iron-deficiency anemia is the primary cause of the pathology we report in the present study.

We believe, then, that iron-deficiency anemia in the Georgia Bight was caused principally by nondietary, nongenetic factors. In particular, closer, more crowded living conditions in mission settings led to a reduction in sanitation, contamination of water sources, and overall decline in quality of life and living circumstances.

The intensification of maize agriculture that has been well documented in this and other settings during the historic period no doubt served to exacerbate the increasingly poor conditions of the mission settings. Increased consumption of maize may have contributed to a reduction in quality of diet and increase in nutritional stress (and see Larsen 1995; various studies in Cohen and Armelagos 1984). While meeting caloric needs, maize is a poor source of protein, and overreliance on it contributes to a variety of health problems, as seen in both past and living populations (Larsen 1995, 1997). Disease and poor nutrition have a synergistic relationship, which thus helps to explain the declines in health observed in this setting.

Our hypothesis that the increase in iron-deficiency anemia in the Georgia Bight is primarily due to parasitism and poor living conditions generally is further substantiated by other indicators of health decline, including increase in nonspecific infectious lesions (periosteal reactions) in long bones (Larsen and Harn 1994), decline in oral health (Larsen et al. 1991), and other negative factors identified in the contact period (see Larsen, Ruff et al. 1992). Decline in human health in the Georgia Bight appears to have begun in the precontact agricultural period, which is related to the consumption of maize and population sedentism (Larsen 1982). Bioarchaeological evidence, however, indicates that the declines in health are more pronounced after the establishment of missions among native populations in the sixteenth and seventeenth centuries.

COMPARISONS WITH OTHER STUDIES
IN THE SPANISH BORDERLANDS

Human remains from other regions of the Spanish borderlands, the broad region on the northern frontier of New Spain extending from Florida to California, are limited. Nevertheless, small skeletal series have been studied by Hill (1996) in west-central Alabama and by Miller (1996) in central Texas. In both regions, late prehistoric populations show low prevalence of porotic hyperostosis, and contact-era populations show high prevalence of porotic hyperostosis. In Alabama, prevalence rises from less than 10 percent to 65 percent, and in Texas, from 0 percent to 40 percent. In the Alabama series, like the Georgia Bight, the severity of expression is also greater. The contact-era remains from Alabama are not from a mission context, but nevertheless the increase in anemia along with other stressors (e.g., infection) attests to the deteriorating conditions following the arrival of Europeans.

The contact-period skeletal remains from Texas are from a mission context, San Juan Capistrano (A.D. 1733–1794), where native populations subsisted on maize, beef, and other domesticates. Their prehistoric predecessors were foragers, depending exclusively on wild plants and nondomesticated animals (Miller 1996). Comparisons of pathology revealed not only an increase in porotic hyperostosis in the mission population but also an increase in infection, dental caries, and other dental conditions in a pronounced manner.

Finally, in the American Southwest, conditions conducive to iron-deficiency anemia appear to have remained high throughout both the late prehistoric and historic periods. That is, in both prehistoric and historic period populations, high prevalence of porotic hyperostosis in a wide range of sites suggests that iron-deficiency anemia was a ubiquitous health burden (Nelson et al. 1994; Stodder 1994, 1996; Stodder and Martin 1992). Some populations living in upland settings and with greater access to animal protein appear to have had relatively low levels of iron-deficiency anemia, such as at Gran Quivira (Stodder and Martin 1992). In populations living in dense, closely crowded settings—such as in cliff dwellings and in pueblos—anemia occurs in high frequencies. Although the arrival of Europeans certainly contributed to poorer health in the American Southwest, iron status in most populations was already poor.

IRON-DEFICIENCY ANEMIA: A BENEFICIAL DISEASE?

The increase in iron-deficiency anemia in the Georgia Bight and elsewhere may have been beneficial for these and other populations in which moderate to high prevalences of porotic hyperostosis have been documented. Clinical and laboratory evidence points to a link between low iron status and decreased microbial activity, representing what Weinberg (1992) has called a type of "nutritional immunity." Weinberg (1992) notes that animal and human studies show that hosts not withholding iron are at increased risk for infection—bacterial, fungal, and protozoan—and conversely, risk of infection decreases with iron withholding (although see Berger et al. 1992; Keusch and Farthing 1986, for alternative perspectives). Pathogens causing infection are dependent on iron that they extract from their human host. If the human host is low in iron stores, then the infection-causing agent cannot survive. Thus, iron-deficiency anemia may be an adaptive response to chronic pathogen loads (Stuart-Macadam 1992).

The relationship between iron withholding and decreased infection seems straightforward. However, iron deficiency comes with a series of functional costs (see Goodman 1994). Even when an individual is only slightly deficient in iron, various key enzymes involved in vital functions (e.g., DNA synthesis) are affected. At the organism level, iron-deficiency anemia has profound negative effects on work capacity, cognition, and the maintenance of a healthy immune system (Goodman 1994). These effects are best seen in children, who respond rapidly to iron depletion (Farley and Foland 1990). Individuals with iron deficiency may have shortened lifespans. A number of bioarchaeological investigators have also reported a strong positive correlation between infection and porotic hyperostosis in archaeological samples and greater mortality in individuals with the lesions (e.g., Mensforth et al. 1978; Huss-Ashmore et al. 1982). Thus, the negative consequences of iron-deficiency anemia appear to outweigh the benefits, leading us to regard the disease as an adjustment rather than an adaptation to increased pathogen loads (and see Goodman 1994).

Summary and Conclusions

Analysis of cribra orbitalia and porotic hyperostosis in archaeological populations from the Georgia Bight reveals increases in prevalence of pathology, but only in the contact period in comparison with precontact populations. This finding lends further support to the hypothesis that iron-deficiency anemia is not linked solely to diet in this region— and to the adoption of maize agriculture in particular—but rather to poor living conditions brought about by population nucleation and sedentism and increased parasitism and water contamination. Maize consumption may well have played a role in increased iron-deficiency anemia—certainly the focus on maize would not have improved iron status. Diet, however, was only one of several players leading to increased population stress. The apparent positive relationship between infection and iron withholding suggests some benefit to mild to moderate iron-deficiency anemia, but the health costs of this anemia are greater than the benefits.

ACKNOWLEDGMENTS

We thank Patricia M. Lambert for her invitation to contribute to this volume this chapter based on the paper delivered in the symposium she organized for the 1996 meetings of the American Association of Physical Anthropologists held in the Research Triangle Park, North Carolina. Jeffry L. Takács assisted in the data analysis. Funding for this research was provided by the National Science Foundation. This chapter is a contribution to the La Florida Bioarchaeology Project.

8 A Comparison of Degenerative Joint Disease between Upland and Coastal Prehistoric Agriculturalists from Georgia

Matthew A. Williamson

One of the fundamental components of bioarchaeological research is the use of pathological skeletal lesions in the study of the interaction between biological and cultural aspects of past populations (Blakely 1977; Buikstra 1977; Buikstra and Cook 1980; Bush and Zvelebil 1991; Grauer 1995; Iscan and Kennedy 1989; Larsen 1987; Larsen and Milner 1994; Powell et al. 1991; Rathbun 1986; Saunders and Katzenberg 1992). Among the various diseases that are a part of this kind of analysis, studies of degenerative joint disease (DJD) have provided some important clues regarding the lifeways of prehistoric populations.

When biological variables such as age and sex are controlled, the frequency of DJD within or between groups can provide useful information on activity patterns and workload (Bridges 1992; Jurmain 1977, 1990; Larsen 1987, 1995; Ortner 1968). In the eastern United States, this approach has been used to examine intrasite differences between sexes (Bridges 1991, 1994; Larsen 1982) and between high and low status agriculturalists (Blakely 1980; Tainter 1980). More abundant are studies that focus on how the transition from hunting and gathering to subsistence agriculture impacted native populations (Bridges 1991, 1992; Larsen 1981, 1982, 1984, 1995). Early research suggested that activity levels, reflected in the frequency of DJD, decreased in accordance with the less strenuous agricultural lifestyle (reviewed in Bridges 1992; Larsen 1995). Work that followed has shown, however, that a distinct pattern associated with changes in subsistence behavior is difficult to identify. For example, in the Caddo culture area of northeast Texas, southwest Arkansas, and southeast Oklahoma, Rose and coworkers (1984) found a decrease in overall DJD during the adoption of agriculture but a subsequent increase in the late prehistoric period. At the same time in the nearby Lower Mississippi Valley, they observed a decrease in osteoarthritis (although osteophytosis increased). Reported DJD frequencies during the transition to intensive agriculture are inconsistent. For example, Goodman and coworkers (1984) observed an increase in Illinois, whereas Larsen (1982) found a decrease on the Georgia coast, and Bridges (1991) found no change at all in Alabama. Indeed, Larsen (1995:200) has concluded that "no definitive pattern relating prevalence and subsistence mode emerges except with regard to specific geographic settings."

Only a few studies have specifically addressed how DJD varies among and between agriculturalists from different geographical settings (e.g., Rose et al. 1984). Even though maize agriculture was widely practiced across the Eastern woodlands, it cannot be assumed that its effects on cultural and biological variables were identical for all populations (Larsen 1995). According to Hally (1994), because of considerable environmental differences within Georgia, the late prehistoric coastal settlement-subsistence pattern probably differed significantly from the type practiced by upland inhabitants. This probably resulted in significant differences in activity patterns between these regions, despite the fact that both were occupied by complex agricultural societies. The purpose of this chapter is to determine if activity patterns, documented through the frequency of degenerative joint disease, varied significantly between late prehistoric (A.D. 1350–1550) Mississippian populations from upland and coastal Georgia, as might be predicted from Hally's model.

Georgia is an excellent location for studying the geographical variation of DJD because it can be divided into separate regions that vary in physical geography and natural resources. These regions are referred to as physiographic provinces and consist of the Cumberland Plateau, Valley and Ridge, Blue Ridge, Piedmont, Coastal Plain, and Coastal Zone (Clark and Zisa 1976) (Figure 8-1). In this study, only the Valley and Ridge, Piedmont, and Coastal Zone are represented by human skeletal remains.

The topography of the Valley and Ridge province ranges from 400–500 m asl in the central Armuchee Ridges District to the relatively flat Great Valley District, which contains a few elevations above 30 m (Clark and Zisa 1976). Relatively nutrient-rich, broad alluvial floodplains are associated with the rivers that flow through the Great Valley District (Hally and Langford 1988). Inhabitants of the Valley and Ridge seem to have exploited riverine and upland resources from permanent

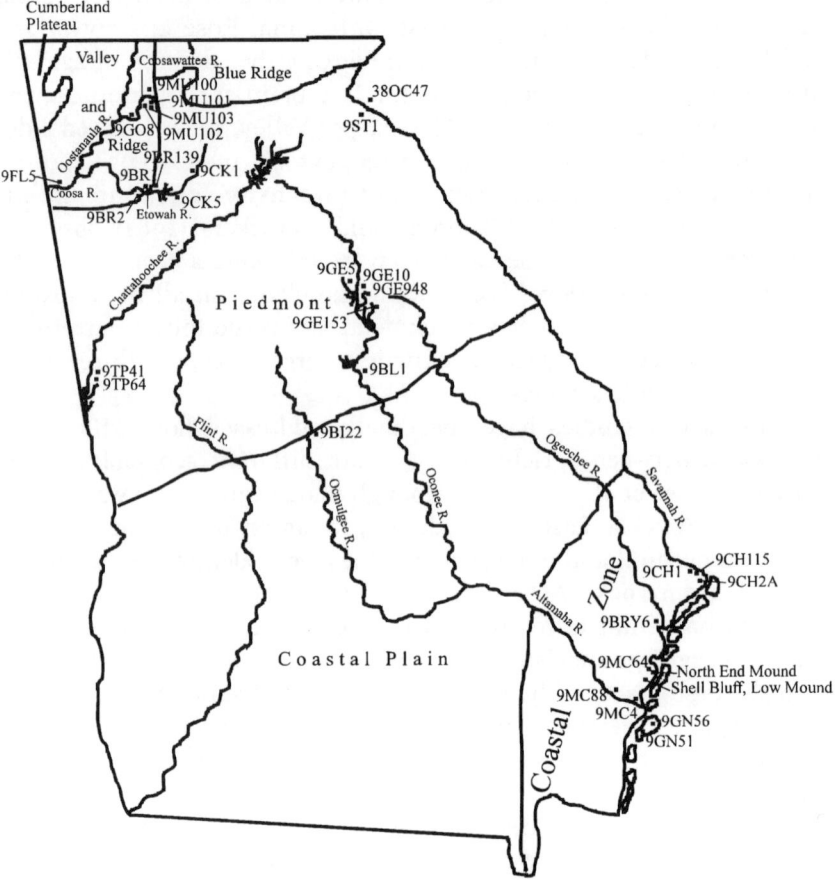

Figure 8-1. Approximate Site Locations.

settlements as well as from temporary camps (Hally and Langford 1988). Subsistence centered on the cultivation of maize, beans, and squash, supplementary hunting and gathering, and exploitation of aquatic resources from river shoals.

The Piedmont Province is bounded by the Valley and Ridge Province to the north and the Coastal Plain to the south (Clark and Zisa 1976). Elevations range from 300 to 450 m asl. The upper region of the Piedmont is characterized by gradually declining hills and ridges and deeply cut streams. The lower region of the Piedmont is defined by rolling hills and broad areas divided by several major rivers. Subsistence in the Piedmont was centered on maize, beans, and squash agriculture, supplemented with numerous wild plants and terrestrial fauna such as deer, turkey, and box turtle (Hally and Rudolph 1986). In addition, aquatic resources were readily available at the river shoals and were easily harvested to supplement the diet (Shapiro 1990).

The Coastal Zone is defined at its western edge by the remnants of a Pleistocene marsh system and to the east by the Atlantic Ocean (Crook 1986). Elevations typically do not rise above 100 m asl. The lagoon-and-marsh section of the zone was probably the most intensively occupied area during the Mississippian period (Crook 1986). According to Larson (1980), the marsh section was probably the most important habitat because of the abundant terrestrial and aquatic faunal species that were present.

The arable land in the interior Coastal Zone contains highland oak forest patches scattered throughout the swamps (Crook 1986). According to Crook, the dispersal of highland areas, as well as limited areas of available soil, would have restricted the size and distribution of agricultural plots. In addition, because the soil nutrients are not renewed by alluvial deposits, these areas can be rapidly depleted. As a result, shifting crops of corn, beans, and squash would have been necessary.

An exception to the typical coastal environment can be found in the area of the Savannah River floodplain where alluvial soil is abundant. In contrast to other areas of the Coastal Zone, this region offered indigenous people the opportunity for permanent settlement and large-scale agriculture (Anderson 1994). Even at sites within the Savannah River floodplain, however, the diet was supplemented with marine foods. Faunal remains recovered from the Irene Mound site (9CH1) included fish and shellfish (Caldwell and McCann 1941).

MATERIALS AND METHODS

Human skeletal remains from upland Georgia were recovered primarily from Middle and Late Mississippian (A.D. 1200–1540) sites (Figure 8-1). Eighty-one males and 81 females were sufficiently complete to allow confident age and sex assignment (Table 8-1). Data regarding the frequency of DJD among coastal Georgia inhabitants were taken from Larsen (1982). Larsen's sample consisted of 340 individuals from eleven Mississippian period sites.

Degenerative joint disease is one of a number of causes of arthritis (joint inflammation). Others include infection, trauma, metabolic disorders (e.g., gout), neoplasms, genetic factors, and bursitis (Ortner and Putschar 1985; Resnick and Niwayama 1988; Steinbock 1976). DJD is usually caused by the mechanical load placed on a joint, although it can be initiated by trauma, and is commonly found on cartilaginous and synovial joints (Jurmain 1977; Resnick and Niwayama 1988).

In order to understand the etiology of DJD, it is necessary to be familiar with joint anatomy because the types of lesions produced by DJD are directly related to the structure of cartilaginous and synovial joints. A cartilaginous joint is united by cartilage, does not have a joint cavity, and exhibits limited movement (Marieb 1992). For example,

Table 8-1. Number of Males and Females from Upland Georgia Sites

Site Number	Site Name	Males	Females
Valley and Ridge			
9BR1	Etowah (Mound B)	0	4
9BR2	Leake	0	1
9BR139	Stamp Creek	1	0
9FL5	King	34	29
9GO8	Baxter	0	1
9MU100	Sixtoe	12	11
9MU101	Bell Field	4	0
9MU102	Little Egypt	16	17
9MU103	Pott's Tract	0	1
Piedmont			
38OC47	Chauga	2	3
9BI22	Draw Bridge	1	0
9BL1	Shinholser	0	1
9CK1	Long Swamp	0	1
9CK5	Wilbanks	0	1
9GE5	Dyar	2	2
9GE153	Ogeltree	0	1
9ST1	Tugalo	0	1
9TP41	Park	4	0
9TP64	Avery	5	7
			Total N
		81	81 162

joints between vertebral bodies are separated by a disk of cartilage that is composed of a semifluid center, called the nucleus pulposus, and a surrounding ring of fibrocartilage, called the annulus fibrosus. A synovial joint exhibits five features: (1) hyaline cartilage that covers the joint surfaces, (2) a joint cavity, (3) an articular capsule composed of an outer fibrous layer and an inner loose connective tissue layer, (4) synovial fluid secreted by the inner layer of the capsule, and (5) supporting ligaments (Marieb 1992). In some cases (e.g., knee), discs of fibrocartilage, called menisci, lie between joint surfaces. The menisci reduce damage to the joint by absorbing shock waves produced by mechanical forces. Synovial joints are freely movable.

Degenerative joint disease of the spine progresses as the fibers of the annulus fibrosus are torn, allowing the nucleus pulposus to protrude through the defect (Schmorl and Junghanns 1971; Steinbock 1976). The gelatinous material then presses against the anterior longitudinal ligament and stimulates subperiosteal bone formation on the margin between the end plate and anterior surface of the centrum (Steinbock 1976). The resulting bony spicules are called osteophytes and the condition is referred to as osteophytosis (OP) or spondylitis deformans (Bridges 1991, 1992; Jurmain 1990; Ortner and Putschar 1985; Schmorl and Junghanns 1971). Severity of this condition ranges from minor lipping of the centrum by small, barely discernible lesions to the merging of osteophytes, superior and inferior to a disc, producing fusion between vertebrae (Ortner and Putschar 1985; Schmorl and Junghanns 1971; Steinbock 1976).

Degenerative joint disease begins in a synovial joint with the breakdown of the articular cartilage. Endochondral bone replacement of cartilage spurs located at the junction of the perichondrium and periosteum subsequently produces lipping on the margins of the joint surface. Even though bone hypertrophy may be extensive, ankylosis (fusion) of synovial joints is very rare. Finally, the cartilage completely erodes allowing contact between the sclerotic subchondral bone of each articular surface, a condition referred to as eburnation (Ortner and Putschar 1985; Steinbock 1976). Classic signs of eburnation are seen as deep grooves in the articular surface and polishing of the subchondral bone. The process of destruction in synovial joints sets up a vicious cycle by altering the mechanical relationship of the bones, which in turn exacerbates the problem. Degenerative joint disease found in the appendicular joints is distinguished from that of the spine by differences in both joint structure and etiology and is therefore referred to as osteoarthritis (OA) (Bridges 1991, 1994; Jurmain 1990; Ortner and Putschar 1985; Steinbock 1976).

For purposes of reducing interobserver error that could result from a comparison to Larsen's published data, the author was personally trained by Larsen in the evaluation of DJD and in the use of the scoring method described by Larsen (1982). DJD was scored as present or absent for each appendicular joint complex: a complex consisted of all the articular surfaces that could be observed for each joint (Table 8-2). For example, the knee joint consists of the distal femur, proximal tibia, and patella. If any one of these bones exhibited osteoarthritis, expressed as marginal lipping, erosive pitting, or eburnation, the condition was scored as present. Only the presence or absence of osteophytosis was recorded for the spinal segments. Cervical, thoracic, and lumbar segments, sacrum, shoulder, elbow, and knee constitute the areas of the skeleton that were examined. Right and left sides were combined.

Because the degeneration of joint surfaces is a natural part of aging, conclusions regarding possible differences in physical activity among or between study samples should control for sex and age. In order to test the effects of sex and age on DJD frequency in the upland sample, the researcher examined 40 males and 41 females with at least six of

Table 8-2. Descriptions of Joint Complexes

Joint	Skeletal Element(s)
Vertebrae	Centrum only
Shoulder	Proximal humerus (head)
	Scapula (glenoid fossa)
Elbow	Distal humerus (trochlea, capitulum)
	Proximal radius (head, radial notch)
	Proximal ulna (trochlear notch)
Knee	Patella (condylar surfaces)
	Distal femur (condyles)
	Proximal tibia (condyles)

the previously described joint complexes present for observation. Affected joints for each individual were added and then divided by the number of joints observed. This produced an arthritis "score" for each individual. The scores for the entire sample were then tested using analysis of variance. Not surprisingly, both sex and age were found to have a significant effect on arthritis score ($p<.05$ for both variables). Therefore, in order to reduce these effects on differences in DJD frequency, males and females were not combined, and each was assigned to one of the following age categories: 20–30 years, 31–40 years, >40 years.

RESULTS

When all upland males are compared to upland females, males tend to have a greater frequency of DJD in all joint complexes (Table 8-3, Figures 8-2 and 8-3). In a few cases along the spinal column, however, females exhibit greater frequencies. For example, 24 percent of females within the 20–30 age range exhibit osteoarthritis on the thoracic segment, compared to 22 percent of males. In the 31–40 age range, 71 percent of females have osteoarthritis on the lumbar segment compared to 60 percent of males. The only statistically significant difference in DJD between upland males and females is the greater frequency of female sacral OP for the 40 age group (53 percent compared to 13 percent; chi-square: $p<.05$).

Although differences between coastal and upland DJD frequency are present, data published in Larsen (1982) were not arranged in age categories, and therefore chi-square tests could not be performed. However, the adult age distributions of upland and coastal samples were not significantly different (Kolmogorov-Smirnov, $p<.05$) (Williamson 1998). Therefore, even though comparisons between upland and coastal males and females were not performed within age categories, observed differences were probably not biased by age differences.

Table 8-3. Frequency of Upland Male and Female Joints Affected by Degenerative Joint Disease Arranged by Age Category

Joint	Female						Male					
	20–30		31–40		41+		20–30		31–40		41+	
	%	N	%	N	%	N	%	N	%	N	%	N
Cervical	15	26	20	5	29	14	22	9	44	16	40	10
Thoracic	24	17	34	6	63	19	22	9	35	20	50	12
Lumbar	17	24	71	7	58	12	17	6	60	15	83	6
Sacrum	3	28	14	7	53*	15	29	7	17	18	13	15
Shoulder	5	42	9	11	9	22	3	31	19	31	10	19
Elbow	0	42	0	10	0	18	0	23	11	28	5	19
Knee	4	46	0	11	13	24	9	23	19	27	29	21

N = number of joints observed.
* = statistically significant ($p < .05$)

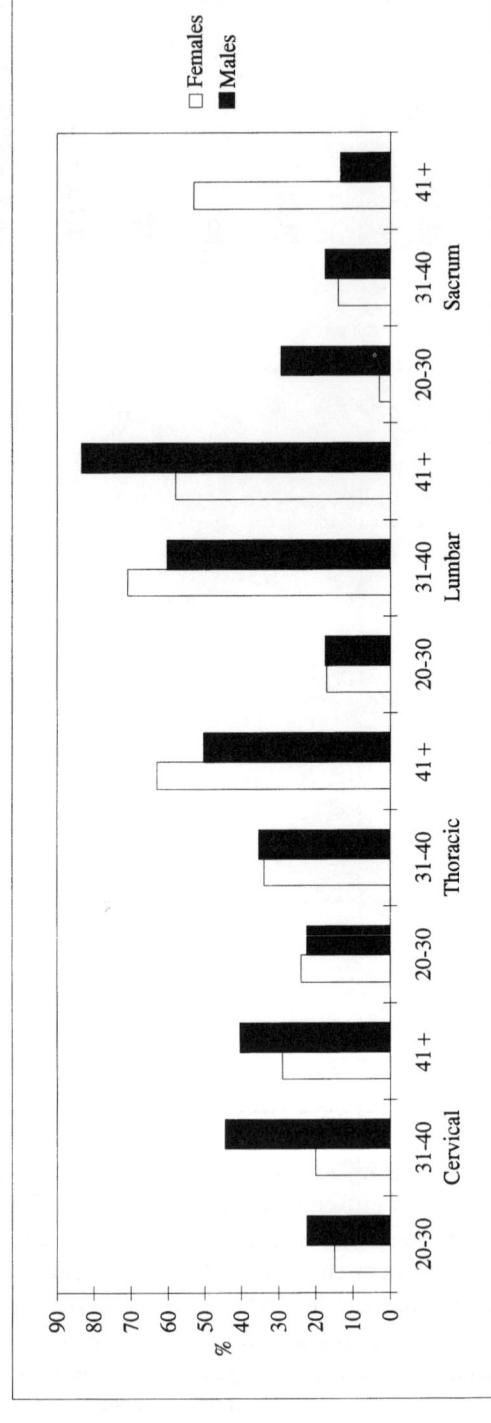

Figure 8-2. Frequency of Upland Female and Male Spinal Segments Affected by Degenerative Joint Disease.

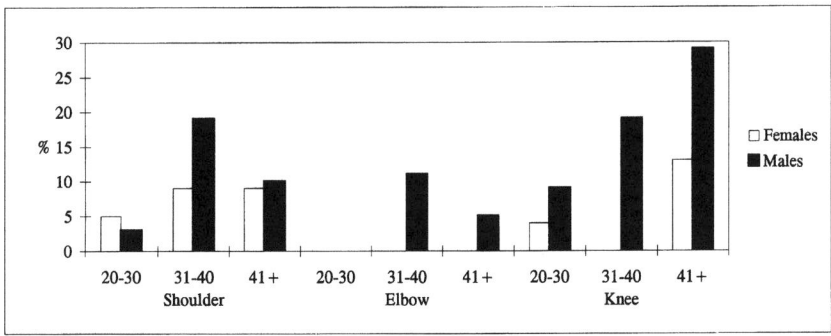

Figure 8-3. Frequency of Upland Female and Male Appendicular Joints Affected by Degenerative Joint Disease.

Table 8-4. Frequency of Upland and Coastal Male and Female Joints Affected by Degenerative Joint Disease

	Males				Females			
	Upland		Coastal		Upland		Coastal	
Joint	%	N	%	N	%	N	%	N
Cervical	24	41	11	53	10	49	1	73
Thoracic	31	48	12	51	37	60	1	72
Lumbar	46	37	28	47	34	59	13	64
Sacrum	19	43	0	33	22	58	6	47
Shoulder	11	81	2	120	7	75	1	144
Elbow	6	70	6	114	0	70	0	167
Knee	18	71	13	111	9	81	3	147

N = number of joints observed.
Coastal data from Larsen (1982).

Except for the elbow, upland males exhibit greater frequencies of osteoarthritis than coastal males for all joint complexes (Table 8-4, Figure 8-4). For example, upland males have greater frequencies of osteoarthritis than coastal males at the thoracic spinal segment (31 percent compared to 12 percent), sacrum (19 percent compared to 0 percent), and shoulder (11 percent compared to 2 percent). Upland females also exhibit greater frequencies of osteoarthritis than coastal females for all joint complexes, except the elbow (Table 8-4, Figure 8-5). Upland females exhibit greater frequencies than coastal females in the cervical (10 percent compared to 1 percent), thoracic (37 percent compared to 1 percent), and lumbar (34 percent compared to 13 percent) spinal segments, the sacrum (22 percent compared to 6 percent), and the shoulder (7 percent compared to 1 percent).

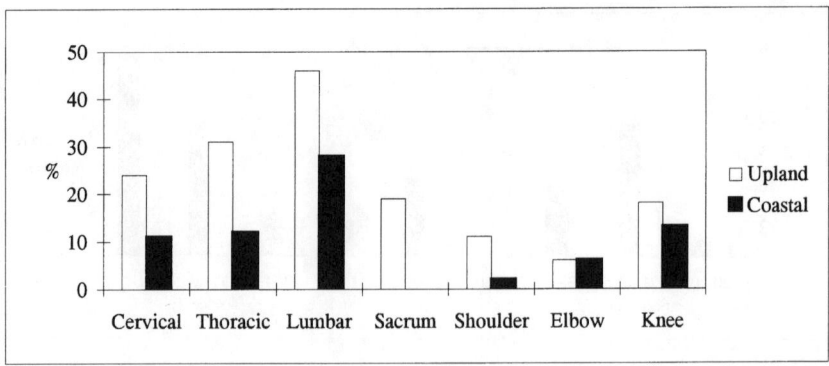

Figure 8-4. Frequency of Upland and Coastal Male Joints Affected by Degenerative Joint Disease.

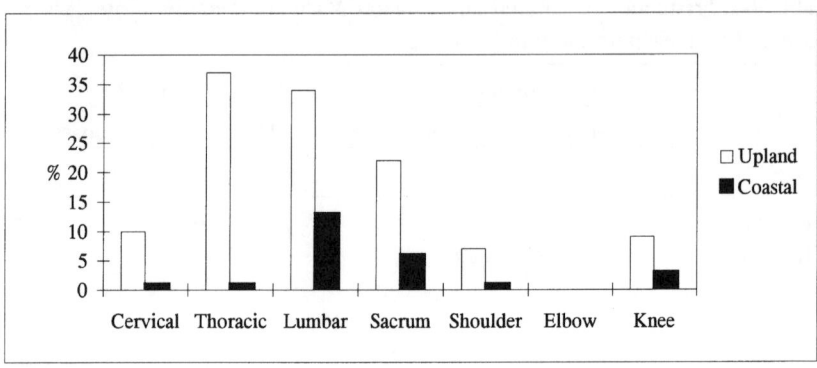

Figure 8-5. Frequency of Upland and Coastal Female Joints Affected by Degenerative Joint Disease.

DISCUSSION AND CONCLUSIONS

Upland Georgia males appear to have experienced greater mechanical stress, particularly in the appendicular skeleton, than females. This conclusion must be viewed as preliminary, however, because of the small sample sizes of many age groups and the fact that only the difference in sacral DJD among older individuals was statistically significant. Still, the results are consistent with the findings of Bridges (1992), who found greater frequencies of DJD among males than females in her review of a variety of prehistoric Southeastern agricultural populations, and with those of Larsen (1982), who observed greater frequencies of DJD for agricultural males than females from the Georgia coast.

Overall, upland males and females appear to have experienced greater mechanical stress than their coastal contemporaries. Although it is tempting to draw conclusions about the specific behaviors of upland Georgia agriculturalists, many researchers warn that doing so would go beyond the current understanding of the relationship between DJD and activity (Bridges 1992; Jurmain 1977, 1990; Larsen 1995; Lovell 1994). Some attempts at reconstructing specific behaviors have relied on studies carried out on living individuals, but these may be inappropriate for use by the paleopathologist. For example, the use of radiographs for the identification of DJD, while not a problem for the clinician, may underrepresent lesion frequency. Subtle osteophytes that might be observed on dry bone specimens typically do not create radiopaque features (Jurmain 1990). Other potential problems include the use of surveys for the collection of data because many cultural factors are not controlled, such as running shoes that absorb mechanical forces (Eichner 1989).

Fortunately, however, while keeping these caveats in mind, general conclusions drawn from population-based data can be illuminating and reliable (Jurmain 1990). The differences observed between upland and coastal individuals suggests that greater terrain relief may have contributed to differences in the frequency of DJD. Perhaps carrying heavy loads up and down hills produced enough stress to account for the relatively high frequency of OP in the upland sample. Similar results have been reported by Rathbun (1984) from studies of DJD in Iran and Iraq. Overall, he observed a higher frequency for the upland Iranian sample relative to the lowland Mesopotamian sample, and he suggests that there may be some correlation between location of residence and frequency of DJD. Larsen and coworkers (1995) compared data on DJD and cross-sectional geometric properties from a prehistoric Western Great Basin sample to other prehistoric North American samples from various topographic settings. Overall, they found that the Great Basin individuals exhibited elevated bone strength and greater frequencies of DJD, both indicating greater mechanical stress. They also interpret these differences as a reflection of the time and effort expended by Great Basin inhabitants on activities in upland zones.

It is probable that the terrain in the Piedmont and Valley and Ridge provinces of Georgia contributed in some way to the mechanical stress experienced by prehistoric agriculturalists. The answer may not be that simple, however. Perhaps coastal populations were less dependent on agricultural production than were upland farmers. Although there is no doubt that the coastal populations grew and consumed maize (see Larsen 1982), recent research suggests that it may not have been as important in the diet of late prehistoric populations as elsewhere in the Southeast. Using stable isotopic data, Larsen, Schoeninger, and coworkers (1992) found a decreased reliance on tropical grasses (e.g., maize) and their consumers and an increased reliance on more indigenous plants and their consumers at the Irene Mound site between A.D. 1150 and 1450. This factor is important because the majority of coastal individuals used in this study of upland and coastal DJD came from the Irene Mound site.

What could have caused the shift in subsistence at the Irene Mound site? Anderson (1994, 1996) has concluded that chiefdoms along the Savannah River experienced widespread collapse by A.D. 1450. In contrast, chiefdoms in upland Georgia were well established during this time (see Hally and Langford 1988; Hally et al. 1990). Although the cause of the collapse is not clear, Anderson argues that the rise of chiefdoms in the Oconee River drainage to the west and the Santee-Wateree drainages to the east in South Carolina was the most important factor. Nevertheless, he adds that decreased rainfall along with diminishing food reserves would have placed significant pressure on the agriculturally based chiefdoms along the Savannah River.

Perhaps the elite from either or both of these competitive polities gained greater control of prestige goods. According to Peregrine (1992), access to prestige goods by members of a Mississippian chiefdom was necessary in order to participate in important social events (e.g., marriage, initiation). To increase their access to such goods, commoners intensified subsistence production so that the elites could participate in competitive exchange. Considering this view, the power of the elite in the Lower Savannah River chiefdom (i.e., Irene Mound) may have declined, and along with it the social pressure to produce significant maize surpluses to support this social class may have declined. Coastal individuals may have then emigrated to the Oconee or Santee-Wateree chiefdoms, where prestige goods were more easily acquired (although there may have been other ways to access such goods—see Muller (1997) for a contrasting view). The departure of this labor force would have resulted in a decrease in agricultural production that could account for their comparatively lower frequencies of degenerative joint disease relative to upland dwellers.

In general, the results of this study are in line with previously expressed views that note an absence of a consistent relationship between patterns of DJD and subsistence, except when specific geographic settings are considered (Bridges 1989, 1991, 1992, 1994; Larsen 1995). Whether related to physiographic differences, political complexity, or both, the levels of physical activity of upland and coastal late prehistoric agriculturalists in Georgia do not appear to have been the same. Life appears to have been more demanding for upland inhabitants.

ACKNOWLEDGMENTS

I would like to thank Clark S. Larsen and David J. Hally for their guidance and for graciously including me in the examination of the human remains collection from the University of Georgia. Leslie E. Sering provided invaluable assistance with the data collection. Stephen P. Nawrocki, Ted A. Rathbun, and Christopher W. Schmidt offered many useful suggestions on earlier drafts of this chapter, and our discussions regarding pathological lesions were particularly helpful. Patricia Lambert and two anonymous reviewers also provided many useful suggestions. Funding for this project was provided by the University of Georgia to Clark S. Larsen.

9 Dental Health and Late Woodland Subsistence in Coastal North Carolina

Elizabeth Monahan Driscoll
David S. Weaver

The North Carolina coastal plain is a region that has not yet been researched extensively by bioarchaeologists. Although many of the human burials have been analyzed by physical anthropologists, primarily from Wake Forest University, University of North Carolina at Chapel Hill, and East Carolina University, little synthesis of the results has been completed. This study addresses the question of Late Woodland subsistence on the North Carolina coast. Specifically, we examine the extent to which maize agriculture was a component of the diet of Late Woodland coastal North Carolina people and the impact of maize agriculture on human health in the region. We then suggest how health differences may be useful for reconstructing cultural differences in the region. Multiple lines of evidence are explored, including dental caries rates, linear enamel hypoplasia, stable carbon and nitrogen isotope ratios, and archaeological evidence of subsistence. We include a preliminary report on six coastal ossuaries and provide a model of dental health in the Late Woodland period. Dental data from six North Carolina sites are compared with data collected by Larsen and coworkers on Georgia coast agricultural and preagricultural populations (Hutchinson and Larsen 1990; Larsen et al. 1991), and previously published data on stable carbon and nitrogen isotopes from Georgia coastal sites (Larsen, Schoeninger, van der Merwe, et al. 1992) are compared with data from one site in North Carolina (Trimble 1996).

The estuarine resource base of the Southeastern coastal plain is particularly rich and diverse, capable of supporting populations of large, sedentary, politically complex hunter-gatherers in some areas (Reitz 1988). Given the richness of estuaries, the question of when, why, and how much use was made of maize horticulture in these regions is intriguing. Here we seek to integrate current information, filling in the gap in the bioarchaeological record between Virginia and South Carolina. An overview of archaeological research on the North Carolina coast is presented to familiarize the reader with the area.

COASTAL NORTH CAROLINA
GEOGRAPHY AND PREHISTORY

The North Carolina coast is part of the Atlantic Coastal Plain, which stretches south and east from the Fall Line from southeastern Virginia to Texas, excluding the southern tip of Florida (Briggs 1974; Reitz 1988). This region also roughly corresponds with the large embayment of the Georgia Bight, which includes the physiographic region from Cape Hatteras, North Carolina, to Cape Canaveral, Florida, and is characterized by rich estuaries and barrier islands for most of its length (Larsen 1982; Reitz 1988). All six of the North Carolina ossuary sites examined for this analysis fall south of Cape Hatteras, North Carolina, and are therefore part of the Georgia Bight and the Atlantic Coastal Plain.

The coastal plain of North Carolina can be divided further into two physiographic regions: the Tidewater and the Inner Coastal Plain. The boundary between the Tidewater and Inner Coastal Plain is the Suffold Scarp, a remnant beach line from the Sangamon Interglacial sea (Bellis et al. 1975). The Tidewater is formed of marine sediments from the Pamlico Terrace. This region includes the Outer Banks, a chain of barrier islands that protects the shallow Albemarle and Pamlico Sounds. These barrier islands are constantly changing location and topology because of wind and wave erosion (Riggs and O'Connor 1975). The northern section of the region is cut by several major rivers with extensive estuaries. Except for the Cape Fear River, the southern section has no large rivers. Consequently, the section has no major estuaries that extend as far inland as in the northern section. There are still significant estuaries lining the coast and barrier islands, however, and many of the food resources Native Americans used (as seen in the archaeological record) came from the estuaries. The six coastal ossuary sites described here are from both the Tidewater and Inner Coastal Plain, and all are located less than a mile from the shore, many on the banks of the rivers flowing into the ocean.

The Inner Coastal Plain consists of the sandy and loamy uplands

with many major rivers, associated floodplains, and swamps. About
10–12,000 years ago the dominant forest was pine (Green 1980). Pine
forest was gradually replaced beginning 6,000 years ago by an oak-
hickory climax forest with abundant resources, including nuts, wood,
mammals, reptiles, fish, shellfish, and birds (Phelps 1983).

Culture History

Early discussions of coastal North Carolina prehistory focus largely on
ceramic taxonomy, reflecting the interests of the time (Haag 1958;
South 1976). Later work explores the reconstruction of behavior, population movement, and diachronic change (Trigger 1989). In more recent
studies, there has been an effort to place the coast in a wider context.
Several authors have divided North Carolina into areas, often based on
cultural assemblages. The most comprehensive work on the region to
date is Phelps's (1983) culture history. He includes the entire North
Carolina coast in a Middle Atlantic region, stretching north from the
Pee Dee River and including the northern part of the South Carolina
coastal plain (Phelps 1983:16). He further divides the Middle Atlantic
into the Northern and Southern Coastal Plains. Temporally, Phelps divides the human occupation of this region into four periods: the Paleo-
Indian, Archaic, Woodland, and Historic. These are the time periods
used by most archaeologists, and the discussion below is based on this
temporal framework.

There have been people living on the Coastal Plain since the Paleo-
Indian period (12,000 B.C.), but it was not until around 2000 B.C., during the Late Archaic period, that the south and north coastal regions
began to emerge as separate areas. The Woodland period followed, ter-
minating in this region only at historic contact. Because the sites analyzed in this study all come from the Late Woodland, we focus on this
period.

The Late Woodland period dates to A.D. 800–1615 in the North
Coastal region and to A.D. 800–1715 in the South Coastal region. After A.D. 800, Phelps relies on protohistoric distributions of linguistic
groups as a model for the regions. The North Coastal region was the
home of Algonkian and Iroquoian language speakers at the time of contact. The Algonkians probably originated in the Great Lakes region
during the Archaic period (Feest 1978) and were exclusively estuarine-
adapted (Phelps 1983). The Iroquoian groups, including the Tuscarora,
Meherrin, and Nottoway, inhabited the Inner Coastal Plain. The South
Coastal region was inhabited by the Siouan Waccamaw at contact.

Phelps (1983) proposes three archaeological phases connected with
these ethnolinguistic groups in the Late Woodland. Colington phase is
associated with the Algonkian-speakers and is characterized by shell-

tempered ware with decorated rims. Large ossuaries containing many robust individuals and few burial goods are characteristic of Algonkian burials. Cashie phase, linked with Iroquoian speakers, is identified by pebble- and sand-tempered ceramics with some rim designs. Ossuaries are also thought to be typical interments. White Oak/Oak Island (Loftfield 1975; Phelps 1983) is connected with the Siouan groups and typified by shell-tempered ceramics, with cord-marked and simple stamped varieties. Multiple burials were often placed in low sand mounds; in some, several individuals were buried in a single depositional event.

ARCHAEOLOGICAL EVIDENCE OF SUBSISTENCE

It is difficult to characterize the subsistence patterns on the coast of North Carolina during the Late Woodland for several reasons. First, the length of the phases is an obstacle. Maize was adopted as a cultigen at some point during the Late Woodland period, but the archaeological phases do not change throughout the period. Therefore, information that classifies a site according to the phase or period does not yield information about subsistence, as it does in some other parts of the coast. For example, on the Georgia coast, the last phases prior to contact are Mississippian, and archaeological manifestations of this period include the use of maize as a cultigen, primarily based on information gathered from human skeletal material (Larsen, Schoeninger, van der Merwe et al. 1992; Reitz 1988). Maize is considered to have been a part of the diet (although not a major contributor) after A.D. 1150 in Georgia and South Carolina (Larsen et al. 1991; Reitz 1988). There is no comparable information available for the North Carolina coast.

Maize is documented on the coast historically through early European explorer accounts and drawings (Hariot 1955; Lawson 1960). Archaeologically, however, there is little direct evidence of maize at any coastal North Carolina Late Woodland ossuary site. The earliest evidence of maize on the coastal plain is from the Late Woodland period. Maize remains have been found at the Flynt site (31On305), Uniflite (31On33) (Glazier 1986, Loftfield 1987), Permuda Island (Loftfield 1985), and Broad Reach (31Cr218) (Mathis 1991, 1993). These sites all date to the latter part of the Late Woodland, however. The largest amount of maize was recovered from a "smudge pit" at Broad Reach. Charcoal from the pit containing charred corncobs has been radiocarbon dated to A.D. intercept 1444 (corrected, see Eastman 1994; Mathis 1991). It is probable that maize was not cultivated on the coast of North Carolina until the middle to latter part of the Late Woodland. Indeed, several of the sites used in this study may actually be preagricultural. Maize was part of the diet of North Carolina coastal people during the Late Woodland, but little is known about the timing and importance of the incorporation of maize agriculture in this region.

Subsistence information available from archaeological sites reveals that the people living along the coast in the Late Woodland relied heavily on resources available from the rich, diverse estuaries nearby. Estuarine adaptation is well documented for the South Carolina and Georgia coast (Reitz 1988), and a similar pattern is evident along the North Carolina coast as well. Faunal analysis at Permuda Island indicates use of estuarine and marine fishes (sea catfish, sheepshead, white basses, and porgies), birds, turtles (land and sea), opossums, rabbits, and white-tailed deer (Loftfield 1985). Studies of middens at Flynt and Uniflite demonstrate the use of similar resources (Glazier 1986). Paleobotanical analyses show that wild plant foods were also important in the diet, including hickory nuts and acorns, as well as cultigens such as sunflower and squash (Loftfield 1987). There is widespread evidence of extensive shell middens all along the North Carolina coast as well, amply demonstrating the use of oysters, clams, and whelks. Other marine invertebrates such as crabs are also present (Loftfield 1985). The wild resources available are rich, and it seems unlikely from archaeological and bioarchaeological evidence that Late Woodland people were ever intensive maize agriculturalists along the North Carolina coast. Nevertheless, the adoption of maize cultivation may have significantly altered seasonal resource scheduling and other aspects of subsistence behavior (Waselkov 1987).

On initial examination, there seems to be little difference between Late Woodland sites in resources used for food on the North Carolina coast, other than the presence/absence of maize and other cultigens such as squash and sunflower. If the resources are similar, then it is plausible to consolidate the information from the North Carolina sites for comparative purposes. The only obstacle to this lumping is the question of the contemporeneity of the sites. A method for dividing the sites into agricultural and preagricultural will allow rough temporal control within the Late Woodland period. One possible method is suggested below.

APPROACH AND RATIONALE

The approach we have chosen to address the question of subsistence and maize use is to collect dental caries and linear enamel hypoplasia (LEH) data from all individuals interred in ossuaries at the six sites and to compare the data to Georgia coast agricultural and preagricultural populations. The Georgia coast has been extensively studied and has a similar resource base, making it a logical case for comparison to the North Carolina coast.

Prior to the adoption of maize, people living along the Georgia coast in the Late Woodland were foragers of wild foods both terrestrial and marine (Larsen 1982; Reitz 1988). Similar resources were used from earlier periods through the Late Woodland. During the Refuge period (1100–400 B.C.), shellfish were not used as heavily as in later periods. Marine and estuarine fish as well as deer, raccoon, rabbit, squirrel, hickory nuts, and acorns constituted the bulk of the diet in the Early Late Woodland (Schoeninger et al. 1990). In the Deptford phase (400 B.C.–A.D. 500), the diet was similar with a heavier use of shellfish and the addition of sea mammals (Thomas and Larsen 1979b). In the Wilmington (A.D. 500–1010) and subsequent St. Catherines (A.D. 1000–1150) phases, even more mollusks were used as a protein source (Larsen 1982). A seasonality study of the shell from middens suggests that populations were mobile (Claassen 1986). Agricultural foods first appear in the diet at the beginning of the Savannah Phase (A.D. 1150–1300) and continue in the Irene Phase (A.D. 1300–1550). Larger, sedentary settlements are seen in the Mississippian times, along with the increasingly heavy use of maize (Caldwell and McCann 1941). In the beginning of the Mississippian, there was actually a rise in shellfish use and a continuation of use of the other marine and terrestrial resources (Larsen 1990). There is no Mississippian phase on the coast of North Carolina, and the data from the Georgia agricultural sample from Irene Mound are included for comparative purposes only.

MATERIALS AND METHODS

Woodland period burials on the North Carolina coastal plain are remarkable in that all three of the ethnolinguistic groups proposed to be present commonly used ossuary interment. Slight differences in mortuary practices are thought to be indicative of cultural differences, but recent study has shown considerable overlap in mortuary practices within and between the proposed ranges for each group (Kakaliouras 1997; Monahan 1994, 1995). Table 9-1 presents the sites used in this study, the minimum number of individuals at each site, and radiocarbon dates, where available.

The minimum number of individuals (MNI) for the individual ossuaries analyzed here ranges from 10 to over 150. The burial sites are all located on the coast or rivers adjacent to estuaries. The populations that contributed to the ossuaries may have been sedentary, but information on settlement patterns is lacking for most of the sites. The sites also lack secure cultural affiliation, due to the lack of firm connec-

Table 9–1. Selected North Carolina Coastal Ossuary Sites

Site	Archaeological Phase	MNI	Radiocarbon Assay	Calibrated intercept	References
McFayden Mound (Bw67)	White Oak/ Oak Island	10	none		South 1962
Cold Morning (Nh 28)	White Oak/ Oak Island	16	1000±80 B.P.	A.D. 984	Coe et al. 1982; Eastman 1994; Ward and Wilson 1980
Garbacon Creek (Cr86)	Colington	31	none		Egloff 1971; Kakaliouras 1997
Broad Reach (Cr218)	Colington	36	670±60 B.P.	A.D. 1168	Eastman 1994; Mathis 1986, 1993; Monahan 1994, 1995
Flynt (On305)	Colington	158	560±60 B.P.	A.D. 1307, 1361, 1379	Bogdan and Weaver 1989; Eastman 1994; Loftfield 1987; Mathis 1986
Piggot (Cr14)	Colington	84	410±50 B.P.	A.D. 1540 (uncorrected)	Truesdell 1995

tions with extant Native American groups and the difficulty of assigning these ossuaries to specific ethnolinguistic groups.

The sites are all dated to the Late Woodland period, either through radiocarbon dates or ceramic types, but the archaeological phases on the coast are quite long, making further statement about them problematic. The current pottery taxonomy does not discriminate variation that would allow finer temporal associations. The series definitions remain the same from A.D. 800 until European contact. The absolute dates for the ossuaries range from early in the Late Woodland to close to European contact. The two undated sites probably fall earlier in the range, and a tentative chronological order (from earliest to latest) of sites is: McFayden Mound (31Bw67), Cold Morning (31Nh28), Garbacon Creek (31Cr86), Broad Reach (31Cr218), Flynt (31On305), and Piggot (31Cr14) (see Table 9-1).

The suggested boundaries of the three ethnolinguistic groups present at contact do not correspond well with archaeological differences in mortuary practices (Kakalioras 1997; Monahan 1994), although pottery types fit the model somewhat better (Phelps 1983). Ossuary interment of the dead is common throughout the North Carolina coastal plain, but there are some broad differences in the numbers buried and possibly the criteria for inclusion in the ossuary. Other differences exist in settlement types and pottery between regions, but several of the ossuaries were excavated as a result of salvage archaeological excavations, and the habitation sites presumably connected with these ossuaries were not excavated. Phelps's reconstruction is widely used at present, however, and is used here to provide an initial framework. Alternative models for assessing these groups have not yet been developed and are beyond the scope of this chapter.

The North Carolina coastal sample has several problems that limit interpretation and consolidation of the sites into a single sample. Two of the sites, McFayden Mound and Garbacon Creek, have not been absolutely dated but are presumed to fall in the early Late Woodland period. There is no universally accepted date for the introduction of maize to the coastal region, so it is unknown which if any of the sites may be preagricultural. At this time it is difficult to determine which sites may be preagricultural for two reasons: (1) little maize has been found archaeologically, but the absence of maize remains at a site is not evidence of the absence of maize in the diet, and (2) the habitation sites related to specific ossuaries have not been excavated for the Piggot, Garbacon Creek, or McFayden Mound sites. Intersite comparisons of dental health reveal an interesting temporal trend in caries rate, providing supporting evidence that the proposed earliest two sites may be preagricultural. Alternately, the results may be due to differences in diet between the northern and southern coastal groups.

Table 9–2. Dental Caries Data for Selected North Carolina Coastal Ossuary Sites

Site	N	Number of Carious Teeth	% Carious teeth
Bw67	216	6	2.8
Nh28	119	6	5.0
Cr86	221	17	7.7
Cr218	224	18	8.0
On305	163	15	9.2
Cr14	629	30	4.7

Table 9–3. Linear Enamel Hypoplasia Data for Selected North Carolina Coastal Ossuary Sites

Site	N	Number of Teeth with LEH	% Teeth with LEH
Bw67	29	12	41.4
Nh28	33	3	9.1
Cr86	56	7	12.5
Cr218	77	37	48.1
On305	60	28	46.7
Cr14	210	23	11.0

Some of the dental samples for the sites are quite small. The total number of teeth is less than 150 each for the McFayden Mound, Garbacon Creek, Broad Reach, and Cold Morning sites. The largest sample comes from the Piggot site, with 629 teeth (see Tables 9-2 and 9-3). Some of the variation between the North Carolina samples is likely caused by the small sample sizes. The ossuary context does not allow comparisons by individuals, only by tooth or tooth type. This means that the dental caries rate may be underestimated because there was a fair amount of antemortem tooth loss in the Garbacon Creek and Flynt site samples, but the rate could not be quantified in a meaningful way due to the presence of loose teeth and the absence of securely identified individuals. The occurrence of dental caries may be higher but masked by this antemortem tooth loss, which often results from this disease process.

There are positive aspects to using ossuary samples in studies that address the diet of a specific population at a certain time. All the ossuaries, with the probable exception of McFayden Mound and possibly Cold Morning, represent a single temporal event. The skeletal remains were disarticulated for the most part, indicating that individuals were processed prior to final deposition in the ossuary, but the time between death and final interment was likely to have been fairly short. The

Huron are known to have performed ossuary burials around every 10 to 15 years (Ubelaker 1974). All the individuals interred in the ossuary died within a relatively short time. Other forms of burial make it more difficult to establish contemporaneity of the individuals, thus leaving open the possibility that temporal differences skew averages.

Dental caries data can be particularly useful in assessing the presence and importance of agricultural foods in the diet (Larsen 1987, 1995; Turner 1979). Dental caries is a disease process that results in demineralization of dental enamel by acids produced by bacterial fermentation of dietary carbohydrates (see review in Hillson 1996; Larsen 1997). Other factors that contribute to dental caries include exposure of tooth surfaces in the mouth and food texture. The less wear a tooth has, the more likely it is that bacteria will aggregate in caries-prone occlusal areas, especially in the deeper grooves between cusps of molar teeth. Agricultural diets tend to be higher in carbohydrates than nonagricultural diets. Agricultural foods are often processed, resulting in less occlusal wear and "sticky" food textures that are more easily caught in occlusal grooves and interproximal surfaces. Maize in particular is a highly cariogenic food (Larsen 1995, 1997), making the presence of maize in the diet readily apparent through studies of dental caries prevalence. In a worldwide survey, nearly all agricultural populations have greater prevalence of dental caries than nonagricultural groups (Turner 1979). The average frequency of teeth affected by carious lesions increases from very low percentages in foragers to 7 percent and higher in agriculturalists (Turner 1979; Larsen 1997). In eastern North America, there is a large increase in dental caries prevalence from the Middle Woodland to the Late Woodland (Larsen et al. 1991). These values can be used as a benchmark of sorts for evaluating the contribution of maize to the diet. We consider the samples with high dental caries frequencies as possible maize agriculturalists, and those with very low frequencies as populations that were not using maize as a part of the diet. We evaluate these possibilities with the available archaeological data. Because the Late Woodland is such a long period in North Carolina, this type of dental health study may help temporally place a site in the chronology. This model must be used with caution, however, as will be discussed below.

All erupted teeth from the ossuaries were examined for dental caries. Unerupted teeth will not have carious lesions, and so were not included in the sample of teeth examined. Pinpoint lesions were included. A percentage of teeth affected by dental caries was determined for each site. It is likely that the dental caries rate was actually underestimated because individual antemortem tooth loss could not be determined due to the nature of the samples of disarticulated, commingled remains. For the same reason, the dental caries rate per individual could not be calculated. On the positive side, ossuary samples are composed of contemporaneous individuals, whose diets were probably similar.

Linear enamel hypoplasia data, or LEH, can be useful in reconstructing nutritional adequacy and health during development (Goodman et al. 1988; Larsen 1995, 1997). Linear enamel hypoplasia is a "deficiency in enamel thickness due to a disruption of ameloblast activity" (Goodman et al. 1980:516). It appears as a visible line or pit in the enamel of a tooth formed during a slowing or cessation of normal enamel deposition during tooth formation. The slowing or cessation is due to a severe episode of stress caused by illness or lack of proper nutrition. The enamel malformation lasts for the duration of the stress and then normal enamel deposition resumes. The result is a defect in the surface of the tooth crown that marks the stage of formation of the tooth crown at the time of the stress. It is therefore possible to determine the age of the individual at the time of the stress (Larsen 1997).

Only canines and incisors were evaluated for LEH. These teeth are more likely to display enamel defects due to the crown morphology and susceptibility to growth disruption (Goodman and Armelagos 1985). A defect was counted as present when it was visible with a 10× hand lens. The distance from the center of the enamel defect to the center of the cemento-enamel junction (CEJ) was measured. Rates of teeth affected by one or more episode of LEH were calculated for all teeth in the sample with fully formed crowns.

Perhaps the best method for determining diet from prehistoric skeletal samples comes from the analysis of stable isotopic signatures of diet. Stable carbon and nitrogen isotope ratios are a direct measure of diet from bone. Stable carbon isotopes ($^{13}C/^{12}C$) reflect consumption of marine and C_3 versus C_4 terrestrial foods in the diet (based on photosynthetic pathways) (Bender et al. 1981; Tieszen et al. 1983). Maize is the only economically important C_4 plant in prehistoric North Carolina. Most other plants eaten were C_3 plants. Carbon isotope ratios are relatively less negative when diets include C_4 plants such as maize ($\delta^{13}C = -15‰$ to $-12‰$) (Schoeninger and Moore 1992). Dietary evidence is not available from all the North Carolina sites, but the range of estuarine resources that have been found at three North Carolina coastal sites from Onslow County (including Flynt) is presented here. The only C_4 plant found thus far at coastal sites is maize. Although some seagrasses have C_4 photosynthetic pathways, no arguments for the dietary use of seagrasses on the coast have been proposed.

Stable nitrogen isotopes ($^{15}N/^{14}N$) are particularly useful for distinguishing the relative contribution of marine and terrestrial components in the diet (Schoeninger and Moore 1992). The $\delta^{15}N$ values in marine plants and animals are more positive than in terrestrial plants and animals (Schwarcz and Schoeninger 1991). Stable nitrogen and carbon isotopes delta values are plotted against each other to clarify the influence of marine foods in the diet, because carbon isotopes are affected by marine components of the diet.

Stable isotope analysis has only been carried out on one of the North Carolina coastal samples, Flynt (Trimble 1996). A problem in comparing the stable isotope data between the North Carolina and Georgia coastal populations is that the isotope values for North Carolina are derived from a single site, and it is unknown whether this site is a representative sample of North Carolina populations. Maize remains were found at the Flynt site.

RESULTS AND INTERPRETATION

Dental Caries

Dental caries data were collected from all deciduous and permanent teeth in the North Carolina samples. An overall percentage was calculated for each site. Only three groups have dental caries rates above the 7 percent mark, which is the critical limit discussed above (see Table 9-3, Figure 9-1). The sites are presented in presumed chronological order. The most recent site, Piggot, shows few carious teeth. This may be because 58 percent of the individuals in the ossuary are subadults (Truesdell 1995). Because dental caries is a progressive degenerative disease, caries rates are often lower in the teeth of younger individuals. The presumed earliest sites show low caries rates. This may indicate that the sites were occupied prior to incorporation of maize in the diet on the North Carolina coast or that they had a different diet. Figure 9-1 demonstrates the clear temporal trend of dental caries prevalence in the ossuaries examined. The presumed temporal trend is not quite as clear when we evaluate dental caries rate for just the molar teeth (Table 9-2). However, the earliest site again shows the fewest carious teeth and the latest site, Flynt, shows the most.

The North Carolina ossuary dental caries rates per tooth type fall consistently between the Georgia preagricultural and agricultural populations (Figure 9-2). The caries rates suggest that the diet of the North Carolina coastal people contained something cariogenic that was not present in the Georgia coast preagricultural population. Maize is likely to have been the source of the higher rates. The dental caries rate is not as high as that for Georgia agriculturalists at Irene Mound, suggesting that maize may not have been as important a dietary component on the North Carolina coast as in Georgia agriculturalists. Alternatively, it could be that the rates for the North Carolina popula-

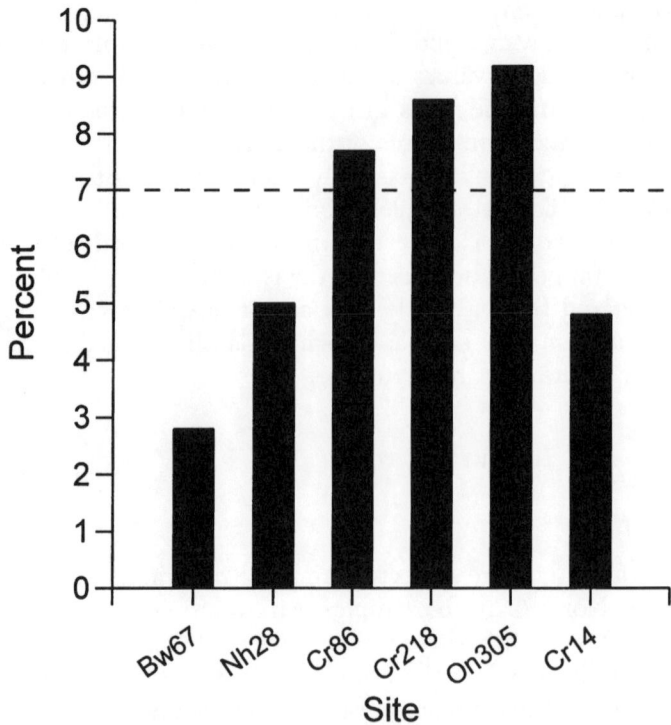

Figure 9-1. Percent of Carious Teeth by Site, Selected North Carolina Coastal Ossuary Sites in Chronological Order. Sites with higher values are likely to have had an agricultural component to the diet.

tion are higher than this chart indicates, if one or more preagricultural North Carolina groups are included, as they probably are. The inclusion of preagricultural samples with the agricultural groups would tend to lower the cumulative dental caries rate because preagricultural groups have fewer carious lesions than agriculturalists. Analysis of the percentage of carious teeth by site supports this hypothesis. When the two earliest sites are removed from the sample, the average dental caries rate for the four later sites is 6.5 percent. Without the Piggot site, the average is 8.2 percent, indicating an agricultural component to the diet for these sites.

Linear Enamel Hypoplasia

There is a great deal of variation in the frequency of deciduous and permanent incisors and canines with at least one episode of LEH in the North Carolina sites. Again, the sites are shown in approximate chronological order (Figure 9-3). The graph is difficult to interpret be-

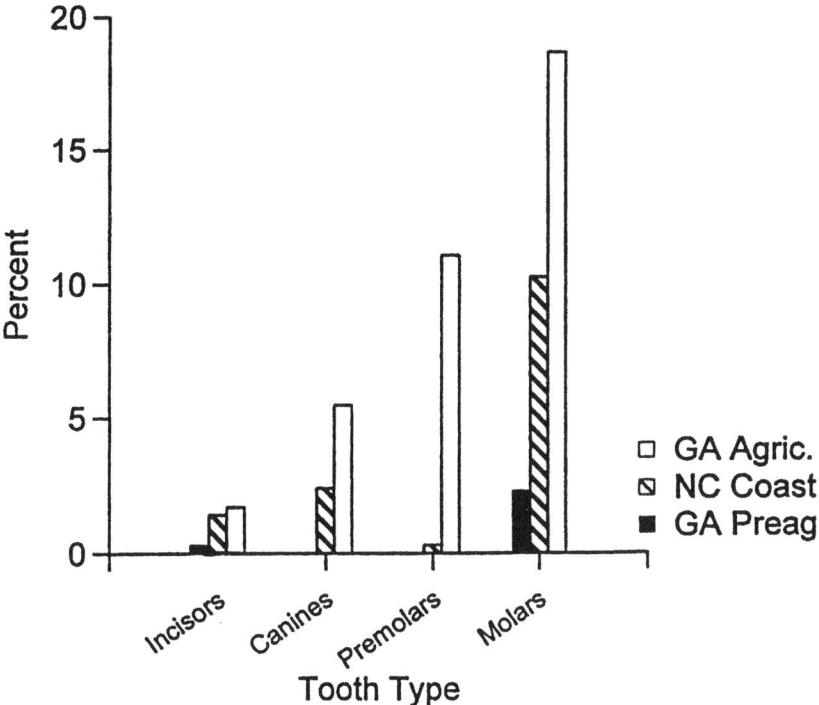

Figure 9-2. Percent of Carious Teeth by Tooth Type, Comparison of Georgia Agriculturalists and Preagriculturalists (Larsen et al. 1991), and Selected North Carolina Coastal Ossuary Sites.

cause the earliest site has a large number of LEH, middle sites have low rates, and the later sites again have higher rates. The exception is the most recent site, Piggot, which has a very low LEH rate. Piggot site data are the most confusing because, although dental caries rates can be influenced by the age distribution of a group, LEH is not affected unless the group contains a large number of edentulous individuals, or individuals with extremely worn teeth. Neither case describes the Piggot site, which is predominantly subadult. It is more likely that the Piggot ossuary contains a larger percentage of children who died before ex-hibiting LEH. Wood and coworkers (1992) caution that LEH and other markers of stress have to be interpreted with care, keeping in mind that only individuals who survive a stress episode will exhibit such markers. Therefore, it seems reasonable to assume that this is the case for Piggot (Truesdell 1995). An alternative explanation to be explored is that the diet of individuals in the Piggot ossuary was different from the diet at the other sites examined. No habitation site associated with

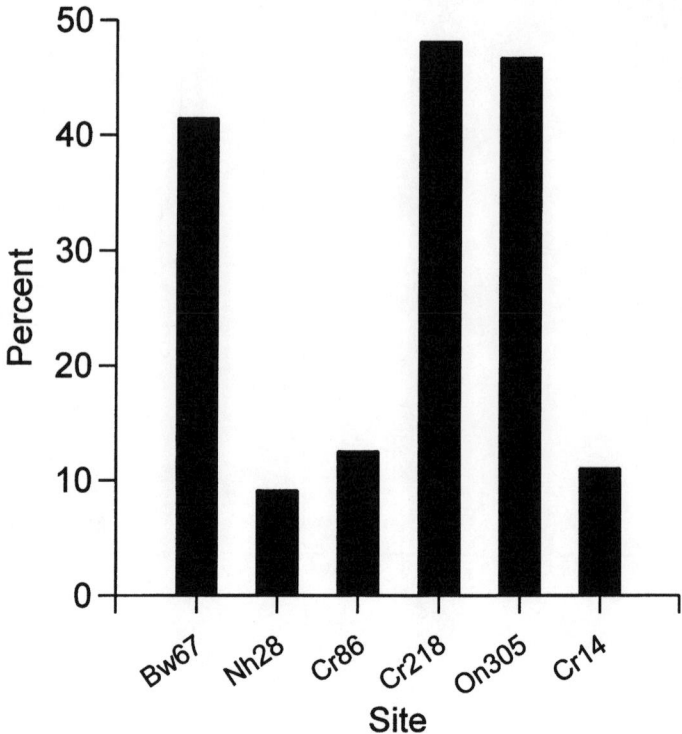

Figure 9-3. Percent of Teeth with at Least One Linear Enamel Defect, Selected North Carolina Ossuary Sites.

Piggot has been excavated, so this possibility cannot be evaluated at present.

Comparison of LEH rates with coastal Georgia samples shows that the North Carolina rates per tooth consistently are lower than those for both agricultural and preagricultural Georgia sites (Figure 9-4). We used a different method for collecting these data, however, which may have introduced interobserver error. How much error might be present is unknown because we did not reevaluate any of the Georgia samples. We scored enamel defects that could be seen with a hand lens, whereas Hutchinson and Larsen (1990) used a microscope (10×). Thus it is possible that the consistent differences could be due to sampling error or differing methodology. At present, however, we will proceed as though the differences we observe are real. The dental caries rates overall suggest that maize was a part of the diet, but LEH indicates that the Cold Morning, Garbacon Creek, and Piggot populations experienced low metabolic stress during dental development. The rates for the rest of the sites were higher but still generally lower than the average for the Georgia samples (Monahan and Weaver 1996).

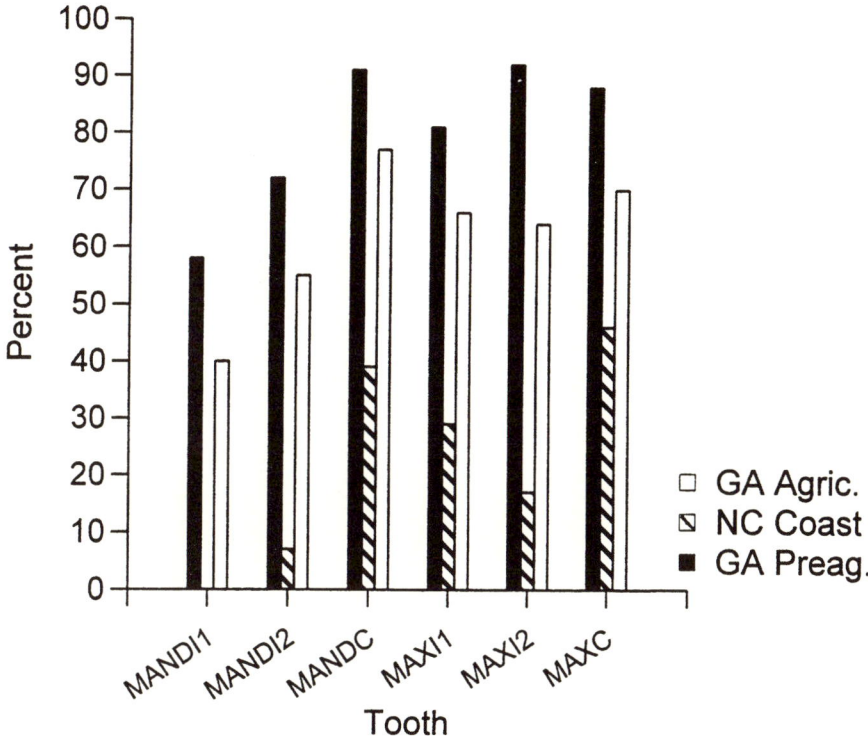

Figure 9-4. Percent of Teeth with at Least One Linear Enamel Defect, Comparison of Georgia Agriculturalists and Preagriculturalists (Larsen et al. 1991), and Selected North Carolina Coastal Ossuary Sites.

Stable Carbon and Nitrogen Isotopes

Stable carbon and nitrogen isotopes were collected from the largest North Carolina coastal sample (Flynt) and analyzed by Trimble (1996). We compared the isotope values to those collected for the Georgia coast material (Figure 9-5) (Schoeninger et al. 1990). The mean isotopic ratios for Flynt are intermediate between the Georgia agricultural and preagricultural samples, but the range is wide enough to encompass the mean values for the Georgia samples (Table 9-4).

The $\delta^{15}N$ values indicate that marine resources were utilized in all three populations, with the heaviest reliance in the Georgia preagricultural sample and the lightest in the Georgia agricultural sample. The North Carolina coastal populations, as represented by the Flynt site, fall between the two Georgia samples in implied reliance on marine resources. The mean $\delta^{13}C$ values for Flynt are virtually identical to the Georgia agricultural sample and only slightly overlap with the preagricultural sample mean, indicating that C_4 plants were more prevalent

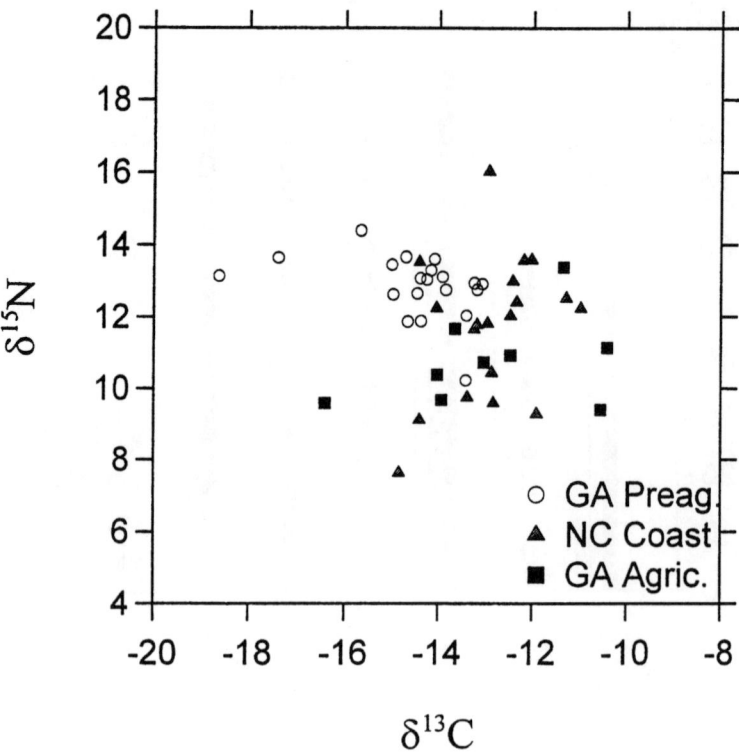

Figure 9-5. Scatterplot Comparison of ^{13}C and ^{15}N Ratios from Georgia
Agriculturalists and Preagriculturalists (Schoeninger et al. 1992) and the
Flynt Site, a Late Woodland North Carolina Coastal Ossuary (Trimble 1996).

Table 9–4. Mean Carbon and Nitrogen Stable Isotope Values

		Mean		± SD	
Context	N	$\delta^{15}N$	$\delta^{13}C$	$\delta^{15}N$	$\delta^{13}C$
GA Preagricultural:[a]					
Refuge-Deptford	8	12.7	−15.1	1.0	1.6
St. Catherines	12	12.8	−14.2	0.6	0.4
NC Coastal:[b]					
Flynt Site (On305)	20	11.7	−12.9	1.9	1.0
GA Agricultural:					
Savannah	9	10.7	−13.0	1.1	2.0

[a]Schoeninger et al. 1990
[b]Trimble 1996

in the diet of North Carolina coastal people than in the Georgia preagricultural sample. A scatterplot of carbon and nitrogen values for each individual sampled supports what the dental caries and LEH data suggest (see Figure 9-5): $\delta^{13}C$ values provide evidence for an agricultural component to the diet of the North Carolina coastal population, but $\delta^{15}N$ values (and archaeological evidence) also indicate that estuarine or marine resources continued to be a significant component of the diet.

CONCLUSIONS

We suggest that the people on the North Carolina coast had incorporated a C_4 plant, probably maize, into their already rich and diverse diet in the Late Woodland but had not sacrificed dietary quality or variety by decreasing emphasis on estuarine resources. This conclusion is supported by the isotope values showing a diet rich in both terrestrial and marine resources, as well as by the low LEH rates indicating less metabolic stress and by a dental caries rate that is consistent with a population utilizing agricultural foods. This hypothesis could be further tested through analysis of other excavated North Carolina coastal ossuaries, including further isotope analysis of both the people and the available resources in the estuarine environment.

The addition of maize horticulture to the subsistence strategy of coastal people in the Late Woodland does not appear to have significantly compromised health and nutrition, as indicated by the linear enamel hypoplasia rates. The LEH pattern varies widely among the sites, with high rates both early and late in the Late Woodland. The incorporation of maize horticulture would have affected the seasonal scheduling of foragers, however, because they would have had to spend time planting and harvesting maize that could have been spent collecting or exploiting other resources. It may also have led to more sedentary settlement patterns, if the groups were not already sedentary.

Waselkov (1987) predicts that horticulture and domestication will lead to rapid abandonment of shellfish gathering when the plant domesticates have a high fat and protein content and thus lower production and utilization costs. Shellfish use does not appear to have diminished even with the addition of maize on the North Carolina coast, fitting this model's predictions that maize is not adequately high in fat and protein to encourage a shift away from shellfish. Mollusks can add a small, continuous amount of protein that can be an essential component of the diet and subsistence strategy. Waselkov states that "decisions regarding the scheduling of shellfish gathering depend not merely on shellfish availability but rather on a continuous reassessment of all potential food resources, constant reappraisal of their present and future relative food values and ease of procurement, and changing estimates of group needs" (1987:111).

Estuarine environments are rich enough that the people living on their fruits do not become reliant on maize horticulture and other domesticates, at least along the North Carolina coast. Precontact Georgia coastal populations never seem to have been intensive maize agriculturists either (Reitz 1988), although they seem to have relied on maize more heavily than did North Carolina groups. Perhaps the difference in dependence is related to the Mississippian emergence in Georgia, which did not reach as far north as the coast of North Carolina. Maize agriculture is part of the cultural repertoire of Mississippian societies. In North Carolina, even after maize becomes a part of the diet, it is difficult to see significant cultural impacts of the addition, except in dental health and archaeological evidence of subsistence. Archaeologists have encountered difficulties in dividing the Late Woodland into smaller time periods in part because of this lack of significant changes. It seems from the archaeological evidence gathered thus far that shifts in settlement pattern or burial practices through time did not occur in the Late Woodland, despite the new subsistence strategy.

Archaeological models of the Late Woodland on the North Carolina coastal plain are difficult to work with primarily because of the long time span of the period. Perhaps a model based on indications of dental health, subsistence, seasonality of resource use (and whether it changes with the addition of maize horticulture), and settlement patterns will prove more fruitful for estimating a site's place in the chronology than ceramic seriation or mortuary practices have thus far. Estimating the dental caries rate may be useful as support for other indications of a site's temporal placement in the Late Woodland. Dental caries rates of less than 7 percent of all erupted teeth of contemporaneous individuals at a site can be the basis for conjecture that the diet of the group did not include maize and therefore probably falls earlier in the Late Woodland. Dental caries rates must be interpreted with caution, however, and be supported by other lines of evidence.

The findings of this study suggest that further work needs to be completed to determine the extent to which maize agriculture was a component of diet of coastal peoples in the Late Woodland in North Carolina. The timing and significance of the adoption of maize agriculture are unclear at this time. It is interesting that the addition of this cultigen does not seem to have had much impact on culture in the Late Woodland in coastal North Carolina. This hypothesis can be further explored through more excavation of habitation sites associated with ossuaries and other burials along the coast. As coastal development and erosion continue in the region, more sites are sure to be exposed. Further information about diet and nutrition can be obtained through additional studies of stable isotope ratios. Although several isolated individual skeletons have been analyzed, only one site (Flynt) has had extensive bone chemistry analysis performed on multiple individuals. The addition of some of the northern coastal plain sites would broaden the range of this study, and comparisons between sites further north and south may prove interesting. Perhaps this type of analysis will prove helpful in answering the regional questions of cultural change in the late prehistoric Southeastern coastal region, forming a more complete backdrop for analysis of the impact of agriculture.

ACKNOWLEDGMENTS

We wish to express our gratitude to Mark Mathis for his insights on North Carolina coastal prehistory, Joe Herbert for his thorough and careful editing of an earlier draft of this chapter, Ann Kakaliouras for her thoughts on the Garbacon Creek site and for her examination of the chapter, Clark S. Larsen for his helpful editing of earlier drafts, and especially Pat Lambert for inviting us to participate in the American Association of Physical Anthropologists symposium, which was the inspiration for this volume, and for her patience and hard work in editing the volume. The human skeletal remains from Broad Reach (31Cr218), Piggot (31Cr14), and Flynt (31On305) sites are housed at Wake Forest University, and the skeletal remains from Cold Morning (31Nh28), Garbacon Creek (31Cr86), and McFayden Mound (31Bw67) are stored at University of North Carolina at Chapel Hill.

I O Life on the Periphery: Health in Farming Communities of Interior North Carolina and Virginia

Patricia M. Lambert

Unlike regions such as the Black Warrior Valley of Alabama described earlier in this volume, North Carolina and Virginia are located on the periphery of the Mississippian cultural sphere. Consequently, this mid-Atlantic region never experienced the same degree of political centralization and population aggregation that characterized Moundville and other Mississippian centers. In the mountains of western North Carolina, cultural attributes such as platform mounds and frontal-occipital deformation document the late and somewhat peripheral participation of Appalachian Summit villages in the South Appalachian Mississippian cultural tradition better known in Tennessee and other points west (Ward and Davis 1999). On the southern piedmont of North Carolina, the relatively sudden appearance of temple mounds, distinct ceramic styles, and pronounced fronto-occipital deformation around A.D. 1200 document the temporally and geographically limited intrusion of immigrants or ideology from Mississippian cultural traditions from the south (Coe 1995; Ward and Davis 1999). On the northern piedmont and in the coastal reaches of North Carolina and Virginia, the lack of material evidence for these cultural attributes suggests an absence of any significant Mississippian influence. Human remains from North Carolina and Virginia thus offer a unique opportunity to assess the extent to which diet and health trends observed at or in proximity to large political centers were paralleled on and beyond the Mississippian periphery.

Because the human skeleton comprises living tissue that responds to various types of environmental stresses experienced by the human body during life, human skeletal remains from this region can provide a wealth of information on the biological costs and constraints of farming these eastern reaches of North America. The consumption of refined high-carbohydrate foods, for example, can result in dental lesions and tooth loss that document the health consequences to teeth of a dietary emphasis on cariogenic foods such as maize. Other chronic bacterial infections cause both abnormal production and destruction of bone, resulting in tell-tale lesions that can be used to document levels of infectious disease. Through the study of the bones of people buried in North Carolina and Virginia archaeological sites, it is therefore possible to identify and explore variability in health risks faced by indigenous farmers of this region. Although all samples included in this study derive from maize agriculturalists, their dependence on this staple food might be expected to have varied from region to region, depending on variables such as micro-climate, population size, access to arable lands and alternative food sources, and unique cultural traditions. Levels of disease might also be expected to have varied according to these parameters. The purpose of this chapter is to explore the extent to which the cultural differences evident in three subregions of the study area were accompanied by concomitant differences in diet and health and to compare general health in this region with health at larger centers such as Moundville in order to assess the costs and benefits of life in the hinterlands relative to that in more productive and populous regions.

REGIONAL PREHISTORY

Prehistorically, North Carolina and southern Virginia followed the agricultural trajectory noted elsewhere in the Southeast: maize agriculture established after A.D. 1000 and the corn-bean-squash triad in place by A.D. 1200 (Smith 1992a, 1992b; Ward and Davis 1999). Botanical and faunal remains recovered from archaeological sites of this region suggest a diverse economy anchored in varying degrees to maize (Ward and Davis 1993, 1999). Analysis of stable carbon and nitrogen isotopes in human skeletal remains from the study area support these interpretations (Trimble 1996). Carbon isotopes values are particularly informative in this regard. Mean ^{13}C values of about −15.8‰ for an earlier agricultural sample from the Donnaha site in North Carolina (A.D. 1040–1480) and −14.6‰ for a somewhat later agricultural sample from the Koehler site in south-central Virginia (A.D. 1300–1400; see Eastman 1994) place late prehistoric piedmont inhabitants between Middle Woodland North Carolinians (−19.1‰) (see Trimble 1996: Table 22) and heavily maize-dependent groups (–7.5‰) such as the Black Mesa Anasazi (Martin et al. 1991: Table 3-6), suggesting a mixed diet that came increasingly to emphasize corn. Although the importance of maize is thought to have increased throughout the late prehistoric period, there is some archaeological evidence for a return to a more mixed economy, perhaps as a result of fur trade activities, in the protohistoric/historic period (Ward and Davis 1993, 1999).

Survey data also suggest that settlement systems underwent organizational changes during the agricultural period. Settlements dating to between A.D. 800–1200 are relatively small, dispersed households and hamlets—the first evidence for sustained sedentary living in this region. In the following three centuries, these dispersed settlements coalesce into compact, fortified villages of approximately 100 to 200 residents. Palisades are a common archaeological feature of villages dating to this time period and provide evidence that intergroup relations were often hostile in nature (Ward and Davis 1999). It was during this period that Town Creek, a relatively large (~550 burials; see Coe 1995:265) Mississippian ceremonial center with cultural attributes reminiscent of Irene Mound in coastal Georgia, flourished on the southern piedmont of North Carolina (Coe 1995; Ward and Davis 1999). Although it has been argued that this center represents the intrusion of culture-bearing immigrants from the south, dental trait analysis comparing human remains from Town Creek and Irene Mound does not support a close genetic relationship (Griffin et al. 2001), and the exact mechanism behind this cultural efflorescence remains obscure. After A.D. 1500, some settlements coalesced and others dispersed as the effects of European contact began to be felt by the native inhabitants. Ultimately, much of the piedmont was abandoned by Siouan groups as people moved north or south to join larger groups for purposes of economy and defense (Swanton 1946; Ward and Davis 1993, 1999).

MATERIALS AND METHODS

The skeletal sample described in this study is composed of 649 individuals, including 282 subadults (<20 years), 366 adults (20+ years), and one unaged individual from thirteen archaeological sites in western and central North Carolina and south-central Virginia (Table 10-1; Figure 10-1). These remains derive from two broad ecological zones: the piedmont region of North Carolina and southern Virginia, occupied historically by Siouan tribes, and the Appalachian Mountains of western North Carolina, traditional homeland of the Cherokee. Included are collections from nine northern piedmont sites, one large southern piedmont site (Town Creek), and three mountain villages. With the excep-

Table 10-1. Frequency of Individuals with Various Pathological Conditions. Arranged by region and time period.

Site	Dates (A.D.)[1]	Ratio Juveniles/ Adults[2]	Dental Caries[3] +/−	Enam. Hypo. Mandib. C.[4] +/−	Cribra Orbitalia[5] +/−	Vertebral Lesions[6] +/−	Diseased Tibiae[7] +/−
Mountains							
Bn-29 (Warren Wilson)	1250–1450	23/34 40.4%	42/2 95.5%	12/10 54.5%	3/10 23.1%	1/25 3.8%	12/19 38.7%
Hw-1/2 (Garden Creek)	1250–1450	15/19 44.1%	25/3 89.3%	11/6 64.7%	2/6 25.0%	0/15 0.0%	3/10 23.1%
Ma-34 (Coweeta Creek)	1600–1700	34/53 39.1%	64/12 84.2%	31/17 64.6%	8/23 25.8%	0/27 0.0%	5/37 11.9%
Southern Piedmont							
Mg-2/3 (Town Creek)	1200–1500	80/115 41.0%	114/24 82.6%	42/17 71.2%	15/45 25.0%	2/47 4.2%	39/67 36.8%
Northern Piedmont							
Vir-150 (Gaston Reservoir)	800–1200	10/17 37.0%	19/5 79.2%	5/6 45.5%	9/8 52.9%	0/22 0.0%	10/10 50.0%
Yd-1 (Forbush Creek)	800–1200	21/33 38.9%	22/7 75.9%	8/1 88.9%	5/21 9.2%	0/11 0.0%	7/21 25.0%
Vir-196 (Hr-1) (Leatherwood Creek)	1200–1400	4/5 44.4%	8/1 88.9%	4/1 80.0%	3/4 42.9%	0/6 0.0%	3/5 37.5%

Table 10-1 continued on next page

Table 10-1. continued

Site	Dates (A.D.)[1]	Ratio Juveniles/Adults[2] +/-	Dental Caries[3] +/-	Enam. Hypo. Mandib. C.[4] +/-	Cribra Orbitalia[5] +/-	Vertebral Lesions[6] +/-	Diseased Tibiae[7] +/-
Vir-231 (Hr-35) (Stockton)	1300–1400	8/18 30.8%	16/3 84.2%	6/3 66.7%	8/13 38.1%	1/16 5.9%	13/9 59.1%
Vir-199 (Hr-4) (Philpott)	1300–1450	6/4 60.0%	6/1 85.7%	1/3 25.0%	2/2 50.0%	0/5 0.0%	4/1 80.0%
Or-11 (Wall)	1400–1500	6/2 75.0%	3/1 75.0%	0/1 0.0%	1/2 33.3%	0/4 0.0%	1/2 33.3%
Sk-1 (Early Upper Saratown) (P/h)	1450–1620	8/4 66.7%	8/3 72.7%	5/1 83.3%	5/3 62.5%	0/8 0.0%	2/7 22.2%
Sk-1a (Upper Saratown)	1670–1710	48/54 47.1%	68/22 75.6%	34/8 81.0%	10/16 38.5%	1/16 5.9%	2/34 5.6%
Or-231 (Occaneechi Town)	1690–1710	8/5 61.5%	11/0 100%	5/2 71.4%	3/6 33.3%	0/6 0.0%	1/6 14.3%
Sk-6 (William Kluttz)	1690–1710	11/3 78.6%	6/4 60.0%	3/0 100.0%	1/3 25.0%	0/5 0.0%	2/4 33.3%
Total	800–1710	282/366 43.5%	412/88 82.4%	167/76 68.7%	75/162 31.6%	5/212 2.3%	104/232 31.0%

Notes: +/− = affected/unaffected. [1]Dates based on R. P. Stephen Davis, pers. comm. 1998; Davis et al. 1997; Research Laboratories of Archaeology 1996; and Ward and Davis 1999; [2]Excludes 1 individual of indeterminate age. Samples include all individuals with at least one scorable [3]tooth, [4]permanent mandibular canine, [5]eye orbit, or [7]tibia (>5 mos.). [6]Sample includes all individuals with at least three scorable vertebrae (most had many more).

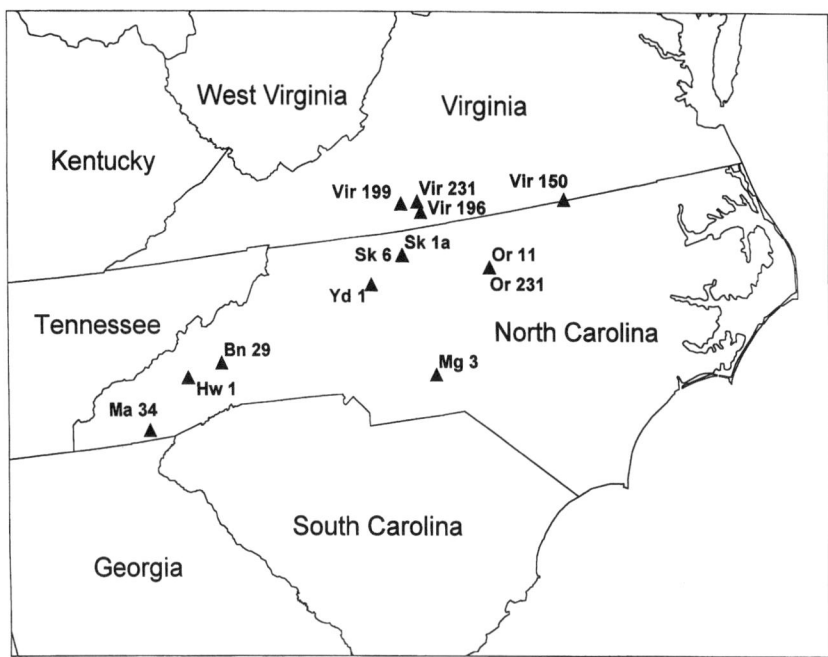

Figure 10-1. Location of Archaeological Sites. (Map generated by R. P. Stephen Davis)

tion of remains from three Virginia sites, this material was recovered by the Research Laboratories of Archaeology at UNC-Chapel Hill during their long history of archaeological reconnaissance and excavation in the area (see Coe 1995; Dickens et al. 1987; Ward and Davis 1993, 1999). The remains from Vir-196 (Leatherwood Creek), Vir-199 (Philpott), and Vir-231 (Stockton) were collected during amateur excavations in the upper Dan River basin and are also curated in the RLA's archaeological repository (Davis et al. 1997; Research Laboratories of Archaeology 1996).

The sample has been combined and partitioned in a number of ways in the following discussion in order to explore both temporal and geographic trends in the health of these eastern agriculturalists. The collections can be divided by geographic and cultural attributes into three broad geographic units: mountain, northern piedmont, and southern piedmont. As indicated previously, cultural attributes such as settlement size, the palisading of village perimeters, and ceramic typologies also suggest several temporal divisions: the early late prehistoric period (ca. A.D. 800–1200), the later half of the late prehistoric period (ca. A.D. 1200–1500), and the protohistoric/historic period (ca. A.D. 1500–1710) (see Ward and Davis 1999).

Patterning in several skeletal indicators of health and disease are explored in this study. These include dental caries, cribra orbitalia, enamel hypoplasia, proliferative (periosteal) lesions of the tibiae, and osteolytic lesions of the spinal column. For purposes of comparison, a few specifics regarding methodology are warranted. In scoring dental caries, teeth were considered carious only if tissue erosion was visible on the tooth surface; discolored lesions were not included in counts of affected teeth. Measures of dental health include frequencies of carious teeth as well as teeth lost during life; the latter are included in some calculations because antemortem tooth loss in these collections strongly correlates with the age-related progression of dental caries. For cribra orbitalia, individuals were scored as affected if multiple foramina and channeling were clearly evident in one or both eye orbits under low power magnification (see Buikstra and Ubelaker 1994). In the scoring of enamel hypoplasia, analysis was limited to the permanent mandibular canines because these are among the most commonly affected teeth in the dentition (e.g., Goodman and Armelagos 1985; Martin et al. 1991); teeth were scored as hypoplastic only if observed lesions could be detected by running a fingernail down the surface of the tooth. Observations of surface texture and nonconformities were used to detect both appositional lesions of tibiae and destructive lesions of the vertebral column. All lesions were scored with the aid of a 10× hand lens under strong, oblique lighting. Observations were made for each individual only if the condition of the remains permitted accurate assessment of the pathological trait under consideration; for this reason, sample sizes for different skeletal indices of health and disease vary by site and region.

The Skeletal Evidence of Diet and Disease

Dental Disease

Data on dental caries and related tooth loss suggest that dental disease was ubiquitous and relatively severe in all of the sampled farming communities of North Carolina and Virginia (Table 10-1). Dental caries is a chronic disease process in which acids produced by the bacterial fermentation of dietary carbohydrates erode tooth enamel (Hunter 1988; Larsen 1997). Modern clinical research has linked these lesions with the consumption of refined carbohydrates, particularly sucrose, but tooth morphology, defective enamel, and lack of oral hygiene can also influence the formation of carious lesions (Harris 1963; Hunter 1988; Infante and Gillespie 1974; Larsen 1983). Numerous bioarchaeological studies have shown that the frequency of carious lesions increased when people made the transition from foraging to farming (Larsen

1987, 1995, 1997). Dental caries rates among modern horticulturalists provide supportive evidence for the importance of corn starch in particular in the production of carious lesions (Milton 1992), although the bioarchaeological record of North America indicates that dependence on other starchy foods can also lead to an increase in the frequency of carious lesions (e.g., Rose et al. 1991; Walker and Erlandson 1986). The high frequency of people with carious dentitions (82.4 percent) is thus consistent with the archaeological and isotopic evidence that refined maize products and probably other starchy foods constituted a significant portion of the diet of these southeastern farmers.

Within the study area, however, differences in the frequency of diseased teeth between regions suggest that the importance of maize as a dietary staple varied geographically (Table 10-2). A comparison of the frequency of carious permanent molars in three late prehistoric North American groups—North Carolina/Virginia farmers, Southwest Puebloan farmers, and California fisherpeople—illustrates the strength of the relationship between diet and dental health and documents the validity of using dental caries as a proxy measure of foods consumed. The frequency of carious molars for prehistoric North Carolina/Virginia farmers (55.6 percent) closely resembles that (52.5 percent) for Puebloan farmers (Martin et al. 1991: Tables 8-12 and 8-13), whereas these differ significantly from frequencies observed in a sample of late prehistoric California fisherpeople (15.4 percent) (Walker and Erlandson 1986: Table 1). This pattern undoubtedly reflects the greater dependence of both farming groups on cariogenic maize foods and of the maritime hunter-gatherers on noncariogenic foods such as fish and sea mammal meat. The differences observed between subregions within the study area in frequency of diseased permanent molars is thus likely to reflect differences in diet that resulted from differences in the availability and use of arable lands and other subsistence-related resources. They may also have been due to cultural factors, such as differing levels of trade or internecine warfare, which could have influenced degree of reliance on storable foods like maize.

The severity of dental disease in prehistoric North Carolina and Virginia samples stands out when these groups are compared to other Southeastern groups. The frequency of carious permanent molars (55.6 percent) in the late prehistoric sample (A.D. 800–1500) is considerably higher than the frequency that Larsen and coworkers (Larsen, Schoeninger, Shavit, and Russell 1990: Table 3) report for a precontact agricultural sample (A.D. 1150–1550) from coastal Georgia (18.8 percent) or that Monahan and Weaver (this volume) report for a late prehistoric sample from coastal North Carolina, which likely reflects the greater dependence of these coastal inhabitants on various noncariogenic marine and estuarine foods. More puzzling, however, is the lower

Table 10-2. Temporal and Geographic Patterns in Diseased (Carious/Lost Antemortem) Permanent Molars by Age (N = 321 individuals, 2605 molars)

Time Period	Age (Years)[1]	Mountains		Southern Piedmont		Northern Piedmont	
		D/T	%	D/T	%	D/T	%
A.D. 800–1200	0–20	–	–	–	–	4/28	14.3
	20–40	–	–	–	–	92/157	58.6
	>40	–	–	–	–	72/102	70.6
A.D. 1200–1500	0–20	77/143	53.8	52/157	33.1	18/31	58.1
	20–40	157/233	67.4	198/295	67.1	108/134	80.6
	>40	71/89	79.8	165/217	76.0	103/107	96.3
A.D. 1500–1710	0–20	34/112	30.4	–	–	56/156	35.9
	20–40	135/269	50.2	–	–	131/230	57.0
	>40	47/79	59.5	–	–	55/66	83.3

[1]Sample excludes individuals that could not be assigned to defined age category. Key: D/T = No. diseased molars / No. molars in sample; % = percent molars diseased.

rate of carious posterior teeth (25.2 percent) reported for Moundville (Powell 1991b: Table 3-9) because ^{13}C values indicate high rates of maize consumption at this site (see Schoeninger et al., this volume). This disparity suggests that the late prehistoric peoples of North Carolina and Virginia obtained a greater proportion of their calories from starchy foods (albeit not necessarily corn) than did residents of Moundville or that residents of Moundville either incorporated more cleansing foods into their diet or consumed corn products prepared in ways less conducive to dental caries. It is also possible that genetic or developmental differences in tooth morphology differentially predisposed indigenous North Carolinians/Virginians to dental disease or that differences in scoring procedures (or inclusion of premolars in the Moundville sample) resulted in the observed disparity.

A rather interesting decline is evident in the frequency of diseased molars from the late prehistoric to the protohistoric/historic period (Table 10-2). Age-based comparisons produce similar results, so these differences cannot be attributed to differences in the age structure of the samples. These data support evidence described above for a return in both mountain and piedmont regions to a more mixed economy in the early days of European contact (Ward and Davis 1993, 1999).

A somewhat curious deviation from this pattern is evident in the increase through time in carious lesions of the permanent maxillary incisors, at least in northern piedmont samples (Figure 10-2). The frequency of carious maxillary incisors is quite high overall in the study area (32.6 percent), ranging from 31 to 35 percent in samples dating between A.D. 1200 and 1500. Comparisons with other prehistoric agriculturalists indicate that these high rates of affected incisors are not a necessary correlate of a maize-dependent diet. For example, despite the close correspondence of carious molar frequencies between prehistoric North Carolina/Virginia and Black Mesa Anasazi samples, Martin and coworkers (1991) report a much lower frequency of carious lesions of the maxillary incisors (5.5 percent). In the Southeast, both Powell (1991b: Table 3-9) and Larsen and coworkers (Larsen, Schoeninger, Shavit, and Russell 1990) also report rates of only 2.5–3.5 percent for broadly contemporaneous prehistoric samples from Moundville and coastal Georgia. This disparity strongly suggests that the native peoples of North Carolina and Virginia were either consuming a unique food or more likely were processing a food in a way that was unique to this region. What could have caused such a pattern in this region? One possibility is the consumption of green corn; the gustatory practice of eating corn "on the cob" leaves particles between the teeth, which can serve to trap foods between the incisors, creating a reservoir of nutrients for caries-causing bacteria. After European contact, the continuing increase in their frequency on the northern piedmont could have

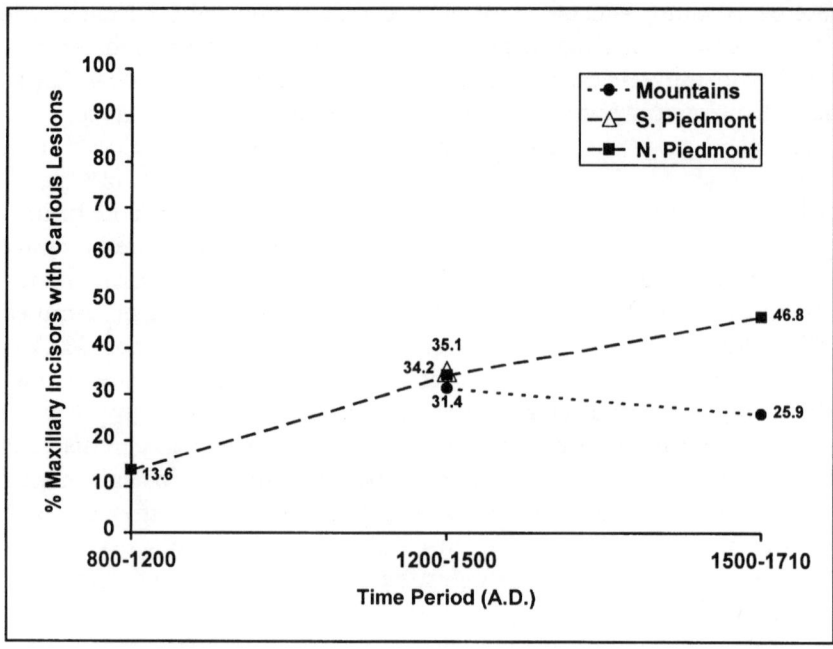

Figure 10-2. Temporal and Geographic Variation in the Frequency of Carious Maxillary Incisors.

related to the introduction of sugar products through trade and other transactions. Introduced sugar products could also in part explain the high frequency of carious maxillary incisors (19.4 percent) in a late contact sample from Mission Santa Catalina de Guale de Santa Maria, although the increase in this case generally correlates with an increase in carious molars and isotopic evidence for increased maize consumption (Larsen, Schoeninger, Shavit, and Russell 1990).

The health consequences of dental disease to people in these Southeastern agricultural communities should not be underestimated. Dental disease is painful, causes bad breath, and in its advanced stages can severely restrict the kinds of foods people are able to consume. Modern clinical research has documented a significant correlation between dental health and nutritional adequacy among the elderly; adequate intake of both micronutrients and fiber appears to be significantly impaired in people with compromised dentitions (Appollonio et al. 1997; Krall et al. 1998). As dental disease progressed with age, people would have come to depend increasingly on cariogenic processed foods such as corn mush that are easy to consume, thus promoting and exacerbating dental disease. Important nutrients available from foods such as red meat and green vegetables that require considerable mastication would have become less accessible, leading to nutritional deficiencies and increased susceptibility to infectious pathogens—particularly those harbored by unrefrigerated prepared foods. It is therefore likely that dental disease ultimately contributed to adult mortality.

Cribra Orbitalia: Skeletal Evidence for Anemia and Scurvy

Cribra orbitalia is another common lesion in the North Carolina/ Virginia collections, with frequencies of affected individuals ranging from about 23 to 63 percent (Table 10-1). A skeletal condition ubiquitous in many prehistoric Native American populations (e.g., Lambert and Walker 1991; Larsen 1987, 1995, 1997; Martin et al. 1991; Walker 1985, 1986), cribra orbitalia refers to sieve-like lesions of the eye orbits. In the bioarchaeological literature, these porous lesions are most commonly attributed to iron-deficiency anemia (see Larsen 1997) and are thought to form in response to anemia when excessive venous vascularization in conjunction with overactive marrow production thins and destroys the orbital plate, resulting in spongy hyperostosis of the orbital roofs (Hengen 1971; Moseley 1974; Stuart-Macadam 1987). Although modern clinical research has implicated a number of different anemic conditions in this physiological response (Moseley 1974; Steinbock 1976), the lack of evidence for congenital anemias in indigenous Native Americans implicates iron-deficiency anemia in the etiology of cribra orbitalia in New World skeletal series (Larsen 1987, 1997). Because cribra orbitalia has been shown to have increased with the transition to maize farming, bioarchaeologists have often linked this condition to nutritional deficiencies associated with the shift to a dietary dependence on maize foods; corn is not a particularly good source of iron and contains phytic acid, a chemical that inhibits the intestinal absorption of iron (Larsen 1987, 1995; Steinbock 1976; Walker 1985). Thus, the cribra orbitalia evidence from sites in this region would certainly be consistent with the dental evidence for high rates of maize consumption.

Nevertheless, recent anthropological research does not support maize as an exclusive explanation for iron-deficiency anemia in indigenous New World populations. The remains of maritime hunter-gatherers from the Santa Barbara Channel area of California, for example, exhibit relatively high rates of cribra orbitalia, despite the heavy dependence of these coastal dwellers on iron-rich animal foods such as sea mammal meat, sardines, and mussels. Iron-deficiency anemia in these west coast communities is instead thought to have resulted from bleeding and nutrient loss associated with bacterial dysentery (Lambert and Walker 1991; Walker 1986)—a common problem today for sedentary agriculturalists in undeveloped countries (Mascie-Taylor 1993;

Mata et al. 1981; Scrimshaw 1964). Thus, although nutritional deficiencies resulting from a dietary dependence on corn may have contributed to anemia in North Carolina and Virginia populations, diarrheal disease resulting from the consumption of contaminated foods and potable water was likely another contributing factor in this disorder.

It is also possible that other conditions were responsible for these lesions. Emerging research suggests that vitamin C deficiency may also cause porous lesions to form in the eye orbits, particularly in the fast-growing bones of infants and children (Ortner 1992; Ortner and Ericksen 1997; Ortner et al. 1999). Unlike in iron-deficiency anemia, orbital lesions associated with scurvy are appositional in nature, resulting from an inflammatory response to chronic hemorrhage. Scurvy interferes with the growth and maintenance of connective tissues, increasing susceptibility to hemorrhage from even minor trauma like normal eye motion. According to Ortner and Ericksen (1997), with healing and remodeling, these lesions may come to resemble milder forms of anemia and thus may be difficult to distinguish from anemic lesions without histological examination.

Orbital lesions were scored using a simple scale of slight, moderate, and severe. Most cases of cribra orbitalia were scored as slight. Following Walker (1986), slight lesions are defined here as a scattering of fine foramina (or shallow channeling) affecting less than a 1 cm^2 area of the upper orbit; moderate and severe lesions are composed of larger pits that affect a greater expanse of the orbital roof. Because mild lesions are particularly subject to inter-observer error (and may not be scored by conservative researchers), results are presented for all lesions (Tables 10-1, 10-2) and for moderate-to-severe lesions only (Figure 10-3). Although overall frequency obviously declines when slight lesions are eliminated from consideration, the general pattern of occurrence remains, supporting the argument that slight lesions are indeed an expression, albeit mild, of the disease condition(s) responsible for porous orbital lesions. Unfortunately, histological examination was not possible at the time of the analysis, so the specific etiology of orbital lesions remains unclear.

Like numerous other skeletal samples, juveniles are more commonly affected than adults in the North Carolina/Virginia sample (Table 10-3), supporting the argument that orbital lesions are indicative of a childhood condition (see also Larsen 1995, 1997; Stuart-Macadam 1985; Walker 1985, 1986). Females are more often affected than males (see also Hengen 1971; Eisenberg 1991; Lambert 1999; Mensforth and Lovejoy 1985; Walker 1986), and Powell (1988) also notes this pattern for the Moundville sample. Although sex differences in the frequency of cribra orbitalia may reflect anemia associated with the greater nu-

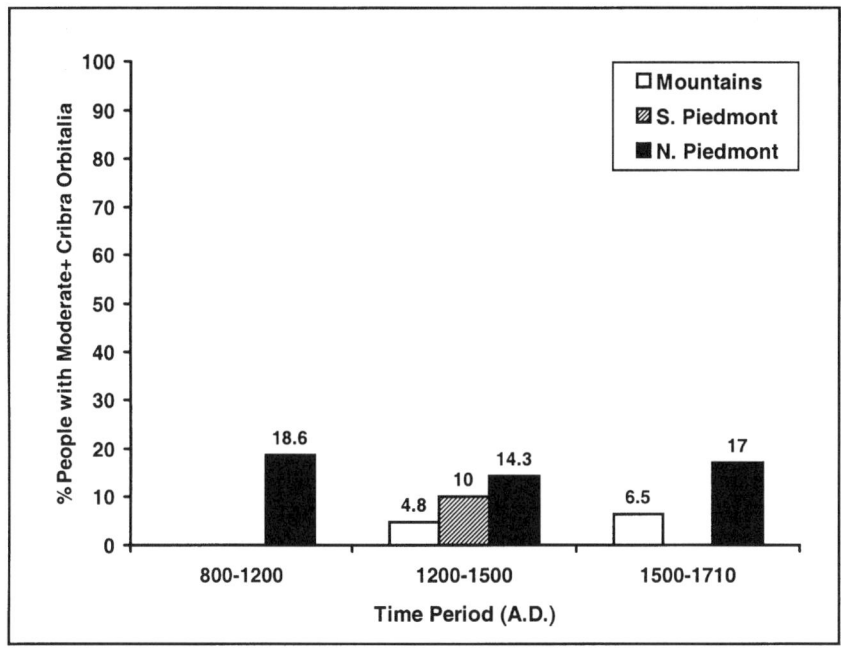

Figure 10-3. Temporal and Geographic Variation in the Frequency of Moderate-to-Severe Cribra Orbitalia.

tritional demands on women resulting from biological differences associated with pregnancy and lactation (Hengen 1971; Mensforth and Lovejoy 1985), this is not an entirely satisfactory explanation for observed results. Clinical and bioarchaeological studies have shown that both anemic and scorbutic lesions tend to form in childhood, due to unique features of skeletal growth and physiology that characterize young children (Lallo et al. 1977; Moseley 1974; Ortner and Ericksen 1998; Stuart-Macadam 1985; Walker 1986). At least one active case of cribra orbitalia was recorded for a young woman, however, so sex differences associated with reproductive biology could in part explain the higher frequency of these lesions in females than in males (see Hengen 1971:69). It is also possible that girls obtained a greater proportion of their calories than boys from maize-based foods, which could have rendered them more susceptible to both iron-deficiency anemia and scurvy.

Although slight temporal variation is evident in the frequency of individuals with cribra orbitalia, geographic setting appears to have been more important in the etiology of this lesion (Tables 10-1, 10-3; Figure 10-3). Orbital lesions are more common in individuals from

Table 10-3. Temporal and Geographic Variation in Cribra Orbitalia by Age (N = 237 individuals)

Time Period A.D.	Age (Years)	Mountains		Southern Piedmont		Northern Piedmont	
		A/T	%	A/T	%	A/T	%
800–1200	0–10	—	—	—	—	5/9	55.6
	10–20	—	—	—	—	2/4	50.0
	>20	—	—	—	—	7/30	23.3
	Total	—	—	—	—	14/43	32.6
1200–1500	0–10	1/1	100.0	4/17	23.5	4/8	50.0
	10–20	0/1	0.0	3/3	100.0	2/2	100.0
	>20	4/19	21.1	8/40	20.0	8/25	32.0
	Total	5/21	23.8	15/60	25.0	14/35	40.0
1500–1710	0–10	2/5	40.0	—	—	8/14	57.1
	10–20	2/2	100.0	—	—	3/6	50.0
	>20	4/24	16.7	—	—	8/27	29.6
	Total	8/31	25.8	—	—	19/47	40.4

Key: A/T = No. affected individuals / No. individuals in sample; % = percent individuals affected.

northern piedmont villages than they are in individuals from either Town Creek or Appalachian Summit villages. Differences in the age structure of these samples may to some extent be influencing results because the age group most susceptible to cribrotic lesions (<10 years) is best represented in the northern piedmont sample. Indeed, age-based comparisons suggest that children were at high risk for the affliction(s) that cause this lesion in both mountain and north piedmont villages, whereas those from the southern piedmont were somewhat better buffered against this health risk (Table 10-3). Unfortunately, the mountain sample is too small (N = 6) for statistically valid conclusions, leaving the question of juvenile susceptibility to conditions causing cribrotic lesions in mountain sites unanswered. The adult sample is larger in all cases, however, and yields results more consistent with, albeit less dramatic than, patterns evident when the sample is taken as a whole (Table 10-3). The data do thus suggest that iron-deficiency anemia and probably scurvy were more of a problem on the northern piedmont than elsewhere in this region.

These differences might be explained by climatic variations (see Hengen 1971:68) such as differences in average temperature or rainfall between the mountains and the piedmont that were more conducive to parasitic infections in the latter. Demographic variables such as settlement size and location could also have been a factor, as could differences in the composition of the diet; certainly, data on dental disease suggest that reliance on maize products was greatest in northern piedmont villages. Whatever the causes, however, the cribra orbitalia data do imply that the probability of being iron deficient or scorbutic in prehistoric North Carolina and Virginia was influenced by where and how people lived.

This is further suggested by comparisons of cribra orbitalia frequencies between locations in the greater Southeast. For example, according to Powell (1990, 1991b), only about 8 percent of prehistoric inhabitants of the Irene Mound site in Coastal Georgia exhibit orbital lesions, and only about 9.3 percent of the Moundville population are thus affected. In addition, a somewhat higher frequency of orbital lesions (~20.0 percent) at the large (888 individuals) Mississippian village of Averbuch in Middle Tennessee (Eisenberg 1991) is similar to that recorded for smaller Appalachian Summit villages in North Carolina (Tables 10-1, 10-3). Although it is likely that differences in scoring techniques account in part for the large discrepancy between low values from Irene Mound and Moundville and those from North Carolina and Virginia, even conservative estimates based on moderate to severe lesions (Figure 10-3) suggest that vitamin deficiency and other causes of porous orbital lesions were a greater problem for inhabitants of relatively small, northern piedmont villages than for larger settlements within and outside the study area.

Enamel Hypoplasia: The Evidence
for Childhood Growth Disruption

Enamel hypoplasia data provide supporting evidence that childhood health was frequently and often severely compromised in these Southeastern farming communities (Table 10-1). Enamel hypoplasia refers to hypocalcification defects that form in tooth crowns when childhood growth is disrupted by systemic metabolic disturbances (e.g., severe infection, starvation) that cause a temporary cessation of ameloblastic activity (Sarnat and Schour 1941). These enamel lesions most commonly appear as linear, horizontal grooves but may also take the form of pits, notches, or vertical grooves in tooth crowns (Giro 1947; Goodman and Armelagos 1985; Sarnat and Schour 1941). Although modern clinical research has implicated a range of health conditions in the etiology of these defects (e.g., Giro 1947; Goodman and Armelagos 1985; Infante and Gillespie 1974; Nikiforuk and Fraser 1981; Ortner and Putschar 1985; Sarnat and Schour 1941), the lesions themselves do not generally differ in appearance according to the particular insult (but see Hutchinson 1909). For this reason, enamel defects provide a good but nonspecific measure of stresses encountered in childhood (Kreshover 1960). The high frequency (69 percent) of individuals in the North Carolina/Virginia sample with enamel hypoplasia of the permanent mandibular canines is evidence that a significant portion of children in these farming communities suffered from at least one systemic condition severe enough to impact normal metabolism and growth.

There is some evidence for both geographic and temporal differences in the distribution of these lesions (Figure 10-4). Rates are relatively consistent between prehistoric mountain and northern piedmont samples, but somewhat higher for the sample from Town Creek, and it may be that the large size of the Town Creek settlement increased exposure of infants and children to acute infections maintained in the larger population. The frequency of individuals with hypoplastic canine teeth in the prehistoric component from North Carolina/Virginia and Moundville (Powell 1991b: Table 3-10) is almost identical (54 percent),[1] however, suggesting a similar rate of childhood stress episodes, despite the much larger size (~3000 people) of the Moundville population (Powell 1988). In contrast, that reported by Hutchinson and Larsen (1990) for Irene Mound, a much smaller site than Moundville (~280 people, see Powell 1990), is somewhat higher (77 percent) than that noted here (64 percent),[2] which could reflect greater susceptibility of these coastal dwellers to the elements but could also be due to scoring

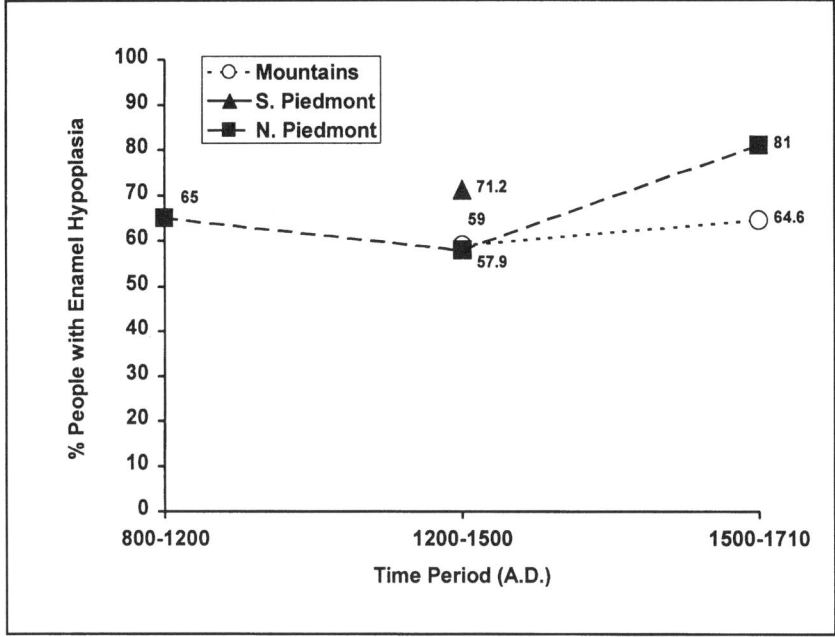

Figure 10-4. Temporal and Geographic Variation in the Frequency of Enamel Hypoplasia of the Mandibular Canines.

differences resulting from the systematic use of a binocular microscope for the Georgia sample.

The increase in frequency of people with affected canines after European contact on the northern piedmont may be related to increased exposure to acute infections introduced by European explorers, traders, and colonists.[3] These findings are consistent with archaeological and historic evidence for depopulation of the northern piedmont after A.D. 1650 and support the argument that epidemic diseases introduced through contacts with European traders played a role in the ultimate demise of these communities (see Ward and Davis 1991). A significant increase in the frequency of hypoplastic canines from the precontact agricultural period to the contact agricultural period was reported for Guale samples from St. Catherines Island, Georgia (Hutchinson and Larsen 1988, 1990), providing corroborating evidence that the prevalence or severity of childhood illness in the Southeast increased after the arrival of Europeans. The absence of a significant increase in the frequency of people with hypoplastic canine teeth in the mountains suggests that contacts with Europeans may have been less common or less devastating in terms of introduced infectious disease, and this observation is also consistent with early historic accounts that describe a thriving seventeenth-century population (Alvord and Bidgood 1912; Ward and Davis 1991).

Proliferative Lesions and Other Skeletal
Evidence for Treponemal Disease

Farming communities of this region were certainly troubled by infectious disease before the arrival of Europeans, but those most troubling to the local populace would have been chronic infections that could be maintained in the relatively low population densities that characterized this region prehistorically. As has been reported for other skeletal series from both coastal and piedmont regions of North Carolina (Bogdan and Weaver 1992; Reichs 1989), lesions characteristic of treponemal disease are readily apparent in these skeletal series and provide additional osteological evidence that some form of treponematosis was endemic in the Southeast before European contact (see also Eisenberg 1991; Powell 1988, 1991a, 1991b, 1992a, 1992b, this volume).

Treponemal disease (e.g., venereal syphilis, endemic syphilis, yaws) is one of the few specific disease syndromes commonly linked with proliferative lesions of the long bones in New World populations (Baker and Armelagos 1988; Lambert 1993; Powell 1988, 1992b, this volume). Although a number of conditions can cause periosteal lesions (see Cook 1976), the overall severity, frequency, and distribution of postcranial lesions in this case is consistent with a diagnosis of treponematosis as the primary (but not exclusive) causal agent. This interpretation is supported by pathognomonic skeletal conditions such as anteriorly bowed ("boomerang") tibiae, gummatous periostitis of the long bones, and cavitating lesions of the cranial vault (Hackett 1967, 1976; Ortner and Putschar 1985; Steinbock 1976) apparent in a number of individuals from these North Carolina/Virginia skeletal series. Indeed, the cranial vaults of six individuals exhibit evidence of late stage infection ranging from discrete cavitation to caries sicca, and those of three others have depressed, circumferential lesions that are more suggestive of cranial syphilis than trauma, indicating a total involvement of approximately 4.5 percent of the observable sample of 201 crania. All are 30+-year-old adults, most from prehistoric sites where tibial lesions are most prominent (Bn-29, Mg-3, Vir-150, Vir-231), and all have affected tibiae. Gross nasal-palatal destruction ("gangosa") that can also accompany tertiary infection (Ortner and Putschar 1985; Steinbock 1976) is absent in these cranial remains, but this could in part be a product of the relatively poor preservation of facial bones in many of these samples. As has been noted for other skeletal series (see Baker and Armelagos 1988; Powell 1988), the absence of evidence for osteochondritis (calcified cartilage at metaphyseal ends of long bones) and

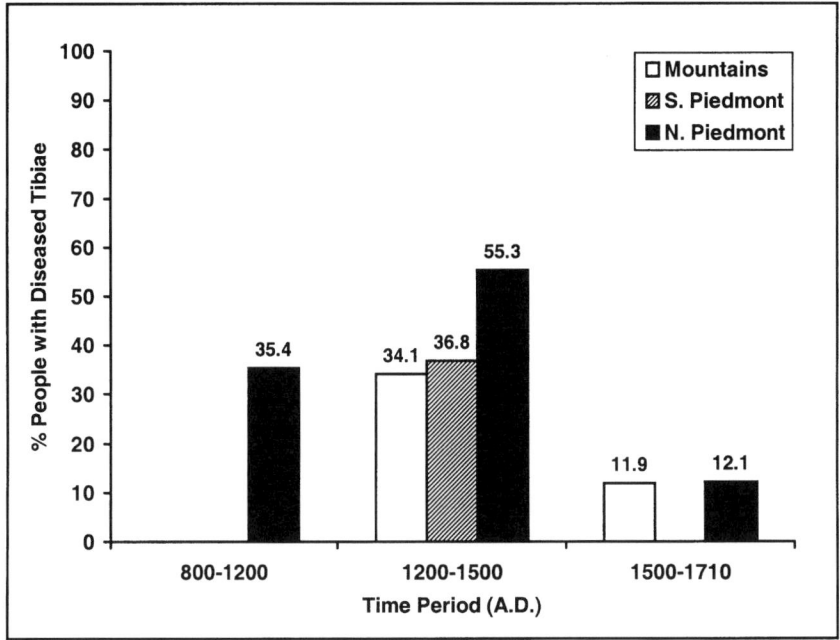

Figure 10-5. Temporal and Geographic Variation in the Frequency of Diseased Tibiae (excludes individuals <6 months; see Lambert 1993). Late prehistoric sample (A.D. 1200–1500) includes 12 individuals with bowed tibiae that lack clearly defined periosteal lesions.

syphilitic dental markers (Hutchinson's incisors, Moon's molars), common characteristics of congenital syphilis (Ortner and Putschar 1985; Powell 1992a, this volume; Steinbock 1976), would tend to implicate a nonvenereal form of the disease. As such, the treponemal syndrome responsible for the observed lesions was likely acquired during childhood through play and other activities that brought children with open sores into intimate contact with those previously uninfected (see Hudson 1965; Ortner 1992).

Comparisons of the frequency of affected tibiae, the bone most likely to exhibit periosteal lesions in cases of treponemal infection (Lambert 1993; Ortner and Putschar 1985; Steinbock 1976) and the long bone most commonly affected with periosteal lesions in the study sample, reveal one distinct geographic variation (Figure 10-5): individuals from later late prehistoric sites (A.D. 1200–1500) on the northern piedmont are more likely to have affected tibiae than individuals from either southern piedmont or mountain villages. This pattern would appear to contradict predictions based on settlement size because northern villages were not larger than villages on the Appalachian Summit and were a good deal smaller than Town Creek. Rates of tibial involvement in some northern piedmont villages (Table 10-1) are quite similar to the rates observed by Powell (1988: Table 33) for the political center at Moundville (50.7 percent) and frequencies recorded by Eisenberg (1991:76) for the large settlement of Averbuch ("over half affected"), but they are much higher than the rates observed by Larsen and Harn (1994: Table 15-1) for late prehistoric agriculturalists from coastal Georgia (15 percent). These data are evidence that a large host population was not essential for the maintenance of high levels of infection in the prehistoric Southeast and provide corroborating evidence that conditions in northern piedmont villages were particularly conducive to the maintenance and spread of disease.

More notable and curious than geographic variations in the North Carolina region is the evidence for a significant decline in the frequency of diseased tibiae from the late prehistoric to the protohistoric/historic period. This is evident in the mountains, where frequencies decline from 34 percent to 12 percent, and even more obviously on the northern piedmont, where a decline from 55 to 12 percent is evident (Figure 10-5).[4] Differences in the age structure of these samples, although present, do not appear to explain this drop in lesion frequency because most affected individuals are adults and comparisons of adults reveal a similar pattern of decline (from 43 to 15 percent). A decline, albeit not as drastic, was also noted by Hogue and Peacock (1995) in skeletal samples from Early and Middle Mississippian times in Oktibbeha County, Mississippi. These data suggest that, after a period of efflorescence associated with the transition to sedentary village living, treponematosis may have begun to decline in severity in some regions of the American Southeast. However, the significant increase in periosteal lesions of the tibiae in missionized populations of the Georgia Bight is evidence that this was not always the case (Larsen and Harn 1994: Table 15-1), and it is equally clear from early eighteenth-century accounts that some form of treponemal disease persisted in the Carolinas well into the historic period (Lawson 1709). It is possible that people in North Carolina and Virginia became more resistant to endemic forms of treponematosis as time progressed, or that less virulent strains of the disease developed through a process of natural selection. Alternately, conditions in the physical environment (e.g., climatic change, particularly cooling) or social environment (e.g., clothing, changes in practices such as sweat baths) may have changed, resulting in conditions less conducive to the spread (or at least, the osteological manifestations) of this nonvenereal infection. Perhaps health improved, but the data on enamel hypoplasia do not support this hypothesis, and it may be that changing patterns of morbidity and mortality had the effect of altering the visibility of this disease osteologically.

According to studies of modern populations, nonvenereal treponematosis does not significantly affect fertility or mortality as does venereal syphilis, and the physical symptoms of ulcers and bone pain are considered by those affected to be "chronic or acute nuisances rather than life-threatening ailments" (Powell 1988:173). A 1988 survey of yaws prevalence in a rural province of Ecuador provides clues to the possible prehistoric prevalence of an endemic form of the disease; in this contemporary South American sample, 90 percent of the population tested seropositive for the pathogen, and more than 10 percent had active lesions (Koff and Rosen 1993). Thus, treponemal disease in the late prehistoric period of this region was likely ubiquitous and troublesome but seldom lethal.

Osteolytic Lesions of the Vertebrae: The Evidence for Tuberculosis

Lesions in human skeletal remains also document the presence of tuberculosis, a more insidious and lethal disease, in indigenous agricultural communities of this region. Both ribs and vertebrae were systematically scored for skeletal signs of this infection (see Buikstra and Cook 1981; Kelley and Micozzi 1984; Ortner and Putschar 1985; Roberts et al. 1994). Unfortunately, ribs were in very poor shape, making it difficult to evaluate prevalence from these skeletal elements.[5] For this reason, the analysis focuses on lesion frequency in vertebral elements.

Osteolytic lesions of the spinal column are present in four prehistoric burials and one historic burial in the study sample. Although such lesions can be caused by a number of pathogenic agents, two pathogenic organisms, *Mycobacterium tuberculosis* and *Blastomyces dermatitidis*, are frequently proffered as causal agents of osteolytic spinal lesions in Southeast skeletal series (see Buikstra and Cook 1981; Eisenberg 1991; Milner 1991; Powell 1988, 1991a, 1991b, 1992a, 1992b, this volume), and together these two diseases probably account for all cases identified here. Both diseases have been identified in skeletal series from Moundville (Powell 1988, 1991a), Irene Mound (Powell 1990, 1991a), and the Averbuch site (Eisenberg 1991), and blastomycosis is known to be endemic to North Carolina (Ortner and Putschar 1985).

In the skeletal material from North Carolina and Virginia, 2.3 percent (5/217) of individuals with 3+ vertebrae exhibit osteolytic activity in one or more spinal elements (Table 10-1). These include two older males (40+ years) and three young adult females (17–25 years). By age and sex, the two males fit the epidemiological profile (30–50 years) for blastomycosis (see Buikstra and Cook 1981; Ortner and Putschar 1985), although their lesions are also consistent with skeletal tuberculosis. One male from Bn-29 has an osteolytic lesion of the first sacral vertebra and extensive remodeling of L4-5. The second male, from Mg-3, has sharply defined osteolytic lesions in the centra of C3, C6, T1, T6,

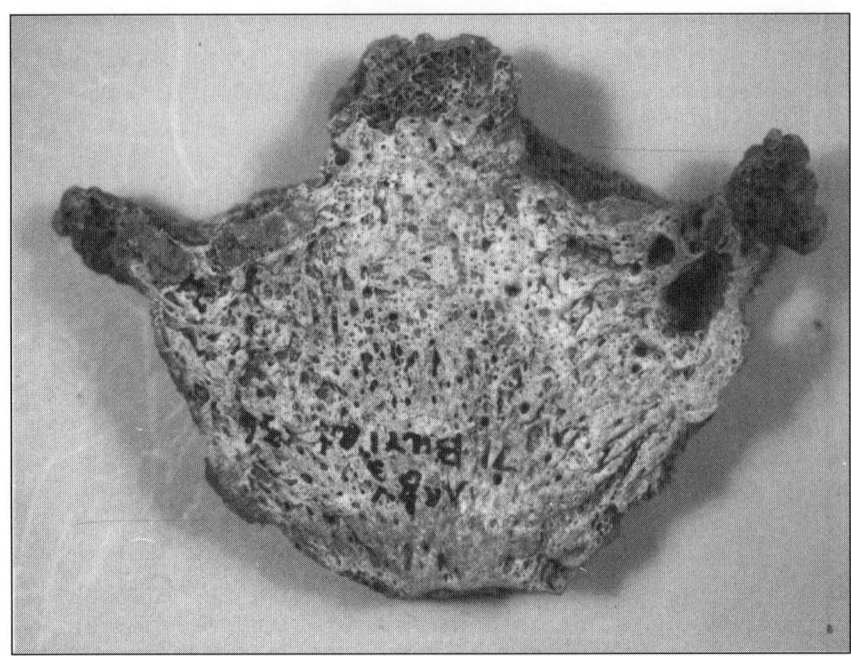

Figure 10-6. Osteolytic Lesions of the manubrium in Burial 46 from Mg-3 (above) and in a vertebra of Burial 5 from Vir-231 (below).

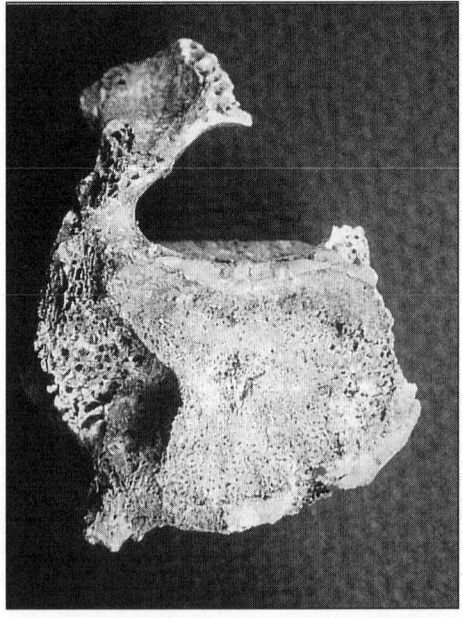

T9, and T12, as well as pathological changes (both osteoblastic and osteolytic) of the manubrium (Figure 10-6). All three females fit the demographic profile for tuberculosis, a disease that favors females over males, particularly during the childbearing years when resistance is reduced due to pregnancy (Youmans 1979:203–204). Their lesions are also consistent with a diagnosis of tuberculosis, being multi-focal in distribution and destructive in nature. A 17-year-old female from Mg-3 has two partially eroded and pathologically fused upper thoracic vertebrae as well as erosive pitting of the acetabular region of both os coxae. A 25-year-old female from Sk-1a has destructive lesions in T-11 and L2-5, and a 21-year-old-female from Vir-231 has osteolytic lesions in L2-S1 (Figure 10-6) as well as in the sternal end of the right clavicle. Given their young age, these three females probably suffered from and likely also died from tuberculosis, and it is quite possible that all five were victims of this disease.

The small size of the affected sample makes it difficult to evaluate geographic and temporal variation in prevalence. No victims are apparent in the early late prehistoric sample, which derives entirely from northern piedmont sites, and it is possible that the disease was absent or uncommon before about A.D. 1200. Epidemiologically, this would be consistent with archaeological evidence that these early agricultural settlements were small and dispersed, demographic conditions less conducive to the maintenance and spread of tuberculosis. Given the low expected frequency of vertebral lesions in tuberculosis (Kelley and Micozzi 1984; Ortner and Putschar 1985), however, it is equally likely that the absence of these lesions in the early sample is simply due to the small size of the early agriculturalist sample. Nonetheless, affected individuals are present in samples from all three regions, which suggests widespread prehistoric occurrence.

Superficially, the lower frequency of tubercular lesions relative to treponemal lesions in these North Carolina and Virginia samples suggests that tuberculosis was the less threatening of the two diseases, and in terms of sheer human misery, this might well be true. In terms of mortality, however, there are reasons to believe that the opposite was the case. As Powell notes earlier in this volume, nonvenereal treponematosis frequently affects but seldom kills infected individuals, whereas tuberculosis is less likely to affect physically but more likely to kill those infected. Archaeologically, these differences in morbidity and mortality would have resulted in the high visibility of treponematosis relative to tuberculosis in mortuary assemblages. An opportunistic infection, tuberculosis also would have targeted and sometimes killed people whose immune systems were compromised by anemia, scurvy, and treponemal disease and might thus have been archaeologically invisible as the killer of these victims. Furthermore,

clinical research indicates that most tubercular infections are pulmonary and do not involve the spinal column (Kelley and Micozzi 1984;
Ortner and Putschar 1985; Roberts et al. 1994), so a frequency of 2.3
percent affected could be indicative of a relatively high rate of overall
infection (see Strouhal 1991). Tuberculosis may thus have been a significant health threat to these agriculturalists and may have been an
important factor in childhood morbidity and mortality.

Summary Discussion

Many of the health problems recorded for human populations throughout the Southeast (e.g., Eisenberg 1991; Hutchinson and Larsen 1988;
Larsen 1983, 1984; Larsen and Harn 1994; Milner 1991; Powell, 1988,
1991a, 1991b, this volume; Reeves, this volume) are evident in human
remains from North Carolina and Virginia. This is good evidence that
political centralization and large settlement size were not always the
most important factors in either the severity or chronicity of diseases
such as dental caries, iron-deficiency anemia, scurvy, treponematosis,
and tuberculosis. Variations within this region further suggest that
variables such as resource distribution, quality of arable land, micro-
climatic variability, and unique cultural practices influenced health
and thus the quality of life in various regions of North Carolina and
Virginia.

Distinct temporal or geographic variations are evident in all of
the health conditions examined in this chapter. Dental disease varies
across both parameters, probably as a result of variability in economic
strategies. Evidence of iron-deficiency anemia, and probably scurvy, is
relatively common overall, but these conditions appear to have been
more of a problem to inhabitants of northern piedmont villages than
to those living elsewhere in the study area. This pattern was probably influenced by differences in subsistence practices but could also
reflect environmental or cultural differences such as unique patterns
of food processing and storage or differences in water supply (spring
versus river) that influenced exposure to gastrointestinal parasites.

Both treponematosis and tuberculosis antedate European contact.
Treponemal disease affects people throughout the temporal sequence,
but it is particularly common in the prehistoric component of the sample; after about A.D. 1500, there is evidence for a decline in the frequency of at least the osteological manifestations of treponematosis,
if not the absolute number of infected individuals. Possibly, improved
diet or sanitation contributed to this decline. Alternately, this pattern
may reflect selection for less virulent strains of the disease. Given the
sensitivity of treponemal organisms to environmental conditions, it is
also possible that climatic change altered the pathogenicity of this dis-

ease. If people were not actually healthier in the early years of European contact, and the data on enamel hypoplasia suggest that they were not, they at least may not have suffered as severely from this familiar endemic disease. Tuberculosis also appears to have been present and likely took its toll, but the spotty, unpredictable distribution of lesions makes interpretations of prevalence difficult.

Life on the periphery was thus fraught with many of the same health problems that plagued more densely settled regions. Indeed, the data presented above suggest that the disease conditions that might be predicted for population centers like Moundville were, at least to some extent, mitigated by the higher overall productivity of these centers— probably in consequence of the greater natural bounty of rich bottomland environments and the greater capacity of their bureaucracies to move resources through the system. Within North Carolina and Virginia, people in smaller agricultural settlements on the northern piedmont appear to have suffered more severely from deprivation and chronic infections than did inhabitants of larger, fortified villages. Once again, this may reflect geographic differences in productivity that constrained population size and viability in the first place, or it may reflect the consequences to health of adopting subsistence strategies that were sub-optimal to the northern piedmont region. In any event, these data support the argument that multiple variables were influencing health in indigenous agricultural communities of this region and further suggest that explanations invoking single-cause explanations in health changes associated with cultural transitions are likely to over-simplify greatly the cause-and-effect relationships in human health and behavior.

NOTES

1. Comparison includes only those individuals with at least two scorable canine teeth; affected individuals exhibit lesions on at least two teeth.

2. Comparison includes all individuals with at least one scorable canine tooth; affected individuals exhibit lesions on at least one tooth.

3. The difference between the prehistoric (A.D. 800–1500) and historic piedmont samples (A.D. 1500–1710) in the frequency of people with at least one affected mandibular canine is statistically significant (X^2=4.518, p=0.034). Confusing this issue, however, are results based on maxillary incisors (although the sample size is smaller): differences in the frequency of hypoplastic incisors are not significant (X^2=.757, p=.384), and affected individuals are actually slightly more common in the prehistoric sample.

4. The difference between prehistoric (mountain/northern piedmont combined) and historic (mountain/northern piedmont combined) samples in the frequency of diseased tibiae is highly significant for both left (X^2=25.054, p<.001) and right (X^2=15.869, p<.001) sides of the bone. Preliminary evaluation

of lesion-frequency for all long bones in samples from the northern piedmont suggests that this pattern is equally strong when all long bones are considered.

5. Seven of 167 individuals that could be scored for rib lesions (despite severe fragmentation in some cases) show signs of either osteoblastic or osteolytic activity. Five of these cases involve visceral rib surfaces: lesions are limited to bone proliferation in two cases and primarily bone destruction in the other three.

ACKNOWLEDGMENTS

I would like to thank Clark Spencer Larsen and Vincais Steponaitis of the Research Laboratories of Archaeology at the University of North Carolina at Chapel Hill for providing me with the opportunity to study the human skeletal remains described in this chapter. R. P. Stephen Davis and Trawick Ward were infinitely patient with my questions on chronology and openly shared information from unpublished texts regarding the location, antiquity, and cultural context of various collections. My thanks to Marianne Reeves, who was great company during the long hours we spent in the archival quarters of the old library studying the collections from North Carolina and Fusihatchee Town, Alabama, and to Elizabeth Monahan, who joined us toward the end of our endeavors and helped in the completion of the North Carolina inventory. Finally, I am grateful for the efforts of two anonymous reviewers, whose thoughtful suggestions greatly improved the quality of this chapter.

I I "Utmost Confusion" Reconsidered: Bioarchaeology and Secondary Burial in Late Prehistoric Interior Virginia

Debra L. Gold

Virginia's best-known prehistoric archaeological excavation took place over 200 years ago, when Thomas Jefferson explored and described a burial mound on his property (Jefferson 1954). Jefferson's work continues to be widely cited as the first example of a careful and problem-oriented excavation strategy in American archaeology (Thomas 1989; Trigger 1989; Willey and Sabloff 1980). As a few recent researchers have noted, this work has not been well recognized for an equally important accomplishment—Jefferson's attempt to interpret the mound in its regional context (Dunham 1994; Hantman and Dunham 1993). Jefferson's mound was one of more than 13 Late Woodland (ca. A.D. 900–1600) accretional burial mounds located in central interior Virginia. This chapter examines mortuary patterning at these mound sites, questioning why large-scale collective secondary burial defined some, but not all, of these burial mounds. I examine the phenomenon of secondary burial and suggest that bioarchaeological analysis can improve our understanding of complex mortuary behavior in past societies.

Jefferson described the burials he uncovered (probably several hundred of them) as "lying in the utmost confusion" (1954:98); it is apparent from his description that he found many collective secondary burial features containing the fragmented and mixed remains of numerous individuals, and these are the only types of burial he describes. Some of the burial areas appear to have contained small amounts of cremated remains in addition to the uncremated bones; others did not contain any evidence of cremation (Jefferson 1954). In this chapter, I want to examine a deceptively simple question: why the mound Jefferson excavated contained these large collective secondary burial features almost exclusively, whereas they are rare or absent in other contemporaneous and culturally affiliated mounds.

In order to address this question, I examine the general nature of secondary burial and argue that bioarchaeological analyses have underexplored utility for the examination of secondary burial. I then present some preliminary results of recent bioarchaeological analysis, comparing collective and noncollective burial features in two late prehistoric Virginia mounds. In the process of examining a question of basic mortuary patterning—how to explain the exclusive occurrence of collective burial features at some Virginia mounds and their absence or limited appearance at others—I present new bioarchaeological information on subsistence and health practices in late prehistoric interior Virginia.

Secondary Burial

Secondary burial is the socially meaningful and prescribed relocation of part or all of a deceased individual from a temporary repository (Metcalf and Huntington 1991). The corpse must be handled by the living at a time removed by weeks or years from the time of death. There is enormous variability in secondary mortuary treatments, and the process may not involve below-ground burial at all, as in cases where remains are elevated or cremated and scattered. In archaeological contexts, secondary burial can be tremendously difficult to identify. Some types of secondary mortuary treatment, especially those with no burial component, leave little or no archaeological trace. Others may be virtually indistinguishable from primary interment, resulting in underreporting of secondary burial and underappreciation of the variety of prehistoric mortuary behavior.

Any definition of secondary burial must include the following characteristics. First, like other forms of ritual, it operates at a number of different levels and may create or transform the social environment as much as, or even more than, it reflects it (Dunham 1994; Jirikowic 1990; Keswani 1989; Metcalf and Huntington 1991). Second, collective secondary burial often requires the collaborative work of large numbers of living individuals. The process frequently involves multiple corpses requiring specific physical treatment and thus brings together the living and the dead in a powerful and protracted way. The secondary processing and interment may include all members of society, or it may be restricted in some way. Finally, the act of secondary burial is typically set in motion by something other than death, and it may be less about the event of death or a single individual's death than about any other type of mortuary treatment (Goldstein 1995). For this reason, analyses that focus exclusively on mortuary behavior may be overlooking important clues to understanding the secondary burial ritual in its larger social context. Bioarchaeological analysis focuses on population characteristics such as diet, health, and genetics that often have more to do with life than with death and thus may be very useful for the interpretation of a mortuary ritual that may also have more to do with life than with death.

There are, of course, some serious limitations to this approach. Bioarchaeological analyses are most powerful when they examine multiple lines of skeletal evidence for any one individual and carefully consider how a burial group relates to an associated living population. In the case of collective secondary burial features where fragmented bones cannot usually be reconstructed to individuals, multiple lines of evidence may be impossible. Nevertheless, analysis based on bioarchaeological examination at the level of the burial population can be tremendously useful in mortuary studies of secondary burial.

ENVIRONMENTAL AND ARCHAEOLOGICAL BACKGROUND

Jefferson's mound was one of at least 13 accretional earthen and earth-stone burial mounds constructed and used in interior Virginia during the Late Woodland period (Figure 11-1). These sites are defined by a series of characteristic traits. They are the only Late Woodland mounds in the area, and all were used for mortuary purposes. All are of earthen or earth and stone construction and are of roughly similar size, and most are located on the floodplains of major rivers or tributaries, many in close proximity to Late Woodland village sites. Ceramic and lithic artifacts deliberately and accidentally included in the mounds suggest temporal and cultural affinity among them (Boyd and Boyd 1992; Dunham 1994; Hantman 1990; MacCord 1986).

Colonial maps and texts (e.g., Barbour 1986) identify interior Virginia as the territory of the Monacan and Mannahoac peoples. Most scholars accept that these were closely related Siouan-speaking peoples, part of a larger Monacan culture in interior Virginia (Mouer 1983; Hantman 1990). All available evidence indicates continuity between the Late Woodland inhabitants who constructed and used the burial mounds and the historically documented Monacan and Mannahoac peoples.

The area in which the mounds are located covers more than 10,000 square miles of central and western Virginia. This area encompasses three distinct physiographic provinces: the Piedmont, Blue Ridge Mountains, and the Ridge and Valley (Figure 11-1). The narrow Blue Ridge

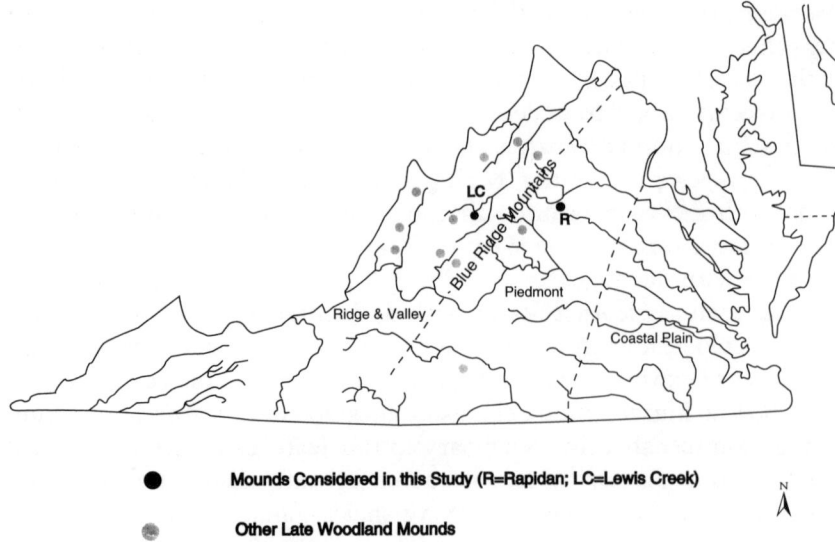

Figure 11-1. Map of Virginia with Physiographic Provinces and Locations of Late Woodland Burial Mounds

Mountain province is approximately 20 miles wide with peaks extending to 4,000 feet above sea level. To the east of the Blue Ridge Mountains is the Piedmont region, consisting of rolling hills at elevations of 300 to 1,500 feet above sea level with fluvial terraces and floodplains. Although only 40 miles wide in northern Virginia, the Piedmont plateau widens considerably at the Virginia/North Carolina border (Fisher 1983). To the west of the Blue Ridge Mountains is the Ridge and Valley Province, characterized by rolling hills and fertile alluvial floodplains. Elevations here range from 1,100 to 1,600 feet above sea level (Dunham 1994; Klein 1994). The Shenandoah, the Rappahanock, and the James are the three major rivers linking the physiographic provinces. These rivers and their tributaries were especially important in Late Woodland times when settlements and subsistence were focused on floodplain locations and resources. These waterways also undoubtedly were an important means of transportation and communication across the mountainous regions of Virginia.

The archaeological record in Virginia shows important changes beginning at approximately A.D. 900 and continuing throughout the Late Woodland period. Prior to this time, native peoples of interior Virginia were primarily hunter-gatherers living in small, seasonally mobile populations. By the Late Middle Woodland period (A.D. 550–900) there is evidence for "incipient sedentism" with seasonal semipermanent settlements and increasing exchange of Middle Atlantic goods, although there is notably little exchange of goods beyond the Mid-Atlantic region (Klein 1994). After A.D. 900, loosely allied permanent settlements were focused on the fertile floodplains of rivers and major tributaries, accompanied by maize horticulture, new technological patterns, and the presence of large communal secondary burial mounds (Barfield and Barber 1992; Dunham 1994; Hantman and Klein 1992). Palisaded villages appear in the Coastal Plain, Shenandoah Valley, and Piedmont regions after approximately A.D. 1200 (Klein 1994; Potter 1993; Walker and Miller 1992).

Hantman has recently examined this evidence and suggested that the late prehistoric inhabitants of this area may have been "an agricultural people, characterized by a dense population, whose mortuary ritual may imply the presence of a centralized and hierarchical sociopolitical system" by the time of European contact in the late sixteenth and early seventeenth centuries (Hantman 1990:684). A rereading of the ethnohistoric documents from the Virginia coastal plain area bolsters the archaeological evidence. On the coast, historical documents describe the Powhatan chiefdom and the workings of its multi-tiered hierarchy in great detail, but the archaeological record thus far contains only limited evidence of this social and political hierarchy (Potter 1993; Turner 1992). It is important to emphasize that researchers who posit some sort of formal ranking recognize great ambiguity in the archaeological and ethnohistoric records and suggest that any such development would have likely occurred late in the Late Woodland period.

VIRGINIA BURIAL MOUNDS

All of the Virginia burial mounds were constructed accretionally, gradually built up over time by the continuous addition of new burial features capped with soil and sometimes also with stone. Despite their similar construction, the mounds present an impressive array of mortuary treatments. Burial treatments present in one or more of the mounds include single and multiple primary interments, cremations, bundle burials, other small secondary interments, and large collective burial features composed of the fragmented and mixed skeletal remains of 30 or more individuals each. Some of the burials were covered by rocks; some, but by no means all, included grave goods. Not all types of interment were used at each mound, but most of the mounds contained several different burial types (Table 11-1). Because of their physical prominence and floodplain locations, the mounds have been affected by looting, land clearing, farming, and erosion for at least 150 years (Dunham 1994).

Because so many of these sites were mostly or completely destroyed without any systematic archaeological excavation, it is difficult to determine patterns in the presence or absence of specific burial

Table 11-1. Mortuary Characteristics of Virginia Mounds

	Primary	Bundle/Sm. Secondary	Cremation	Collective Burial Features	Rock-Covered Burial Features	Deliberate/ Included Artifacts
Bell #1 (44RB7)		X			X	
Bowman (44RM281)		X	X	X	X	X
Brumback (44SH129)	X	X	X	X	X	X
Clover Creek (44HD9)		X	X	X	X	X
Hayes Creek (44RB2)	X		X			X
John East (44AU35)	X	X	X		X	X
Leesville (44CP8)			X		X	X
Lewis Creek (44AU20)	X	X	X			X
Rapidan (44OR1)		X	X	X		
Rivanna (44AB15)		X		X	X	
Withrow #1 (no site number)		X	X	X	X	

Adapted from MacCord 1986

Note: In several cases, the burial mounds were destroyed prior to any archaeological examination, and accounts of mortuary treatment are anecdotal. For this reason, features not marked as present (X) may actually have occurred in these sites.

treatments at the various sites. One distinction, however, is relatively apparent from both recent archaeological research (MacCord 1986; Dunham 1994) and historic descriptions of mound excavations (Jefferson 1954; Fowke 1893, 1894). This is the fact that the large collective burial features were predominant at the two sites in the Piedmont region yet occurred only sporadically in mounds to the west. This is not an insignificant distinction. Mortuary ritual tends to be highly regulated within societies (Morris 1992; O'Shea 1984), and construction of these features required the participation of a large number of living individuals over an extended period of time. Although the burial mounds were built up accretionally over hundreds of years, the large collective burial features within them were used within very short periods of time (most likely days; Gold 1999) and thus would have required a significant investment of labor. In attempting to explain the occurrence of these burial features, I examine a couple of interrelated questions: How does an understanding of the nature of secondary collective burial help explain mortuary patterning in late prehistoric Virginia and, more specifically, why were collective secondary burial features apparently used exclusively at Piedmont mound sites but only sporadically at mounds to the west?

RAPIDAN AND LEWIS CREEK MOUNDS

In order to examine collective secondary burial in the Virginia mound sites, I have studied two different mounds in some detail. The first is Rapidan Mound, located in the Piedmont on the floodplain of the Rapidan River, a major tributary of the Rappahannock. The other is Lewis Creek Mound, adjacent to Lewis Creek in the Ridge and Valley province (Figure 11-1). Rapidan is the only known Piedmont mound other than the one excavated by Thomas Jefferson. Jefferson's mound has never been found again, nor do any collections from it survive, although he did describe his findings in his *Notes on the State of Virginia* (Jefferson 1954), and it is from this description that I and others (e.g., Boyd and Boyd 1992; Dunham 1994; Hantman and Dunham 1993) suggest strong similarities between Jefferson's Mound and Rapidan Mound.

A century of sporadic excavations at Rapidan concluded with the excavation of the last remaining portion of the mound by the University of Virginia in the late 1980s. This excavation revealed two previously undisturbed collective secondary burial features, which were labeled Mound Feature 9 and Mound Feature 10, as well as parts of previously disturbed but otherwise similar features (Figure 11-2). The minimum number of individuals in Mound Feature 9 was 34 and in Mound Feature 10 was 32. There was no evidence for deliberately in-

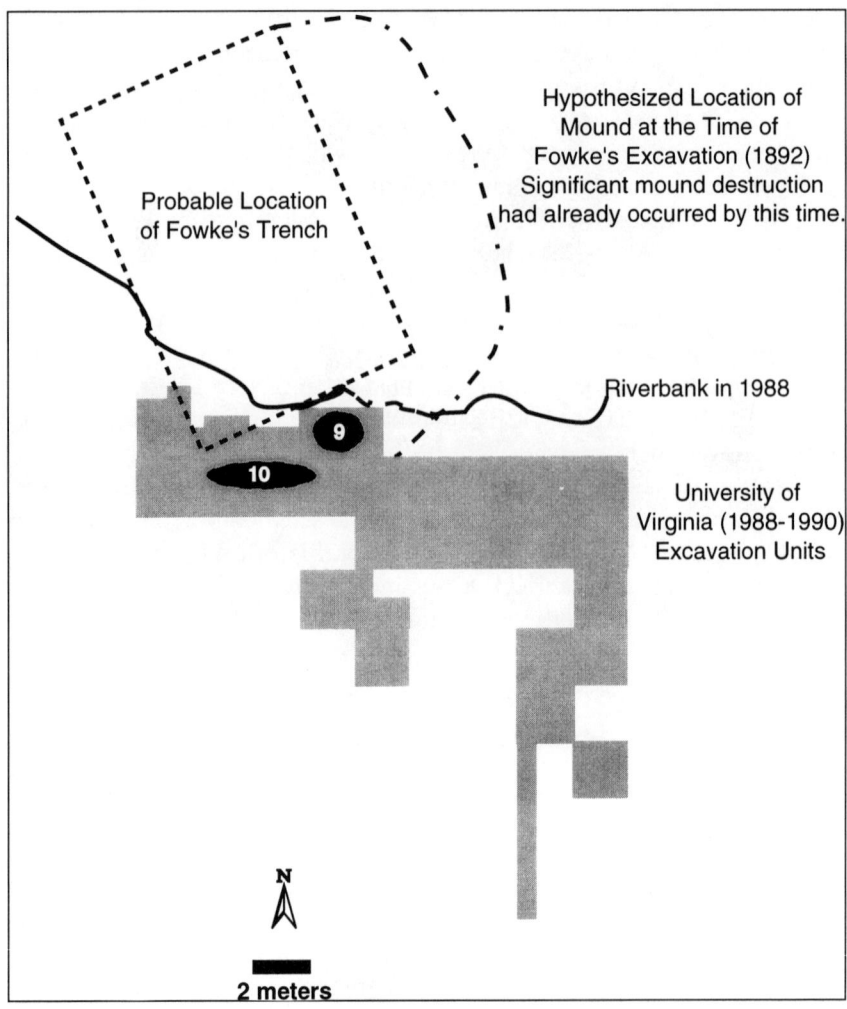

Figure 11-2. Plan View of Rapidan Mound (44OR1)

cluded grave goods with any of the burials or burial features at Rapidan. Small amounts of cremated bones were found in most of the collective burial features (Dunham 1990, 1994; Holland et al. 1983). Radiocarbon dates indicate that these features were constructed and used in the fourteenth and early fifteenth centuries.[1]

Lewis Creek Mound's estimated original size and shape are about the same as Rapidan Mound. Lewis Creek Mound was heavily looted throughout the late nineteenth and early twentieth centuries. When the remnant site was excavated by the Archaeological Society of Virginia in 1964, only the outer edge of the mound remained undisturbed

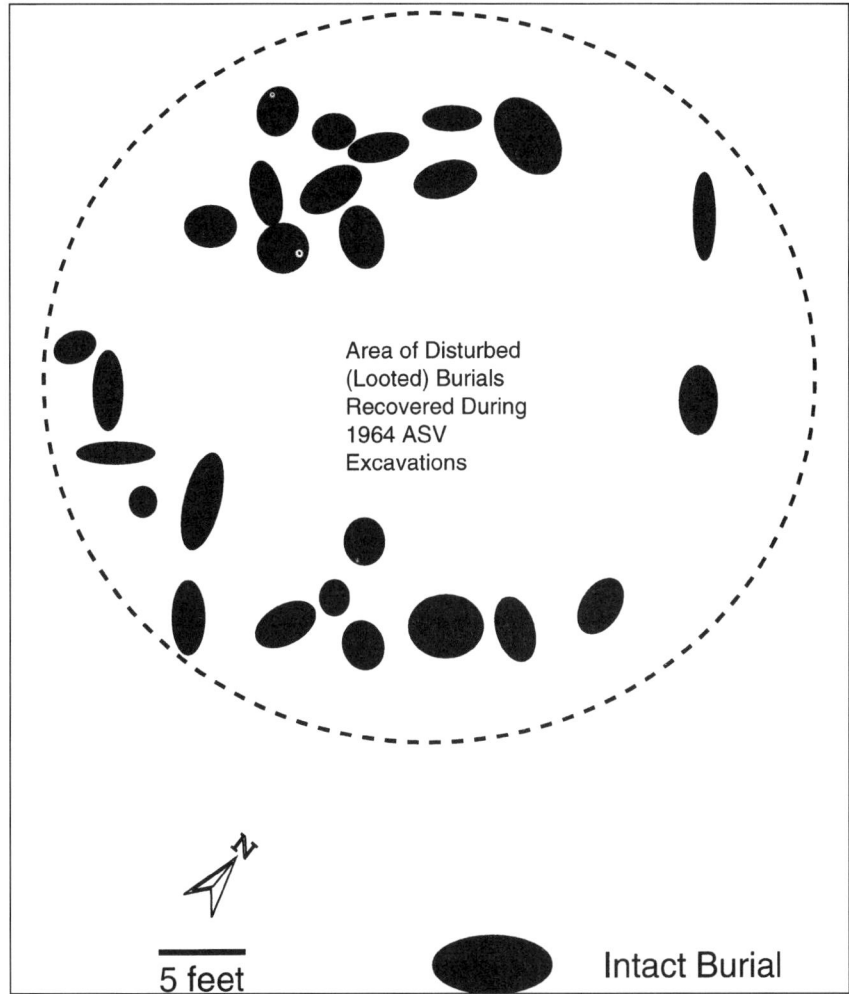

Area of Disturbed
(Looted) Burials
Recovered During
1964 ASV
Excavations

5 feet

Intact Burial

Figure 11-3. Plan View of Lewis Creek Mound (44AU20)

(MacCord and Valliere 1965; MacCord 1986). In this area, the excavators uncovered 26 separate burials containing the remains of 37 individuals. Artifacts, including projectile points, shell beads, and clay and
stone pipes, were found with several of the burials. The excavators also
collected a large number of well-preserved bones and bone fragments
representing a minimum of 124 individuals left by the looters in the
disturbed center portion of the mound (Figure 11-3). Radiocarbon dates
indicate that both areas of the mound date from approximately A.D.
1000 to 1225.[2]

The extant skeletal remains from Rapidan and Lewis Creek Mounds are the most complete and best preserved of the five Virginia mound sites for which such collections exist. The two collections each contain remains of at least 150 individuals, yet these represent only a small fraction, both by number of individuals and by mound volume, of the original sites; the other collections are far more fragmentary. Unfortunately, future discovery of new mounds or additional skeletal collections from any of the known mounds is extremely unlikely.

The preceding discussion has highlighted the differences between Lewis Creek and Rapidan Mounds by describing them in the context of the complex of Late Woodland accretional burial mounds in interior Virginia. Three general hypotheses may be suggested to account for the differences in burial practices between Lewis Creek and Rapidan Mounds, specifically the use of large collective burial features at Rapidan Mound and the absence of such features at Lewis Creek Mound. These hypotheses are:

- The mounds, and the burial features within them, were created and used by populations that were culturally distinct from one another.
- The mounds were created and used by culturally linked populations, but epidemic disease or other widespread social problems necessitated mass burial in the specific case of Rapidan Mound.
- The differences represent a chronological shift within a region composed culturally related populations. The change in burial practices over time is linked to social factors.

The following discussion of bioarchaeology will examine these three general hypotheses. The results of the bioarchaeological study, combined with archaeological and ethnohistorical information from the region, allow us to rule out hypotheses one and two. The bioarchaeology and archaeological data do support hypothesis three, which is discussed in greater detail in the concluding sections of this chapter.

DEMOGRAPHY

Over the years there have been widely varying interpretations of the total number of individuals in the Virginia mounds, with estimates ranging from the low hundreds to the low thousands. A combination of current osteological analysis and historical description may provide the best estimate for the number of individuals interred at Rapidan. Fowke (1894) reported finding 18 distinct collective burial features during his late nineteenth-century trench excavation at Rapidan. From Fowke's brief description of the features he found, they appear to have been very similar in size and composition to the two complete collective burial features excavated by the University of Virginia. Fowke estimated that his trench explored one-quarter of the original mound. If he was correct in this estimation, if the entire mound contained the same density of burials, and if these features were similar in composition to those excavated by the University of Virginia, the original number of burials would have been approximately 2,160[3] (Gold 1996, 1999). Dunham (1994), using a somewhat different set of assumptions, arrives at an estimated minimum mound population of approximately 1,000 individuals. Unfortunately refinement of these figures is not possible with the data currently available; for purposes of this study, it is sufficient to note that Rapidan Mound, and most likely Jefferson's Mound as well, originally contained between 1,000 and 2,000 individuals. There were probably fewer individuals at Ridge and Valley mounds such as Lewis Creek where there was much less collective burial and, consequently, a lower ratio of individuals to mound volume for similarly sized mounds.

Life-table-based reconstruction of demographic patterns was not possible at either Rapidan or Lewis Creek, although for different reasons. Ideally, reconstruction of sex and age at death proceeds from examination and comparison of multiple cranial and post-cranial skeletal markers (Bass 1987; Ubelaker 1989; White 1991). In practice, researchers are frequently forced to make the best of incomplete skeletal remains but still need fair bone preservation and comparable skeletal elements. At Rapidan, the burial features each consisted of the fragmentary, disarticulated, and thoroughly mixed remains of more than 30 individuals. These diverse skeletal elements could not be reconstructed to individuals, and many diagnostic skeletal features were poorly preserved. At Lewis Creek the bulk of the skeletal material was recovered from the central portion of the remnant mound, an area that had been repeatedly disturbed by looters. Although these unprovenienced bones were in an excellent state of preservation, there is no way to rearticulate the individual skeletal elements. Thirty-seven individuals were recovered in situ at the outer edges of the mound, but it is impossible to extrapolate the relationship of these undisturbed fringe burials to the rest of the mound.

Although demographic quantification was not possible, certain qualitative observations can be made. All burial areas at both sites contained both male and female adults. The skeletal remains of all categories of subadults, including infants, were found in the looted area of Lewis Creek Mound. At Rapidan, however, there is evidence to suggest the deliberate exclusion of many subadults, especially infants, from some interment in the mounds. Infants and children were not excluded from the site altogether but do seem to have been included only very rarely. Thomas Jefferson's description of the mound he excavated also suggests very few subadult skeletal remains, and elsewhere I have suggested that this was a characteristic of the Late Woodland burial mounds in the Virginia Piedmont, though not of the burial mounds to the west in the Ridge and Valley province (Gold 1999). The combination of collective burial features with the deliberate exclusion of certain individuals (subadults) occurring only at the western, later mound sites suggests a change in some of the social factors governing mound burial.

SKELETAL EVIDENCE OF SUBSISTENCE

Captain John Smith wrote that the native peoples of interior Virginia were "barbarous . . . living for the most part of wild beests and fruits" (Barbour 1986:165). Smith's descriptions of interior Virginia lifeways were based primarily on hearsay (Hantman 1990), but they have been remarkably persistent. Although recent researchers (Hantman 1990; Mouer 1983) have provided linguistic, historical, and archaeological evidence that Smith was both misinformed and misunderstood, the archaeological evidence for plant cultivation in prehistoric interior Virginia is scanty. Skeletal and dental analyses indicate a mixed subsistence pattern including collection of seasonally available wild plant and animal foods and aquatic resources and cultivation of both native weedy plants and maize (Gold 1994). Skeletal data provide clear evidence for consumption of starchy carbohydrate plant food—maize—throughout late prehistoric interior Virginia. These data and their implications are explored in detail in the following sections.

Stable Isotope Analysis

Trimble (1996) analyzed the stable carbon and nitrogen isotopes extracted from the teeth and bones of more than 130 individuals from all regions of Late Woodland Virginia. Her data indicate that maize was incorporated into the diet during Late Woodland times in all regions. Her Piedmont samples showed that C_4 plants formed no more than 50 percent of the diet. Ridge and Valley samples indicated dietary patterns similar to those of the Piedmont, although perhaps less diverse and more reliant on C_4 plants. Coastal Plain samples showed evidence of the importance of marine resources in the diet, but this was not the case in the Piedmont or Appalachian Valley samples she examined. Trimble also noted that the Piedmont sites in her study showed the greatest evidence of dietary diversity, whereas the Appalachian Valley sites showed the least evidence of dietary diversity. Table 11-2 presents the carbon isotope data for Rapidan and Lewis Creek Mounds. These figures show that most of the Rapidan Mound samples had $^{13}C/^{12}C$ ra-

Table 11-2. Carbon Isotope Data

Sample Number	Feature/ Area of Site	Age	Sex	^{13}C Value (‰)
Rapidan				
OR–1–198C	MF 4	Adult	?	−13.9
OR–1–308C	MF 10	Adult	?	−17.7
OR–1–32C	MF 9	Adult	?	−19.3
OR–1–332C	MF 10	Adult	?	−16.5
OR–1–71C	MF 9	Adult	?	−15.9
OR–1–79C	MF 10	Adult	?	−16.7
Or–1–81	1979 Exc.	Adult	?	−18.9
OR–1–98C	MF 9	Adult	?	−16.9
Lewis Creek Looted				
SI–382.013A		Adult	?	−9.9
SI–382.013B		Adult	?	−14.4
SI–382.013C		Adult	?	−15.3
SI–382.013D		Adult	?	−10.6
SI–382.013E		Adult	?	−11.7
SI–382.014A		Child	?	−12.9
SI–382.014B		Child	?	−12.5
SI–382.014C		Child	?	−13.5
SI–382.014D		Child	?	−10.6

Note: All sites were analyzed by Trimble (1996).

tios indicative of a diet composed of 30 to 50 percent maize, although a few values indicate higher maize consumption. Most of the Lewis Creek Mound samples had ^{13}C/^{12}C ratios indicative of a diet composed of 60 to 80 percent maize consumption.

Dental Caries

Dental caries is the progressive demineralization of dental hard tissues as a result of production of oral bacteria. Untreated dental caries leads to cavities of increasing size and severity, but the progression is typically slow. Carious lesions are most prevalent on posterior teeth because their deeper pits and fissures both trap soft foods and are less easily cleansed by natural means (Hillson 1996; Larsen 1995; Lukacs 1989).

Numerous studies of modern and archaeological populations have demonstrated a link between dental caries and dietary patterns (e.g.,

Larsen 1997). All common types of dietary sugar are associated with increased cariogenicity, as are starches. Diets heavy in sticky-textured, high-carbohydrate foods are the ones most clearly associated with high dental caries rates, and these tend to be agricultural diets. In Eastern North America, maize is the cultigen most clearly associated with high caries rates (Larsen 1987, 1995; Powell 1985).

The method for scoring dental caries in this study is that recommended by Lukacs (1989). All lesions were assigned to one of four size categories: (1) pit/small fissure; (2) medium to large carious lesion (constituting less than half of the tooth crown); (3) large carious lesion (more than half of the tooth crown destroyed), and (4) tooth crown completely destroyed by dental caries with only the root remaining.

One or more carious lesions were present on 18.2 to 29.3 percent of the teeth in this study (Table 11-3). Researchers in the Eastern Woodlands typically report dental caries rates of less than 8 percent of all teeth in prehistoric hunter-gatherer populations and rates of 10 to 50 percent of all teeth in agricultural populations (Larsen 1987). Dental caries rates from Late Woodland Virginia clearly indicate consumption of sticky carbohydrates, and all available archaeological and ethnohistoric evidence suggests that much of this plant food intake would have been in the form of maize.

All carious lesions were categorized according to their severity, as determined by the size of the lesion. Dental caries is a progressive disease, so to a certain extent the size of a lesion is a factor of age, but lesion size also provides a rough indication of the importance of starchy carbohydrates in the diet. "Severe" lesions are defined here as those in which more than half of the tooth crown has been destroyed. Severe carious lesions are extremely infrequent in the Virginia mound samples, occurring on less than 3.0 percent of the molars and in some cases not occurring at all (Table 11-3).

Dental Wear

Except in the most severe cases, attrition of the dental enamel is not a disease process. Rather, it is natural outcome of mastication and of nonalimentary uses of the teeth (Powell 1985:308). Dental wear rates are highly correlated with subsistence practices, both in terms of type of food consumed and food preparation techniques. Generally speaking, hunter-gatherer groups show significantly higher levels of dental wear than do agricultural groups. Dental wear in the Eastern Woodlands tends to decrease with the shift to agriculture due to reduced consumption of hard and abrasive foods, as well as extended cooking made possible by ceramic technology. Food preparation techniques must be examined, however, because in some areas increased use of

Table 11–3. Dental Data

	Rapidan MF 9	Rapidan MF 10	Lewis Creek Intact Burials	Lewis Creek Looted Burials
Total number teeth	374	409	86	2997
Caries frequency (all teeth)	28.2% (N=295)	18.2% (N=356)	29.3% (N=75)	24.8% (N=2745)
Caries frequency (molars)	53.1% (N=111)	38.4% (N=133)	57.7% (N=26)	59.9% (N=1011)
Frequency of severe caries (all teeth)[1]	0%	.8%	1.3% (N=26)	1.4% (N=1011)
Frequency of severe caries (molars)	0%	.8%	0%	2.9%
Frequency of severe wear (all teeth)[2]	8.25% (N=315)	5.00% (N=360)	29.87% (N=77)	13.21% (N=2771)
Frequency of Severe Wear (Molars)	5.50% (N=109)	5.97% (N=134)	19.23% (N=26)	6.27% (N=1021)
Frequency of Severe Wear (Incisors)	9.09% (N=44)	0 (N=49)	12.5% (N=8)	9.34% (N=439)
Frequency of one or more Enamel Defect (Incisors & Canines)	73.4% (N=79)	76.3% (N=97)	69.6% (N=20)	58.2% (N=716)

[1]Severe Caries defined as one-half or more of tooth crown destroyed
[2]Severe Wear defined as score of six or higher on scale developed by Smith (1984)

grinding stones to process maize resulted in increased rates of dental wear (Larsen 1995; Hillson 1996). There is little evidence for food preparation techniques in Late Woodland interior Virginia. Ethnohistoric accounts indicate that the coastal Powhatan peoples used wooden mortars by the early seventeenth century. Other preparation and serving dishes were made of wood as well, although stone implements also appear in the archaeological and ethnohistoric records (Rountree 1989).

All teeth in this study were scored for degree of dental wear based on the eight-stage system developed by Smith (1984). This procedure assigns the continuous variable wear to one of eight discrete categories based on the amount of cusp enamel that has been removed and the amount of dentine exposed on the tooth surface.

It is difficult to find comparative data for dental attrition rates scored by percentage of all teeth rather than by individual. By any measure, however, the amount of dental attrition at both Rapidan and Lewis Creek was low. The percentage of molars with severity of wear scored as six or higher ranged from 5.0 percent to 6.1 percent.[4] Because dental wear is age progressive, low rates of dental attrition may indicate a particularly young burial population. As noted above, the fragmentary and jumbled nature of the skeletal remains at these sites precludes accurate reconstruction of age-at-death patterns. Skeletal evidence is present, however, to indicate that neither of the skeletal collections in this study represents unusually young burial populations. Cranial sutures span the expected range of closure for prehistoric Native American populations (Gold 1994). Furthermore, the frequency of vertebral arthritis in these populations (see below) indicates that the burial population is not skewed toward younger individuals. Similar to the pattern of dental caries, these frequencies seem to be consistent with an interpretation of horticultural resources as a moderately important part of a diet composed of a combination of cultivated and noncultivated foods.

The isotope and macroscopic data presented here do not show exactly the same pattern. The isotope data described are part of a much larger study of stable carbon and nitrogen isotopic composition of bone at many sites spanning approximately 1,600 years in coastal and interior Virginia and North Carolina (Trimble 1996). My examination of the dental data suggests that the apparent greater use of maize in the Ridge and Valley may actually be a result of the small number of mound samples in this overall study. The macroscopic skeletal data indicate that maize cultivation became an important but not exclusive dietary component sometime before A.D. 1100 throughout interior Virginia and remained a consistent dietary staple for the next several centuries. Contemporaneous groups in interior Virginia consumed varying amounts of maize, but there is no apparent temporal trend of increasing or decreasing maize consumption.

SKELETAL EVIDENCE OF HEALTH

Although overall health of the mound populations appears to have been fairly good, the health patterns do vary from site to site. The burial population interred at Rapidan Mound is by most measures the healthiest; these individuals present both the fewest types of pathological lesions and the overall mildest profile of these lesions. Individuals interred at Rapidan exhibited a very low level of skeletal fractures and other traumas as well, although this may be at least partly due to the fragmentary nature of the skeletal remains from this site. Descriptions of the frequency and severity of specific paleopathological lesions are provided in the following sections.

Nutritional Deficiency

Skeletal markers of specific nutritional deficiencies are extremely rare in the Virginia mound collections. The only occurrence of such skeletal pathologies is the presence of mild porotic hyperositis on the posterior cranial vaults of two adult individuals from the undisturbed portions of Lewis Creek and mild cribra orbitalia on the superior eye orbits of one subadult individual from the same area of the same site (Table 11-4). These lesions have multiple etiologies but are commonly indicative of iron-deficiency anemia in the Eastern Woodlands (Larsen 1987). In this case, their low frequency and mild form indicate that anemia was not a significant problem for most of the individuals at these sites. The fragmentary nature of the looted skeletal remains from Lewis Creek Mound and all of the remains from Rapidan Mound may have obscured some evidence of nutritional deficiency. It is also possible that the lack of subadults in the burial populations may account for the low frequency of cribra orbitalia. In general, however, the skeletal evidence suggests that it is unlikely that either iron loss or underconsumption of iron and other essential minerals or vitamins was a significant problem for the populations interred in the mound sites.

Enamel Hypoplasia

Enamel hypoplasia is a condition resulting in linear grooves or pits that form during the development of tooth enamel (i.e., during infancy and childhood). Enamel hypoplasia results from stress sufficient to interrupt normal growth during the years of tooth crown formation. These enamel defects may occur following prolonged nutritional deficiency and/or infectious disease. Although hypoplastic lesions are formed when crown formation resumes after a period of stress-induced inactivity and thus may not appear if an individual died as a result of the stress, they are an excellent indicator of childhood dietary and disease stress (Goodman and Armelagos 1985).

Table 11–4. Paleopathology Data

Pathology	Rapidan MF 9	Rapidan MF 10	Lewis Creek Intact Burials	Lewis Creek Looted Burials
Frequency of Periosteal Lesions (Tibiae)	17.3% (N = 75)	20% (N = 65)	52.9% (N = 34)	60.9% (N = 176)
Periosteal Lesion Severity (Tibiae)	76.9% Mild 23.1% Moderate	61.5% Mild 38.5% Moderate	77.8% Mild 16.7% Moderate 5.6% Severe	50.5% Mild 43% Moderate 6.5% Severe
Osteoarthritis (Vertebral Bodies)	16.9% (N = 83)	8.8% (N = 57)	38.5% (N = 13)	13.2% (N = 517)
Porotic Hyperostosis[1]	None	None	Mild lesions on the posterior crania of 2 out of 13 adult individuals with observable crania	None
Cribra Orbitalia[1]	None	None	Mild lesions of the superior eye orbits of 1 out of 13 subadult individuals	None

[1]Because of the fragmentary nature of the skeletal remains from Rapidan Mound and the Lewis Creek Mound looted area, no total number of observable specimens is provided.

Most of the teeth included in this study were not associated with a particular individual or even with other teeth, so it was often not possible to check for the presence of enamel defects on multiple teeth of one individual. In order to avoid overestimating the occurrence of this defect, I recorded only those lesions that consisted of lines or grooves that covered most or all of a tooth crown circumference, or deep, repeated pitting that was clearly not the result of postmortem processes. All teeth were examined for enamel hypoplasia using a 10× hand lens under a strong light. The frequency of enamel hypoplasia on adult incisors and canines combined varied from 58 percent to 76 percent (Table 11-3).

Periostitis

Periostitis is an inflammation of the periosteum that can result in bony lesions. It may be a response to trauma or infection (White 1991) but usually reflects a chronic, non-life threatening infection rather than a life-ending illness. Periosteal lesions occur most frequently on the long bone shafts, especially the tibia and fibula (Chase 1988). As is true of most archaeological cases, periosteal lesions are by far the most common markers of disease in the Virginia burial mound populations. All periosteal lesions were assigned to one of three stages of severity. Mild periosteal lesions are characterized by raised cortical striations and a few healed lesions. Moderate periosteal lesions are characterized by more frequent lesions, both active and healed. Significant proliferative reactions and involvement (active and healed lesions) of large portions of the bone characterize severe periosteal lesions. At Rapidan, periosteal lesions are visible on 17.3 percent of the tibiae from Mound Feature 9 and 20 percent of the tibiae from Mound Feature 10. Two-thirds to three-quarters of these lesions were categorized as mild, whereas the remaining cases were classified as moderate; none could be considered severe (Table 11-4).

At Lewis Creek, the periosteal lesions were observed on 60.9 percent of the right tibiae from the looted area and over 52.9 percent of all individuals in the in situ area. At this site, mild cases comprised more than 50 percent of the observations. Most of the rest were classified as moderate, but severe lesions were visible on over 6.5 percent of tibiae from the looted area and 5.6 percent of the in situ individuals (Table 11-4).

Osteoarthritis

Mild osteoarthritis of the cervical and thoracic vertebral bodies is fairly frequent at these sites. At Rapidan Mound, 16.9 percent of all vertebral bodies in Mound Feature 9 and 8.8 percent of all vertebral bodies in Mound Feature 10 displayed evidence of mild to moderate osteoarthritic lipping and (in rare cases) partial collapse of the vertebral body. At Lewis Creek Mound, 13.2 percent of the vertebrae recovered from the looted area and 38.5 percent of the vertebrae from intact individuals displayed evidence of mild to moderate osteoarthritis (Table 11-4).

The presence of osteoarthritic lesions in other areas of the body (especially the joints of the appendicular skeleton) is more difficult to quantify because of the fragmentary nature of the skeletal remains. Such lesions are present at both sites, although they appear to be fairly rare. The pattern of osteoarthritis at both Rapidan and Lewis Creek seems consistent with an interpretation of gradual, age-progressive development resulting from repeated minor loading stresses to the back.

In summary, although subsistence patterns remained stable in the study area, health patterns did not. The skeletal evidence indicates that overall population health in the region was good, especially compared to some other areas of the late prehistoric Southeast (e.g., Eisenberg 1991; Milner 1995). The population interred at Rapidan Mound shows less evidence of chronic infection and nutritional disease than the population interred a few centuries earlier at Lewis Creek Mound.

TRAUMA

Three of the crania from Rapidan Mound show evidence of healed, depressed fractures (ca. 1.5–2.0 cm. in diameter) on the frontal and parietal regions.[5] These are the clearest indications of violence among at least a subset of this population. It is important to note that there are no indications of this or any other type of violent trauma in the skeletal remains from Lewis Creek Mound, but the evidence at this point is insufficient to conclude that there was an increase in violence late in the Late Woodland period.[6]

SUMMARY

A variety of evidence suggests that the populations interring their dead at mounds in the Piedmont region invested heavily in burial treatment emphasizing group collectivity over individual identity, especially compared to Ridge and Valley mound sites. The collective burial features are the most obvious sign of this to the modern archaeological eye, but there are more subtle pieces of evidence as well. These include the probable interment of a greater number of corpses in the Piedmont mounds and the underrepresentation of infants and children, who at death may not have reached the appropriate age of inclusion within the group. The absence of grave goods in the Piedmont mounds may indicate a conscious rejection of symbols of individual identity in the communal burial ritual, especially since artifacts were deliberately included in many Ridge and Valley mound interments. What does all of this mean in terms of the central question of this study, that is, how do we explain the fact that, despite close cultural affiliation with the Ridge and Valley, Piedmont populations were apparently the only ones emphatically and consistently engaging in collective mortuary treatment in their accretional burial mounds?

Osteological study allows us to rule out several possibilities. Reconstruction of dietary patterns indicates that the subsistence economy of all of the populations in the mound area was very similar. Although there were regional variations in the amounts of maize and other dietary components, there is no discernible temporal trend within the period of mound use. This study supports the conclusion of previous researchers that the mounds were constructed and used by culturally related populations, even over hundreds of kilometers and hundreds of years (Boyd and Boyd 1992; Dunham 1994; Hantman 1990, 1993, 1998; MacCord 1986). There is no evidence for epidemic disease or similar social problems that might have necessitated or encouraged group burial for the sake of expediency. The exclusion of most subadults from the collective burial argues against expedient burial, as does the overall healthy profile of the Rapidan population, the low level of traumatic lesions observable in these populations, and the complete absence of perimortem trauma.

In summary, the bioarchaeological data indicate an overall similarity in subsistence and health patterns across Late Woodland interior Virginia. The differences that do exist tend to be quantitative rather than qualitative; they are insufficient to explain differences in mortuary patterning between the Piedmont and Ridge and Valley physiographic provinces. I suggest that to understand the predominance of collective secondary burial in Piedmont mound sites we need to look to the culturally related mound sites not only to the west but also to the east and to the Coastal Plain of Virginia.

In 1607, when the English established their first settlement at what became known as Jamestown, the Algonquian-speaking native peoples of coastal Virginia were loosely allied under the paramount chief Powhatan. These people were referred to by the English as the Powhatans, a practice that continues to the present although the Powhatans actually consisted of more than 30 distinct groups dispersed over more than 6,500 square miles (Rountree 1993).

Although Chief Powhatan's power was far from absolute, it was substantial. Powhatan obtained and maintained his power through a combination of physical conquest and intimidation. The relationship of the Powhatans with their neighbors, especially their neighbors to the west, is worthy of consideration here. English colonial texts describe the Monacans[7] most often as the adversaries of the Powhatans. For example, in 1607 a Powhatan guide claimed that "the Monanacah was his Enimye, and that he came Downe at the fall of the leafe and invaded his Countrye" (Archer 1969:88; see Hantman 1993 for a more complete account of descriptions of the relationship between the Powhatan and Monacan peoples).

Archaeological evidence suggests that a cultural boundary between what became the Powhatan and Monacan areas first developed around or before A.D. 900 and was maintained into the seventeenth century (Egloff 1985; Hantman 1993). During this same period, the archaeological evidence indicates some sort of cultural affiliation among the native peoples of the Virginia Piedmont and Ridge and Valley (Hantman 1990). How then do we account for the variety of mortuary treatments evident in Monacan area burial mounds, especially the prevalence of large collective secondary burial features in the Piedmont mounds? I have suggested that to answer this question we must examine secondary burial in general and the specific context of secondary burial in the eastern Monacan area. The large multiple burial features would have served to reinforce notions of group identity both through the collective nature of the mortuary treatment itself and through the necessity of periodically bringing together large numbers of living people to process and re-inter thirty or more corpses at one time (Brown 1995). This emphasis on the collective group appears to have been both stronger and in need of more continuous reinforcement in the east than in populations interring their dead in mounds farther west. Bioarchaeological analysis rules out catastrophic health problems or great differences in subsistence as a possible explanation for these differences. I suggest instead that this emphasis on collective identity may have been related to real or perceived threats to the east, although not necessarily in a one-sided way.

Concluding Remarks

In this chapter I have argued that understanding biological patterns of diet, health, and demography adds depth to any study of the cultural phenomenon of secondary burial, and I have attempted to apply bioarchaeological analysis to the study of collective secondary burial through one very specific case study. I have suggested that bioarchaeological information allows us to rule out certain hypotheses for regional differences in Late Woodland burial mounds in interior Virginia. Bioarchaeological analysis further suggests that the differences may be attributable to social and political factors related to the development and maintenance of a cultural boundary between the Native peoples of the Virginia Piedmont and Coastal Plain.

The construction and use of the mounds in Virginia apparently spans the 700-plus years of the Late Woodland period. Although it is unlikely that most mounds were in use for that entire time, most of them do seem to have been built over hundreds of years and to be intertwined with the social and political changes that took place throughout late prehistoric Virginia (Dunham 1994; Gold 1999; MacCord 1986). Archaeological data suggest that boundaries formed during the early part of the Late Woodland period persisted into the early seventeenth century, and it is on this basis that I have been able to argue that regional differences in mound construction and use may be related to social tensions associated with these boundaries.

Future research needs include a better understanding of the relationship between the mounds and associated village sites, additional bioarchaeological information, and more precise dating of the mounds and the features within them. Despite the preliminary nature of both the data and the specific conclusions I have drawn here, I hope that I have demonstrated the more general utility of bioarchaeological analysis in interpretations of prehistoric mortuary behavior at the regional level.

Acknowledgments

Osteological analysis of the Rapidan Mound was supported by the Virginia Department of Historic Resources, the University of Virginia Department of Anthropology, the University of Virginia College of Arts and Sciences, and the H. H. Rackham Graduate School at the University of Michigan. Osteological analysis of the Lewis Creek Mound was supported by a Smithsonian Predoctoral Fellowship, Department of Anthropology, National Museum of Natural History. Funding for radiocarbon dates was provided by Sigma Xi, a dissertation grant from the Department of Anthropology, University of Michigan, and a Turner Award from the Department of Geology, University of Michigan. For their assistance with so many parts of this work I thank David Hazzard, E. Randolph Turner, Keith Egloff, and Catherine Slusser at the Virginia Department of Historic Resources; Jeffrey Hantman and Stephen Plog at the University of Virginia; Gary Dunham at the University of Nebraska Press; Douglas Ubelaker and David Hunt at the Smithsonian Institution; and Richard Ford, John Speth, Henry Wright, and Milford Wolpoff at the University of Michigan. The comments of Patricia Lambert and two anonymous reviewers are also greatly appreciated.

Notes

1. Based on AMS dates of human bone collagen. The date obtained for Mound Feature 9 is cal A.D. 1295–1400 (one sigma). The date obtained for Mound Feature 10 is cal A.D. 1300–1430 (one sigma).

2. Based on AMS dates of human bone collagen. Two dates were obtained for the intact burials at Lewis Creek: cal A.D. 990–1160 (one sigma) and cal A.D. 1030–1160 (one sigma). One date was obtained for the looted portion of the mound: cal A.D. 1010–1160 (one sigma).

3. This calculation uses an average figure of 30 individuals per collective burial feature.

4. The rate for individuals from the Lewis Creek non-looted area is 19.2 percent, but this is an exceptionally small sample and so presents questionable results.

5. These healed fractures were not found on cranial fragments from Mound Features 9 and 10 but rather were from a collection of skeletal remains excavated from the site in 1979 by the Archaeological Society of Virginia (Holland et al. 1983). These skeletal remains are from a different mound feature, but one that was apparently very similar in all characteristics to Mound Features 9 and 10 (Gold 1995, 1999).

6. Healed, depressed cranial fractures are also found on the frontal bones of three out of sixteen skulls excavated from Linville Mound in the northern Ridge and Valley. This site was excavated in the late nineteenth century (Fowke 1894). The collection of skeletal remains from this site is small, and there are no radiocarbon dates for this site (Gold 1999).

7. Following the lead of researchers such as Hantman (1990, 1993) and Mouer (1983) I use the term *Monacan* to refer to all of the Colonial-era Native peoples of the north-central Piedmont and Ridge and Valley of Virginia. This includes the groups labeled as Monacan and Mannahoac in John Smith's 1608 Map of Virginia (Barbour 1986). For a complete discussion of Mannahoac-Monacan interaction and unity, see Hantman (1993).

References

Adair, J.
1930 *History of the American Indians*, edited by S. C. Williams. Watauga Press, Johnson City, Tennessee.

Allan, M. J.
1996 Tennessee Valley Rock Art Portraying Mississippian Maces. *Southeastern Archaeological Conference Bulletin* 39:17 (abstract).

Alland, D., G. E. Kalkut, A. R. Moss, R. A. McAdam, J. A. Hahn, W. Bosworth, E. Ducker, and B. R. Bloom
1994 Transmission of Tuberculosis in New York City, an Analysis by DNA Fingerprinting and Conventional Epidemiologic Methods. *New England Journal of Medicine* 330: 1710–1716.

Allison, M. J., E. Gerszten, J. Munizaga, C. Santoro, and D. Mendoza
1981 Tuberculosis in Pre-Columbian Andean Populations. In *Prehistoric Tuberculosis in the Americas*, edited by J. E. Buikstra, pp. 49–62. Northwestern University Archaeological Program, Scientific Papers No. 5, Evanston.

Allison, M. J., D. Mendoza, and A. Pezzia
1973 Documentation of a Case of Tuberculosis in Pre-Columbian America. *American Review of Respiratory Diseases* 107:985–991.

Alvord, C. W., and L. Bidgood (editors)
1912 *The First Explorations of the Trans-Allegheny Region by the Virginians, 1650–1674.* Arthur H. Clark Co., Cleveland.

Ambrose, S. H.
1987 Chemical and Isotopic Techniques of Diet Reconstruction in Eastern North America. In *Emergent Horticultural Economies of the Eastern Woodlands*, edited by W. F. Keegan, pp. 78–107. Southern Illinois University Press, Carbondale.
1990 Preparation and Characterization of Bone and Tooth Collagen for Isotopic Analysis. *Journal of Archaeological Science* 17:431–451.

Ambrose, S., and L. Norr
1993 Experimental Evidence for the Relationship of the Carbon Isotope Ratios of Whole Diet and Dietary Protein to Those of Bone Collagen and Carbonate. In *Molecular Archaeology of Prehistoric Human Bone*, edited by J. Lambert and G. Grupe, pp. 1–37. Springer-Verlag, Berlin.

Anderson, D. G.
1994 *The Savannah River Chiefdoms: Political Change in the Late Pre-*

historic Southeast. University of Alabama Press, Tuscaloosa, Alabama.

1996 Chiefly Cycling and Large-Scale Abandonments as Viewed from the Savannah River Basin. In *Political Structure and Change in the Prehistoric Southeastern United States,* edited by J. F. Scarry, pp. 150–191. University Press of Florida, Gainesville.

Angel, J. L.
  1966 Porotic Hyperostosis, Anemias, Malarias, and Marshes in the Prehistoric Eastern Mediterranean. *Science* 153:760–763.
  1974 Patterns of Fractures from Neolithic to Modern Times. *Anthropologiai Kozlemanyek* 18:9–18.

Appollonio, I., C. Carabellese, A. Frattola, and M. Trabucchi
  1997 Influence of Dental Status on Dietary Intake and Survival in Community-Dwelling Elderly Subjects. *Age and Ageing* 26(6):445–456.

Archer, G.
  1969 [1607] Relayton of the Discovery of our River. In *The Jamestown Voyages Under the First Charter,* edited by P. L. Barbour, pp. 80–98. Hakluyt, Cambridge.

Ash, J. E., and S. Spitz
  1945 *Pathology of Tropical Diseases.* American Registry of Pathology, Washington D.C.

Aufderheide, A. C., and C. Rodriguez-Martin (editors)
  1998 *The Cambridge Encyclopedia of Human Paleopathology.* Cambridge University Press, Cambridge.

Baker, B. J., and G. J. Armelagos
  1988 The Origin and Antiquity of Syphilis. *Current Anthropology* 29(5):703–737.

Barbour, P. L. (editor)
  1986 *The Complete Works of Captain John Smith (1580–1631).* Vols. 1–3. University of North Carolina Press, Chapel Hill.

Barfield, E. B., and M. B. Barber
  1992 Archaeological and Ethnographic Evidence of Subsistence in Virginia During the Late Woodland Period. In *Middle and Late Woodland Research in Virginia: A Synthesis,* edited by T. R. Reinhart and M. E. N. Hodges, pp. 225–248. Dietz Press, Richmond, Virginia.

Baron, H., S. Hummel, and B. Herrmann
  1996 *Mycobacterium tuberculosis* Complex DNA in Ancient Human Bones. *Journal of Archaeological Science* 23:667–671.

Bass, W. M.
  1987 *Human Osteology: A Laboratory and Field Manual.* 3rd edition.

Special Publication No. 2, Missouri Archaeological Society, Columbia.

1995   Human Osteology. Missouri Archaeological Society, Columbia.

Baynes, R. D., and T. H. Bothwell

1990   Iron Deficiency. *Annual Review of Nutrition* 10:133–148.

Bellis, V., M. P. O'Connor, and S. R. Riggs

1975   *Estuarine Shoreline Erosion in the Albemarle-Pamlico Region of North Carolina.* University of North Carolina Sea Grant Publication Sg-75-29, Raleigh.

Bender, M. M.

1968   Mass Spectrometric Studies of Carbon-13 in Corn and Other Grasses. *Radiocarbon* 10:468–472.

Bender, M. M., D. A. Baerreis, and R. L. Steventon

1981   Further Light on Carbon Isotopes and Hopewell Agriculture. *American Antiquity* 46:346–353.

Benenson, A. S. (editor)

1995   *Control of Communicable Diseases in Man.* American Public Health Association, Washington, D.C.

Berger, J., D. Schneider, J.-L. Dyck, A. Joseph, A. Aplogan, P. Galan, and S. Hercberg

1992   Iron Deficiency, Cell-Mediated Immunity and Infection among 6–36 Month Old Children Living in Togo. *Nutrition Research* 12:39–49.

Berti, P. R., and M. C. Mahaney

1995   Conservative Scoring and Exclusion of the Phenomenon of Interest in Linear Enamel Hypoplasia Studies. *American Journal of Human Biology* 7:313–320.

Blakey, M. L., T. E. Leslie, and J. P. Reidy

1994   Frequency and Chronological Distribution of Dental Enamel Hypoplasia in Enslaved African Americans: A Test of the Weaning Hypothesis. *American Journal of Physical Anthropology* 95:371–383.

Blakely, R. L.

1977   Sociocultural Implications of Demographic Data from Etowah, Georgia. In *Biocultural Adaptation in Prehistoric America*, edited by R. L. Blakely, pp. 45–66. Southern Anthropological Society Proceedings No. 11. University of Georgia Press, Athens.

1978   Resorptive Lesions in the Prehistoric and Historic Skeletal Samples from Etowah, Georgia (Abstract). *American Journal of Physical Anthroplogy* 48(3):382.

1980   Sociological Implications of Pathology Between the Village Area and Mound C Skeletal Remains from Etowah, Georgia.

In *The Skeletal Biology of Aboriginal Populations in the South-eastern United States*, edited by P. Willey and F. H. Smith, pp. 28–38. Miscellaneous Papers 5. Tennessee Anthropological Association, Knoxville.

Blakely, R. L., and D. S. Mathews

1986   What Price Civilization? Tuberculosis, for One. In *The Burden of Being Civilized, An Anthropological Perspective on the Discontents of Civilization*, edited by M. Richardson and M. C. Webb, pp. 11–23. Southern Anthropological Society Proceedings No 18. University of Georgia Press, Athens.

Blitz, J. H.

1988   Adoption of the Bow in Prehistoric North America. *North American Archaeologist* 9:123–145.

1993   *Ancient Chiefdoms of the Tombigbee.* University of Alabama Press, Tuscaloosa.

Bogdan, G., and D. S. Weaver

1989   Report on the Human Skeletal Remains from the Flynt Site 31 On 305. Wake Forest University Physical Anthropology Laboratory, Winston-Salem, N.C. Ms. on file.

1992   Pre-Columbian Treponematosis in Coastal North Carolina. In *Disease and Demography in the Americas*, edited by J. W. Verano and D. H. Ubelaker, pp. 155–163. Smithsonian Institution Press, Washington, D.C.

Boyd, D. C., and C. C. Boyd

1992   Late Woodland Mortuary Variability in Virginia. In *Middle and Late Woodland Research in Virginia: A Synthesis*, edited by T. R. Reinhart and M. E. N. Hodges, pp. 249–276. Dietz Press, Richmond, Virginia.

Braun, D., D. C. Cook, and S. Pfeiffer

1998   DNA from the *Mycobacterium tuberculosis* Complex Identified in North American, Pre-Columbian Human Skeletal Remains. *Journal of Archaeological Science* 25(3):271–278.

Braund, K. E. H.

1990   Guardians of Tradition and Handmaidens of Change: Women's Roles in Creek Economic and Social Life During the Eighteenth Century. *American Indian Quarterly* (Summer):239–258.

Bridges, P. S.

1985   *Changes in Long Bone Structure with the Transition to Agriculture: Implications for Prehistoric Activities.* Ph.D. dissertation, Department of Anthropology, University of Michigan, Ann Arbor.

1989   Changes in Activities with the Shift to Agriculture in the Southeastern United States. *Current Anthropology* 30:385–394.

1991   Degenerative Joint Disease in Hunter-Gatherers and Agricultu-
        ralists from the Southeastern United States. *American Journal
        of Physical Anthropology* 85:379–391.
1992   Prehistoric Arthritis in the Americas. *Annual Review of An-
        thropology* 21:67–91.
1994   Vertebral Arthritis and Physical Activities in the Prehistoric
        Southeastern United States. *American Journal of Physical An-
        thropology* 93:83–94.
1996   Warfare and Mortality at Koger's Island, Alabama. *Interna-
        tional Journal of Osteoarchaeology* 6:66–75.

Briggs, J.
1974   *Marine Zoogeography.* McGraw-Hill, New York.

Brothwell, D. R.
1970   The Real History of Syphilis. *Science Journal* 6(9):27–33.

Brothwell, D. R., and R. Burleigh
1975   Radiocarbon Dates and the History of Treponematoses in
        Man. *Journal of Archaeological Science* 2:393–396.

Brown, J.
1995   On Mortuary Analysis—with Special Reference to the Saxe-
        Binford Research Program. In *Regional Approaches to Mortuary
        Analysis,* edited by L. A. Beck, pp. 3–28. Plenum Press, New
        York.

Brues, A.
1957   Skeletal Material from the Nagle Site. *Bulletin of the Okla-
        homa Anthropological Society* 5:93–99.
1958   Skeletal Material from the Horton Site. *Bulletin of the Okla-
        homa Anthropological Society* 6:27–32.
1959   Skeletal Material from the Morris Site (Ck-39). *Bulletin of the
        Oklahoma Anthropological Society* 7:63–70.

Buikstra, J. E.
1977   Biocultural Dimensions of Archaeological Study: A Regional
        Perspective. In *Biocultural Adaptation in Prehistoric America,*
        edited by R. L. Blakely, pp. 67–84. Southern Anthropological
        Society Proceedings No. 11. University of Georgia Press,
        Athens.
1981   *Prehistoric Tuberculosis in the Americas* (editor) Northwestern
        University Archaeological Program, Scientific Papers No. 5.
        Evanston.
1991   Out of the Appendix and Into the Dirt: Comments on Thir-
        teen Years of Bioarchaeological Research. In *What Mean These
        Bones?,* edited by M. L. Powell, P. S. Bridges, and A. M. W.
        Mires, pp. 172–188. University of Alabama Press, Tuscaloosa.
1992   Diet and Disease in Late Prehistory. In *Disease and Demogra-*

phy in the Americas, edited by J. W. Verano and D. H. Ubelaker, pp. 87–101. Smithsonian Institution Press, Washington, D.C.

Buikstra, J. E., W. Autry, E. Breitburg, L. Eisenberg, and N. van der Merwe

1988   Diet and Health in the Nashville Basin: Human Adaptation and Maize Agriculture in Middle Tennessee. In *Diet and Subsistence: Current Archaeological Perspectives,* edited by B. V. Kennedy and G. M. LeMoine, pp. 243–269. University of Calgary Archaeological Association, Calgary, Alberta.

Buikstra, J. E., and D. C. Cook

1978   Pre-Columbian Tuberculosis: An Epidemiological Approach. *Medical College of Virginia Quarterly* 14:32–44.

1980   Paleopathology: An American Account. *Annual Review of Anthropology* 9:433–470.

1981   Pre-Columbian Tuberculosis in West-central Illinois: Prehistoric Disease in Biocultural Perspective. In *Prehistoric Tuberculosis in the Americas,* edited by J. E. Buikstra, pp. 161–172. Northwestern University Archaeological Program, Scientific Papers No. 5. Evanston.

Buikstra, J. E., and J. H. Mielke

1985   Demography, Diet, and Health. In *The Analysis of Prehistoric Diets,* edited by R. I. Gilbert, Jr., and J. H. Mielke, pp. 359–422. Academic Press, Orlando.

Buikstra, J. E., and G. R. Milner

1991   Isotopic and Archaeological Interpretations of Diet in the Central Mississipi Valley. *Journal of Archaeological Science* 18:319–329.

Buikstra, J. E., and D. H. Ubelaker (editors)

1994   *Standards for Data Collection from Human Skeletal Remains.* Arkansas Archaeological Survey Research Series No. 44. Fayetteville.

Buikstra, J. E., and S. Williams

1991   Tuberculosis in the Americas: Current Perspectives. In *Human Paleopathology: Current Syntheses and Future Options,* edited by D. J. Ortner and A. C. Aufderheide, pp. 161–172. Smithsonian Institution Press, Washington, D.C.

Bullen, A. K.

1972   Paleoepidemiology and Distribution of Prehistoric Treponemiasis (Syphilis) in Florida. *Florida Anthropologist* 25:133–175.

Bush, H., and M. Zvelebil (editors)

1991   *Health in Past Societies: Biocultural Interpretations of Human Skeletal Remains in Archaeological Contexts.* BAR International Series 567. British Archaeological Reports, Oxford.

Bushnell, A. T.
    1994   *Situado and Sabana: Spain's Support System for the Presidio and
            Mission Provinces of Florida.* Anthropological Paper No. 74.
            American Museum of Natural History, New York.
Butler, C. S.
    1936   *Syphilis Sive Morbus Humanus—A Rationalization of Yaws So-
            Called.* Science Press Printing Co., Lancaster.
Caldwell, J., and C. McCann
    1941   *Irene Mound Site, Chatham County, Georgia.* University of Geor-
            gia Press, Athens.
Carlson, D. S., G. J. Armelagos, and D. P. Van Gerven
    1974   Factors Influencing the Etiology of Cribra Orbitalia in Prehis-
            toric Nubia. *Journal of Human Evolution* 3:405–410.
Cassidy, C. M.
    1972   *A Comparison of Nutrition and Health in Preagricultural and
            Agricultural Amerindian Skeletal Populations.* Ph.D. disserta-
            tion, Department of Anthropology, University of Wisconsin,
            Madison.
    1984   Skeletal Evidence for Prehistoric Subsistence Adaptation in the
            Central Ohio River Valley. In *Paleopathology at the Origins of
            Agriculture,* edited by M. N. Cohen and G. J. Armelagos, pp.
            307–345. Academic Press, Orlando.
Chase, J. W.
    1988   *A Comparison of Signs of Nutritional Stress in Prehistoric Popu-
            lations of the Potomac Piedmont and Coastal Plain.* Ph.D. disser-
            tation, American University. University Microfilms, Ann
            Arbor.
Child, A. M., D. E. Minnikin, A. M. S. Ahmed, M. S. Copley, and A.
Chamberlain
    1997   Mycolic acids—biomarkers for Ancient Tuberculosis. Paper
            presented at the International Congress, "The Evolution and
            Paleoepidemiology of Tuberculosis," Szeged, Hungary.
Chulay, J. D.
    1990   Treponema Species (Yaws, Pinta, Bejel). In *Principles and Prac-
            tice of Infectious Diseases,* edited by G. L. Mandell, R. G.
            Douglas, Jr., and J. E. Bennett, pp. 1808–1816. Churchill
            Livingstone, New York.
Claassen, S.
    1986   Shellfishing Seasons in the Prehistoric Southeastern United
            States. *American Antiquity* 51:21–37.
Clark, G. A., M. A. Kelley, J. M. Grange, and M. C. Hill
    1987   The Evolution of Mycobacterial Disease in Human Popula-
            tions: A Reevaluation. *Current Anthropology* 28:45–62.

Clark, W., and A. Zisa
  1976 Physiographic Map of Georgia. Georgia Department of Natural
        Resources, Atlanta.
Cockburn, T. A.
  1963 The Origins of the Treponematoses. *Bulletin of the World
        Health Organization* 24:221–228.
Coe, J. L.
  1995 *Town Creek Indian Mound.* University of North Carolina
        Press, Chapel Hill.
Coe, J. L., M. Ward, H. T. Graham, L. Navey, S. H. Hogue, and J.
Wilson
  1982 Archeological and Paleo-osteological Investigations at the Cold
        Morning Site, New Hanover, NC. Research Laboratories of An-
        thropology, University of North Carolina at Chapel Hill. Ms.
        on File.
Cohen, M. N., and G. J. Armelagos (editors)
  1984 *Paleopathology at the Origins of Agriculture.* Academic Press,
        Orlando, Florida.
Cole, G., and C. H. Allbright
  1983 Summerville I–II Fortifications. In *Excavations in the Lubbub
        Creek Archaeological Locality.* Vol. I of *Prehistoric Agricultural
        Communities in West Central Alabama,* edited by C. S. Peebles,
        pp. 140–196. University of Michigan, Ann Arbor.
Cook, D. C.
  1976 *Pathologic States and Disease Process in Illinois Woodland Popu-
        lations: An Epidemiologic Approach.* Ph.D. dissertation, Univer-
        sity of Chicago, Chicago.
  1984 Subsistence and Health in the Lower Illinois Valley: Osteologi-
        cal Evidence. In *Paleopathology at the Origins of Agriculture,* ed-
        ited by M. N. Cohen and G. J. Armelagos, pp. 237–270. Aca-
        demic Press, Orlando.
  1990 Epidemiology of Circular Caries: A Perspective from Prehis-
        toric Skeletons. In *A Life in Science: Papers in Honor of J.
        Lawrence Angel,* edited by J. E. Buikstra, pp. 64–84. Center for
        American Archaeology, Kampsville.
  1994 Dental Evidence for Congenital Syphilis (and its Absence) Be-
        fore and After the Conquest of the New World. In *L'Origine
        de la Syphilis en Europe, avant ou après 1493?,* edited by O.
        Dutour, G. Palfi, J. Berato, and J.-P. Brun, pp. 169–175. Edi-
        tions Errance, Paris.
  1998 Syphilis. Not Quite: Paleoepidemiology in an Evolutionary
        Context in the Midwest. Paper presented at the 67th Annual
        Meeting of the American Association of Physical Anthropolo-
        gists, Salt Lake City, Utah.

Cook, D. C., and J. E. Buikstra
    1979   Health and Differential Survival in Prehistoric Populations:
            Prenatal Dental Defects. *American Journal of Physical Anthro-
            pology* 51:649–664.
Cook, F. C.
    1966   *The 1966 Excavations at the Lewis Creek Site.* University of
            Georgia, Laboratory of Archaeology, Research Manuscript No.
            274.
    1970   *The 1970 Excavation at the Townsend Mound.* University of
            Georgia, Laboratory of Archaeology, Research Manuscript No.
            275.
    1978   *The Kent Mound: A Study of the Irene Phase on the Lower Geor-
            gia Coast.* M.A. thesis, Florida State University, Tallahassee.
Cook, F. C, and C. E. Pearson
    1973   *Three Late Savannah Burial Mounds in Glynn County, Georgia.*
            University of Georgia, Laboratory of Archaeology, Research
            Manuscript No. 276.
Crook, M. R., Jr.
    1984   Evolving Community Organization on the Georgia Coast. *Jour-
            nal of Field Archaeology* 11:247–263.
    1986   *Mississippi Period Archaeology of the Georgia Coastal Zone.* Uni-
            versity of Georgia, Laboratory of Archaeology Series, Report
            No. 23.
Crosby, A. W., Jr.
    1969   The Early History of Syphilis: A Reappraisal. *American Anthro-
            pologist* 71:218–227.
Cushing, F. H.
    1897   Exploration of Ancient Key Dwellers' Remains on the Gulf
            Coast of Florida. *Proceedings of the American Philosophical Soci-
            ety* 25:329–432.
Daly, M.
    1989   Anemia in the Elderly. *American Family Physician* 39:129–136.
Dannenberg, A. M., Jr.
    1994   Pathogenesis and Immunology: Basic Aspects. In *Tuberculosis,*
            3rd edition, edited by D. Schlossberg, pp. 17–40. Springer-
            Verlag, Berlin.
Davis, R. P. S., J. Eastman, and T. O. Maher
    1997   *Archaeological Investigations at the Stockton Site in Henry
            County, Virginia.* Research Report No. 14, Research Laborato-
            ries of Anthropology, University of North Carolina, Chapel
            Hill.
DeJarnette, D. L., and C. S. Peebles
    1970   The Development of Alabama Archaeology: The Snow's Bend
            Site. *Journal of Alabama Archaeology* 16:77–119.

DeNiro, M.
   1985   Postmortem Preservation and Alteration of In Vivo Bone Colla-
          gen Isotope Ratios in Relation to Paleodietary Reconstruction.
          Nature 317:806–809.
DeNiro, M., and S. Epstein
   1978   Influence of Diet on the Distribution of Carbon Isotopies in
          Animals. *Geochimica et Cosmochimica Acta* 42:495–506.
   1981   Influence of Diet on the Distribution of Nitrogen Isotopes in
          Animals. *Geochimica et Cosmochimica Acta* 45:341–351.
DePratter, C. B.
   1976   Settlement Data from Skidaway Island: Possible Implications.
          Paper presented at the Annual Meeting of the Southern An-
          thropological Society.
   1978   Prehistoric Settlement and Subsistence Systems, Skidaway
          Island, Georgia. *Early Georgia* 6:65–80.
   1979   Ceramics. In *The Anthropology of St. Catherines Island: 2. The
          Refuge-Deptford Mortuary Complex*, edited by D. H. Thomas
          and C. S. Larsen, pp. 109–132. Anthropological Papers of the
          American Museum of Natural History 56 (part 1).
   1991   *W.P.A. Archaeological Excavations in Chatham County, Georgia:
          1937–1942.* University of Georgia, Laboratory of Archaeology
          Series, Report No. 29.
   n.d.   An Archaeological Survey of Ossabaw Island, Chatham
          County, Georgia. Unpublished manuscript.
Desowitz, R. S.
   1997   *Who Gave Pinta to the Santa Maria? Torrid Diseases in a Temper-
          ate World.* W. W. Norton and Co., New York.
Despommier, D., R. Gwadz, and P. J. Hotez
   1995   *Parasitic Diseases.* 3rd edition. Springer-Verlag, Berlin, Ger-
          many.
Dickens, R. S., H. T. Ward, and R. P. S. Davis, Jr.
   1987   *The Siouan Project: Seasons I and II.* Monograph Series 1, Re-
          search Laboratories of Anthropology, University of North Caro-
          lina, Chapel Hill.
Dimmick, F. R.
   1989   A Survey of Upper Creek Sites in Central Alabama. *Journal of
          Alabama Archaeology* 35:1–86.
Dockall, H. D., and D. G. Steele
   1995   Occurrence of Treponemal Lesions among Prehistoric Hunters
          and Gatherers of the Western Margin of the Gulf of Mexico.
          Paper presented at the 64th Annual Meeting of the American
          Association of Physical Anthropologists, Oakland.
Dunham, G. D.
   1990   Excavations at 44-OR-1, 1988–1990: Ritual Patterning at a

Late Woodland Burial Mound. Report on File, Virginia Department of Historic Resources, Richmond.

1994 *Common Ground, Contesting Visions: The Emergence of Burial Mound Ritual in Late Prehistoric Central Virginia.* Ph.D. dissertation, University of Virginia. University Microfilms, Ann Arbor.

Dunn, F. L.
1965 On the Antiquity of Malaria in the Western Hemisphere. *Human Biology* 37:385–393.

Dunn, M. E.
1981 Botanical Remains from the Cemochechobee Site. In *Cemochechobee: Archaeology of a Mississippian Ceremonial Center on the Chattahootchee River,* by F. T. Schell, V. J. Knight, Jr., and G. S. Schnell, pp. 252–255. University of Florida Press, Gainesville.

Duray, S. M.
1990 Deciduous Enamel Defects and Caries Susceptibility in a Prehistoric Ohio Population. *American Journal of Physical Anthropology* 81:27–34.

Dutour, O., G. Palfi, J. Berato, and J.-P. Brun (editors)
1994 *L'Origine de la Syphilis en Europe, avant ou après 1493?* Editions Errance, Paris.

Dye, D. H.
1990 Warfare in the Sixteenth-Century Southeast: The de Soto Expedition in the Interior. In *Columbian Consequences: Archaeological and Historical Perspectives on the Spanish Borderlands East,* vol. 2, edited by D. H. Thomas, pp. 211–222. Smithsonian Institution Press, Washington, D.C.

Eastman, J. M.
1994 The North Carolina Radiocarbon Date Study, Parts 1 and 2. *Southern Indian Studies* 42.

Egloff, B. J.
1971 *Methods and Problems of Mound Exploration in the Southern Appalachian Area.* M.A. thesis, University of North Carolina, Chapel Hill.

Egloff, K. T.
1985 Spheres of Cultural Interaction Across the Coastal Plain of Virginia in the Woodland Period. In *Structure and Process in Southeastern Archaeology,* edited by R. S. Dickens, Jr., and H. T. Ward, pp. 229–242. University of Alabama Press, Tuscaloosa.

Eichner, E. R.
1989 Does Running Cause Osteoarthritis? *The Physician and Sports Medicine* 17(3):147–154.

Eisenberg, L. E.
1986 The Patterning of Trauma at Averbuch: Activity Levels and

Conflict During the Mississippian Period. Paper presented at the 55th Annual Meetings, American Association of Physical Anthropologists, Albuquerque.

1991 Mississippian Cultural Terminations in Middle Tennessee: What the Bioarchaeological Evidence Can Tell Us. In *What Mean These Bones?*, edited by M. L. Powell, P. S. Bridges, and A. M. W. Mires, pp. 70–88. University of Alabama Press, Tuscaloosa.

El-Najjar, M. Y.
1979 Human Trepomenatosis and Tuberculosis: Evidence from the New World. *American Journal of Physical Anthropology* 51:599–618.

Ensor, B. E., and J. D. Irish
1995 Hypoplastic Area Method for Analyzing Dental Enamel Hypoplasia. *American Journal of Physical Anthropology* 98:507–517.

Ezzo, J. A., C. S. Larsen, and J. H. Burton
1995 Elemental Signatures of Human Diets from the Georgia Bight. *American Journal of Physical Anthropology* 98:471–481.

Farer, L. S., A. M. Lowell, and M. P. Meador
1979 Extrapulmonary Tuberculosis in the United States. *American Journal of Epidemiology* 109:205–209.

Farley, J.
1993 Schistosomiasis. In *The Cambridge World History of Human Disease*, edited by K. F. Kiple, pp. 992–997. Cambridge University Press, Cambridge, England.

Farley, P. C., and J. Foland
1990 Iron Deficiency Anemia. *Postgraduate Medicine* 87:89–101.

Feest, C. F.
1978 North Carolina Algonquians. In *Handbook of the North American Indians.* Vol. 15 (Northeast), edited by B. G. Trigger, pp. 271–281. Smithsonian Institution Press, Washington, D.C.

Filon, D., M. Faerman, P. Smith, and A. Oppenheim
1995 Sequence Analysis Reveals a B-Thalassaemia Mutation in the DNA of Skeletal Remains from the Archaeological Site of Akhziv, Israel. *Nature Genetics* 9:365–368.

Fisher, H. G.
1983 The Virginia Piedmont—A Definition: A Review of the Physiographic Attributes and Historic Land Use of this Region. In *Piedmont Archaeology*, edited by J. M. Wittkofski and L. E. Browning, pp. 2–8. Archaeological Society of Virginia Special Publication No. 10.

Fowke, G.
1893 Aboriginal Remains of the Piedmont and Valley Region of Virginia. *American Antiquity* 6:415–422.

1894   *Archeologic Investigations in the James and Potomac Valleys.* Bureau of American Ethnology Bulletin 23. U.S. Government Printing Office, Washington, D.C.

Fritz, G. J.

1993   Early and Middle Woodland Period Paleoethnobotany. In *Foraging and Farming in the Eastern Woodlands*, edited by C. M. Scarry, pp. 39–56. University Press of Florida, Gainesville.

Fundaburk, E. L., and M. D. Foreman

1957   *Sun Circles and Human Hands: The Southeastern Indians—Art and Industries.* E. L. Fundaburk, Luverne, Alabama.

Gardner, W. M.

1966   The Waddells Mill Pond Site. *Florida Anthropologist* 19:43–64.

Garten, A. M. A.

1997   *Skeletal Evidence for Tuberculosis and Treponematosis in a Fort Ancient Population.* M.A. thesis, Department of Anthropology, University of Kentucky, Lexington.

Giro, C. M.

1947   Enamel Hypoplasia in Human Teeth: An Examination of Its Causes. *American Dental Association Journal* 34:310–317.

Glazier, E. W., Jr.

1986   Late Woodland Plant Food Utilization Along the Central North Carolina Coast. Paper Presented at the Annual Meeting of the Southern Anthropological Society, April.

Goggin, J. M., and W. T. Sturtevant

1964   The Calusa: A Stratified Nonagricultural Society (with notes on sibling marriage). In *Explorations in Cultural Anthropology: Essays in Honor of George Peter Murdock*, edited by W. Goodenough, pp. 179–219. McGraw-Hill, New York.

Gold, D. L.

1994   Late Prehistoric Subsistence in Piedmont Virginia: Evidence from the Rapidan Mound Site. Paper presented at the 51st annual meeting of the Southeastern Archaeological Conference, Lexington, Kentucky.

1995   Late Prehistoric Sociopolitical Organization in Piedmont Virginia. Paper presented at the 60th annual meeting of the Society for American Archaeology, Minneapolis, Minnesota.

1996   "Persons Fallen in Battle or . . . the Common Sepulcher of a Town?": Interpreting Late Woodland Demography in Interior Virginia. Paper presented at the 53rd annual meeting of the Southeastern Archaeological Conference, Birmingham, Alabama.

1999   *Subsistence, Health and Emergent Inequality in Late Prehistoric Interior Virginia.* Ph.D. dissertation, University of Michigan, Ann Arbor.

Goldstein, L. G.
    1995   Landscapes and Mortuary Practices: A Case for Regional Per-
           spectives. In *Regional Approaches to Mortuary Analysis*, edited
           by L. A. Beck, pp. 101–124. Plenum Press, New York and
           London.
Goldstein, M. S.
    1957   Skeletal Pathology of Early Indians in Texas. *American Jour-
           nal of Physical Anthropology* 15:299–312.
Goodman, A. H.
    1991   Stress, Adaptation, and Enamel Developmental Defects. In *Hu-
           man Paleopathology: Current Syntheses and Future Options*, ed-
           ited by D. J. Ortner and A. C. Aufderheide, pp. 280–287.
           Smithsonian Institution Press, Washington, D.C.
    1994   Cartesian Reductionism and Vulgar Adaptationism: Issues
           in the Interpretation of Nutritional Status in Prehistory. In
           Paleonutrition: The Diet and Health of Prehistoric Americans, ed-
           ited by K. D. Sobolik, pp. 163–177. Southern Illinois Univer-
           sity at Carbondale, Center for Archaeological Investigations,
           Occasional Paper No. 22.
Goodman, A. H., and G. J. Armelagos
    1985   Factors Affecting the Distribution of Enamel Hypoplasias
           Within the Human Permanent Dentition. *American Journal of
           Physical Anthropology* 68:479–493.
Goodman, A. H., G. J. Armelagos, and J. C. Rose
    1980   Enamel Hypoplasias as Indicators of Stress in Three Prehis-
           toric Populations from Illinois. *Human Biology* 52:515–528.
Goodman, A. H., D. L. Martin, G. J. Armelagos, and G. Clark
    1984   Indicators of Stress from Bone and Teeth. In *Paleopathology at
           the Origins of Agriculture*, edited by M. N. Cohen and G. J.
           Armelagos, pp. 13–49. Academic Press, Orlando.
Goodman, A. H., and J. C. Rose
    1990   Assessment of Systemic Physiological Perturbations from Den-
           tal Enamel Hypoplasias and Associated Histological Struc-
           tures. *Yearbook of Physical Anthropology* 33:59–110.
Goodman, A. H., R. B. Thomas, A. C. Swedlund, and G. J. Armelagos
    1988   Biocultural Perspectives on Stress in Prehistoric, Historical,
           and Contemporary Population Research. *Yearbook of Physical
           Anthropology* 31:169–202.
Grange, J. M., and M. D. Yates
    1994   Zoonotic Aspects of *Mycobacterium bovis* Infection. *Veterinary
           Microbiology* 40:137–151.
Grauer, A. L. (editor)
    1995   *Bodies of Evidence: Reconstructing History Through Skeletal
           Analysis.* Wiley-Liss, New York.

Green, M. D.
   1982   *The Politics of Indian Removal: Creek Government and Society in Crisis.* University of Nebraska Press, Lincoln.
Green, P. R.
   1980   Holocene Environmental Change and the Nature of Coastal Settlement: An Assessment from Southeastern Virginia. *Southeastern Archaeological Conference Bulletin* 23:26–32.
Gremillion, K.
   1995   Comparative Paleoethnobotany of Three Native Southeastern Communities from the Historic Period. *Southeastern Archaeology* 14:1–16.
Griffin, J. B.
   1985   Changing Concepts of the Prehistoric Mississippian Cultures of the Eastern United States. In *Alabama and the Borderlands: From Prehistory to Statehood*, edited by R. Badger and L. Clayton, pp. 40–63. University of Alabama Press, Tuscaloosa.
Griffin, M. C., P. M. Lambert, and E. I. Monahan
   2001   An Assessment of Biological Relationships for Native American Populations of Spanish Florida. In *Bioarchaeology of La Florida: Human Biology in Northern Frontier New Spain*, edited by C. S. Larsen (in press). University Press of Florida, Gainesville.
Grin, E. I.
   1953   *Epidemiology and Control of Endemic Syphilis: Report on a Mass-Treatment Campaign in Bosnia.* World Health Organization Monograph Series, No. 11. Geneva.
   1956   Endemic Syphilis and Yaws. *Bulletin of the World Health Organization* 15:959–973.
Haag, W. G.
   1958   *The Archaeology of Coastal North Carolina.* Louisiana State University Press, Baton Rouge.
Hackett, C. J.
   1951   *Bone Lesions of Yaws in Uganda.* Blackwell Scientific Publications, Oxford.
   1963   On the Origin of the Human Treponematosis. *Bulletin of the World Health Organization* 29:7–41.
   1967   The Human Treponematoses. In *Diseases in Antiquity*, edited by D. Brothwell and A. T. Sandison, pp. 152–169. Charles C. Thomas, Springfield, Ill.
   1976   *Diagnostic Criteria of Syphilis, Yaws, and Treponarid (Treponematoses) and of Some Other Diseases in Dry Bones.* Springer-Verlag, Berlin.
Haddy, A., and A. Hanson
   1982   Nitrogen and Fluorine Dating of Moundville Skeletal Samples. *Archaeometry* 24:37–44.

Haldane, J.
    1949   The Rate of Mutations of Human Genes. *Hereditas* (Supplement) 35:267–273.

Hallberg, L.
    1981   Bioavailability of Dietary Iron in Man. *Annual Review of Nutrition* 1:123–147.

Hally, D. J.
    1994   An Overview of Lamar Culture. In *Ocmulgee Archaeology: 1936–1986*, edited by D. J. Hally, pp. 144–221. University of Georgia, Athens.

Hally, D. J., and J. B. Langford
    1988   *Mississippi Period Archaeology of the Georgia Valley and Ridge Province.* Laboratory of Archaeology Series Report No. 25. University of Georgia, Athens.

Hally, D. J., and J. L. Rudolph
    1986   *Mississippi Period Archaeology of the Georgia Piedmont.* Laboratory of Archaeology Series Report No. 24. University of Georgia, Athens.

Hally, D. J., M. T. Smith, and J. B. Langford
    1990   The Archaeological Reality of DeSoto's Coosa. In *Columbian Consequences: Archaeological and Historical Perspectives on the Spanish Borderlands East,* vol. 2, edited by D. H. Thomas, pp. 121–138. Smithsonian Institution, Washington, D.C.

Haltom, W. L., and A. R. Shands
    1938   Evidences of Syphilis in Mound Builders' Bones. *Archives of Pathology* 25:228–242.

Hann, J. H.
    1990   Summary Guide to Spanish Florida Missions and *Visitas,* with Churches in the Sixteenth and Seventeenth Centuries. *The Americas* 56:417–513.

Hantman, J. L.
    1990   Between Powhatan and Quirank: Reconstructing Monacan Culture and History in the Context of Jamestown. *American Anthropologist* 92:676–690.
    1993   Powhatan's Relations with the Piedmont Monacans. In *Powhatan Foreign Relations 1500–1722,* edited by H. C. Rountree, pp. 94–111. University Press of Virginia, Charlottesville and London.
    1998   Ancestral Monacan Society: Cultural and Temporal Boundedness in American Indian History in Virginia. Paper presented at the 63rd annual meeting of the Society for American Archaeology, Seattle.

Hantman, J. L., and G. H. Dunham
    1993   The Enlightened Archaeologist. *Archaeology* 16(3):44–49.

Hantman, J. L., and M. J. Klein
   1992   Middle and Late Woodland Archaeology in Piedmont Virginia.
          In *Middle and Late Woodland Research in Virginia: A Synthesis*,
          edited by T. R. Reinhart and M. E. N. Hodges, pp. 137–164.
          Dietz Press, Richmond, Virginia.
Hardham, J. M., J. G. Frye, N. R. Young, and L. V. Stamm
   1997   Identification and Sequences of the *Treponema pallidum* flhA,
          flhF, and or f304 genes. *DNA Sequence* 7:107–116.
Hariot, T.
   1955   *A Briefe and True Report of the New Found Land of Virginia.*
          Dover Press, New York.
Harris, R.
   1963   Biology of the Children of Hopewood House, Bowral, Austra-
          lia. IV. Observations of Dental Caries Experience Extending
          Over Five Years (1957–1961). *Journal of Dental Research*
          42:1387.
Hengen, O. P.
   1971   Cribra Orbitalia: Pathogenesis and Probable Etiology. *Homo*
          22:57–75.
Henschen, F.
   1961   Cribra Cranii, a Skull Condition Said to Be of Racial or Geo-
          graphical Nature. *Pathologia and Microbiologia* 24:724–729.
Hill, M. C.
   1981   Analysis, Synthesis and Interpretation of the Skeletal Mate-
          rial Excavated for the Gainesville Section of the Tennessee-
          Tombigbee Waterway. *Biocultural Studies in the Gainesville
          Lake Area of the Tennessee Tombigbee Waterway.* Vol. 4. Report
          of Investigations 14. Office of Archaeological Research, Univer-
          sity, Alabama.
   1996   Protohistoric Aborigines in West-Central Alabama: Probable
          Correlations to Early European Contact. In *Bioarchaeology of
          Native American Adaptation in the Spanish Borderlands*, edited
          by B. J. Baker and L. Kealhofer, pp. 17–37. University Press of
          Florida, Gainesville.
Hill-Clark, M. C.
   1981   The Mississippian Decline in Alabama: A Biological Analysis.
          American Journal of Physical Anthropology 54:233.
Hillson, S.
   1996   *Dental Anthropology.* Cambridge University Press, Cambridge.
Hoeprich, P. D. (editor)
   1977   *Infectious Diseases, a Modern Treatise on Infectious Processes.*
          2nd edition. Harper and Row, New York.
Hogue, S. H., and E. Peacock
   1995   Environmental and Osteological Analysis at the South Farm

236   References

Site (22OK534), a Mississippian Farmstead in Oktibbeha County, Mississippi. *Southeastern Archaeology* 14:31–45.

Holl, A.
1993   Community Interaction and Settlement Patterning in Northern Cameroon. In *Spatial Boundaries and Social Dynamics*, edited by A. Holl and T. E. Levy, pp. 39–62. Ethnoarchaeological Series 2 International Monographs in Prehistory, Ann Arbor.

Holland, C. G., S. Speiden, and D. Van Roijen
1983   The Rapidan Mound Revisited: A Test Excavation of a Prehistoric Burial Mound. *Archaeological Society of Virginia Quarterly Bulletin* 38(1):1–42.

Hoshower, L.
1992   *Bioanthropological Analysis of a Seventeenth-Century Native American Spanish Mission Population: Biocultural Impacts on the Northern Utina*. Ph.D. dissertation, University of Florida, Gainesville.

Hoshower, L., and J. T. Milanich
1993   Excavations in the Fig Springs Mission Burial Area. In *The Missions of La Florida*, edited by B. G. McEwan, pp. 217–243. University Press of Florida, Gainesville.

Hotez, P. J., and D. I. Pritchard
1995   Hookworm Infection. *Scientific American* 272(6):68–74.

Howell, N.
1982   Village Composition Implied by a Paleodemographic Life Table: The Libben Site. *American Journal of Physical Anthropology* 59:263–269.

Hoyme, L. E., and W. Bass
1962   *Human Skeletal Remains from the Tollifero (Ha6) and Clarksville (Mc14) Sites, John H. Kerr Reservoir Basin, Virginia*. Bureau of American Ethnology Bulletin 182:329–400. Smithsonian Institution, Washington, D.C.

Hrdlička, A.
1909   Tuberculosis Among Certain Indian Tribes of the United States. *Bureau of American Ethnology Bulletin* 42. Washington, D.C.

1922   The Anthropology of Florida. *Publications of the Florida State Historical Society*, 1.

Hudson, C.
1976   *The Southeastern Indians*. University of Tennessee Press, Knoxville.

1997   *Knights of Spain, Warriors of the Sun: Hernando de Soto and the South's Ancient Chiefdoms*. University of Georgia Press, Athens.

Hudson, C., M. T. Smith, and C. B. DePratter
1990   The Hernando de Soto Expedition: From Mabila to the Missis-

sippi River. In *Towns and Temples Along the Mississippi*, edited by D. H. Dye and C. A. Cox, pp. 181–207. University of Alabama Press, Tuscaloosa.

Hudson, E. H.
1946   *Treponematosis*. Oxford University Press, Oxford.
1958   *Non-venereal Syphilis, a Sociological and Medical Study of Bejel.* E. and S. Livingstone, Edinburgh.
1961   Endemic Syphilis—Heir of the Syphiloids. *Archives of Internal Medicine* 108:1–4.
1963   Treponematosis and Pilgrimage. *American Journal of the Medical Sciences* 246(6):645–656.
1965   Treponematosis and Man's Social Evolution. *American Anthropologist* 67:885–901.
1968   Christopher Columbus and the History of Syphilis. *Acta Tropica* 25(1):1–16.

Hulse, F. S.
1941   The People Who Lived at Irene: Physical Anthropology. In *Irene Mound Site, Chatham County, Georgia*, edited by J. Caldwell and C. McCann, pp. 57–68. University of Georgia Press, Athens.

Hulton, P.
1984   *America 1585: The Complete Drawings of John White.* University of North Carolina Press and British Museum Publications, London.

Hunter, P. B.
1988   Risk Factors in Dental Caries. *International Dental Journal* 38:211–217.

Huntington, R., and P. Metcalf
1979   *Celebrations of Death: The Anthropology of Mortuary Ritual.* Cambridge University Press, Cambridge.

Huss-Ashmore, R., A. H. Goodman, and G. J. Armelagos
1982   Nutritional Inference from Paleopathology. *Advances in Archaeological Method and Theory*, vol. 5, edited by M. G. Schiffer, pp. 395–474. Academic Press, New York.

Hutchinson, D. L.
1991   *Postcontact Native American Health and Adaptation: Assessing the Impact of Introduced Diseases in Sixteenth Century Gulf Coast Florida.* Ph.D. dissertation, University of Illinois, Champaign-Urbana.
1993a   Treponematosis in Regional and Chronological Perspective from Central Gulf Coast Florida. *American Journal of Physical Anthropology* 92:249–261.
1993b   Analysis of Skeletal Remains from the Tierra Verde Site, Pinellas County, West-Central Florida. *The Florida Anthropologist* 46(4):263–276.

Hutchinson, D. L., and C. S. Larsen
    1988   Determination of Stress Episode Duration from Linear Enamel
           Hypoplasias: A Case Study from St. Catherines Island, Geor-
           gia. *Human Biology* 60:93–110.
    1990   Stress and Lifeway Change: The Evidence from Enamel Hy-
           poplasias. In *The Archaeology of Mission Santa Catalina de
           Guale: 2. Biocultural Interpretations of a Population in Transi-
           tion*, edited by C. S. Larsen, pp. 50–65. Anthropological Papers
           of the American Museum of Natural History 68. New York.
Hutchinson, D. L., C. S. Larsen, M. J. Schoeninger, and L. Norr
    1998   Regional Variation in the Pattern of Maize Adoption and Use
           in Florida and Georgia. *American Antiquity* 63:397–416.
Hutchinson, D. L., C. S. Larsen, M. Williamson, and V. D. Green Clow
    1998   Temporal and Spatial Variation in the Patterns of Treponema-
           tosis in *La Florida*. Paper presented at the 67th Annual Meet-
           ing of the American Association of Physical Anthropologists,
           Salt Lake City, Utah.
Hutchinson, D. L., and L. Norr
    1991   Corn and Subsistence in Central Gulf Coast Florida: The Evi-
           dence from Stable Isotope Analysis. Paper Presented at the
           56th Annual Meeting of the Society for American Archaeol-
           ogy, New Orleans.
    1994   Late Prehistoric and Early Historic Diet in Gulf Coast Florida.
           In *In the Wake of Contact: Biological Responses to Conquest*, ed-
           ited by C. S. Larsen and G. R. Milner, pp. 9–20. Wiley-Liss,
           New York.
    1998   Unpublished data on file at Department of Anthropology, East
           Carolina University, Greenville, N.C.
Hutchinson, J.
    1909   *Syphilis*. New and enlarged edition. Cosell, London.
Infante, P. F., and G. M. Gillespie
    1974   An Epidemiologic Study of Linear Enamel Hypoplasia of De-
           ciduous Anterior Teeth in Guatemalan Children. *Archives of
           Oral Biology* 19:1055–1061.
Iscan, M.-Y., and K. A. R. Kennedy (editors)
    1989   *Reconstruction of Life from the Skeleton*. Alan R. Liss, New
           York.
Iscan, M. Y., and P. Miller-Shaivitz
    1985   Prehistoric Syphilis in Florida. *Journal of the Florida Medical As-
           sociation* 72:109–113.
Jackson, B. E., J. L. Boone, and M. Henneberg
    1986   Possible Cases of Endemic Treponematosis in a Prehistoric
           Hunter-Gatherer Population on the Texas Coast. *Bulletin of the
           Texas Archeological Society* 57:183–193.

Jacobi, K. P., P. S. Bridges, and M. L. Powell
1996 Healing Stages of Scalping in Prehistoric Remains. *American Journal of Physical Anthropology* Supplement 22:130–131.
Jacobi, K., D. C. Cook, R. S. Corruccini, and J. S. Handler
1992 Congenital Syphilis in the Past: Slaves at Newton Plantation, Barbados, West Indies. *American Journal of Physical Anthropology* 89:145–158.
Jefferson, T.
1954 *Notes on the State of Virginia,* edited by W. Peden, pp. 98–100.
[1787] W. W. Norton, New York and London.
Jenkins, N., and B. Ensor
1981 The Gainesville Lake Area Excavations. *Archaeological Investigations in the Gainesville Lake Area of the Tennessee-Tombigbee Waterway.* Vol. 1. Report of Investigations 11. Office of Archaeological Research, University, Alabama.
Jirikowic, C.
1990 The Political Implications of a Cultural Practice: A New Perspective on Ossuary Burial in the Potomac Valley. *North American Archaeologist* 11(4):353–374.
Johannessen, S.
1984 Paleoethnobotany. In *American Bottom Archaeology,* edited by C. Bareis and J. Porter, pp. 197–214. University of Illinois Press, Urbana.
1993 Farmers of the Late Woodland. In *Foraging and Farming in the Eastern Woodlands,* edited by C. M. Scarry, pp. 57–77. University of Florida Press, Gainesville.
Johannessen, S., and L. A. Whalley
1988 Floral Analyses. In *Late Woodland Sites in the American Bottom Uplands,* edited by C. Bentz, D. McElrath, F. Finney, and R. Lacampagne, pp. 265–288. American Bottom Archaeology FAI-270 Site Reports No. 18. University of Illinois Press, Urbana.
Johnson, W. D.
1993 Tuberculosis. In *The Cambridge World History of Human Disease,* edited by K. F. Kiple, pp. 1059–1068. Cambridge University Press, Cambridge.
Jones, B. C.
1982 Southern Cult Manifestations at the Lake Jackson Site, Leon County, Florida: Salvage Excavation of Mound 3. *Midcontinental Journal of Archaeology* 7:3–44.
Jones, B. C., R. Storey, and R. Widmer
1991 The Patale Cemetery: Evidence Concerning the Apalachee Mission Mortuary Complex. In *San Pedro y San Pablo de Patale: A Seventeenth-Century Spanish Mission in Leon County, Florida,* edited by B.C. Jones, J. Hann, and J. F. Scarry. Florida Archaeol-

ogy No. 5. Florida Bureau of Archaeological Research, Talla-
hassee.

Jones, G. D.
  1978 The Ethnohistory of the Guale Coast through 1684. In *The An-
        thropology of St. Catherines Island: Natural and Cultural History,*
        edited by D. H. Thomas, G. D. Jones, R. S. Durham, and C. S.
        Larsen. Anthropological Papers of the American Museum of
        Natural History 55(2):178–210.

Jones, J.
  1876 *Explorations of the Aboriginal Remains of Tennessee.* Smith-
        sonian Contributions to Knowledge 22(259).

Jurmain, R. D.
  1977 Stress and the Etiology of Osteoarthritis. *American Journal of
        Physical Anthropology* 46:353–366.
  1990 Paleoepidemiology of a Central California Prehistoric Popula-
        tion from CA-ALA-329: II. Degenerative Disease. *American
        Journal of Physical Anthropology* 83:83–94.
  1991 Paleoepidemiology of Trauma in a Prehistoric Central Califor-
        nia Population. In *Human Paleopathology: Current Syntheses
        and Future Options,* edited by D. J. Ortner and A. C. Aufder-
        heide, pp. 241–248. Smithsonian Institution Press, Washing-
        ton, D.C.

Kakaliouras, Ann
  1997 Patterns of Health and Disease at the Garbacon Creek Site
        (31Cr86). Ms. on file, Department of Anthropology, University
        of North Carolina, Chapel Hill.

Katzenberg, M. A.
  1977 An Investigation of Spinal Disease in a Midwest Aboriginal
        Population. *Yearbook of Physical Anthropology* 20:349–355.

Katzenberg, M. A., H. P. Schwarcz, M. Knyf, and J. Melbye
  1995 Stable Isotope Evidence for Maize Horticulture and Paleodiet
        in Southern Ontario, Canada. *American Antiquity* 60:335–
        350.

Keegan, W. F., and M. J. DeNiro
  1988 Stable Carbon- and Nitrogen-Isotope Ratios of Bone Collagen
        Used to Study Coral-Reef and Terrestrial Components of Pre-
        historic Bahamian Diet. *American Antiquity* 53:320–336.

Kelley, M. A.
  1980 *Disease and Environment: A Comparative Analysis of Three
        Early American Indian Skeletal Collections.* Ph.D. dissertation,
        Department of Anthropology, Case Western Reserve Univer-
        sity, Cleveland.

Kelley, M. A., and L. E. Eisenberg
  1987 Blastomycosis and Tuberculosis in Early American Indians: A

Biocultural View. *Midcontinental Journal of Archaeology* 12(1):89–116.

Kelley, M. A., and M. S. Micozzi
  1984 Rib Lesions in Chronic Pulmonary Tuberculosis. *American Journal of Physical Anthropology* 65:381–386.

Kent, S.
  1986 The Influence of Sedentism and Aggregation on Porotic Hyperostosis and Anaemia: A Case Study. *Man* 21:605–636.
  1992 Anemia through the Ages: Changing Perspectives and Their Implications. In *Diet, Demography, and Disease: Changing Perspectives on Anemia*, edited by P. Stuart-Macadam and S. Kent, pp. 1–30. Aldine de Gruyter, New York.

Keswani, P. S.
  1989 *Mortuary Ritual and Social Hierarchy in Bronze Age Cyprus.* Vols. 1 and 2. Ph.D. dissertation, University of Michigan.

Keusch, G. T., and M. J. G. Farthing
  1986 Nutrition and Infection. *Annual Review of Nutrition* 6:131–154.

Kiple, K. F.
  1994 The Treponematoses. In *The Cambridge World History of Human Disease*, edited by K. F. Kiple, pp. 1053–1055. Cambridge University Press, Cambridge.

Klein, M. J.
  1994 *An Absolute Seriation Approach to Ceramic Chronology in the Roanoke, Potomac and James River Valleys, Virginia and Maryland.* Ph.D. dissertation, University of Virginia. University Microfilms, Ann Arbor.

Klepinger, L. L.
  1982 Tuberculosis in the New World: More Possibilities, Probabilities, and Predictions (Abstract). *American Journal of Physical Anthropology* 57:203.

Knight, V. J., Jr.
  1992 Preliminary Report on Excavations at Mound Q, Moundville. Paper presented at the 49th Annual Southeastern Archaeological Conference, Little Rock, Arkansas.
  1994 Evidence for the Dating of Mounds A, B, P, R, and S, Moundville. Paper presented at the 51st Annual Southeastern Archaeological Conference, Lexington, Kentucky.

Knight, V. J., Jr., and V. P. Steponaitis
  1998a A New History of Moundville. In *Studies in Moundville Archaeology*, edited by V. J. Knight, Jr., and V. P. Steponaitis, pp. 1–25. Smithsonian Series in Archaeological Inquiry. Smithsonian Institution Press, Washington, D.C.
  1998b *Studies in Moundville Archaeology.* Smithsonian Institution Press, Washington, D.C.

Koff, A. B., and T. Rosen
  1993   Nonvenereal Treponematoses: Yaws, Endemic Syphilis, and
         Pinta. *Journal of the American Academy of Dermatology*
         29(4):519–535.
Krall, E., C. Hayes, and R. Garcia
  1998   How Dentition Status and Masticatory Function Affect Nutri-
         ent Intake. *Journal of the American Dental Association*
         129:1261–1269.
Kreshover, S. J.
  1960   Metabolic Disturbances in Tooth Formation. *New York Acad-
         emy of Sciences Annal* 85, Article 1:161–167.
Lallo, J.
  1973   *The Skeletal Biology of Three Prehistoric American Indian Socie-
         ties from Dickson Mounds.* Ph.D. dissertation, Department of
         Anthropology, University of Massachusetts, Amherst.
Lallo, J. W., G. J. Armelagos, and R. P. Mensforth
  1977   The Role of Diet, Disease, and Physiology in the Origin of
         Porotic Hyperostosis. *Human Biology* 49:471–483.
Lambert, P. M.
  1993   Health in Prehistoric Populations of the Santa Barbara Chan-
         nel Islands. *American Antiquity* 58:509–521.
  1999   Human Remains. In *Environmental and Bioarchaeological Stud-
         ies of the Ute Mountain Ute Piedmont,* edited by B. R. Billman.
         Soil Systems Publications in Archaeology No. 22, vol. 5.
         Phoenix.
Lambert, P. M., and P. L. Walker
  1991   Physical Anthropological Evidence for the Evolution of Social
         Complexity in Coastal Southern California. *Antiquity* 65:963–
         973.
Larsen, C. S.
  1981   Skeletal and Dental Adaptations to the Shift to Agriculture on
         the Georgia Coast. *Current Anthropology* 22:422–423.
  1982   *The Anthropology of St. Catherines Island: 3. Prehistoric Human
         Biological Adaptation* (editor). Anthropological Papers of the
         American Museum of Natural History 57, part 3.
  1983   Behavioral Implications of Temporal Change in Cariogenesis.
         Journal of Archaeological Science 10:1–8.
  1984   Health and Disease in Prehistoric Georgia: The Transition to
         Agriculture. In *Paleopathology at the Origins of Agriculture,* ed-
         ited by M. N. Cohen and G. J. Armelagos, pp. 367–392. Aca-
         demic Press, Orlando.
  1987   Bioarchaeological Interpretations of Subsistence Economy and
         Behavior from Human Skeletal Remains. In *Advances in Ar-*

chaeological Method and Theory, edited by M. Schiffer, pp. 339–445. Academic Press, Orlando.

1990a Biological Interpretation and the Context for Contact. In *The Archaeology of Mission Santa Catalina de Guale: 2. Biocultural Interpretations of a Population in Transition*, edited by C. S. Larsen, pp. 11–25. Anthropological Papers of the American Museum of Natural History No. 68.

1990b *The Archaeology of Mission Santa Catalina de Guale: 2. Biocultural Interpretations of a Population in Transition* (editor). Anthropological Papers of the American Museum of Natural History No. 68.

1993 On the Frontier of Contact: Mission Bioarchaeology in La Florida. In *The Spanish Missions of La Florida*, edited by B. G. McEwan, pp. 322–356. University Press of Florida, Gainesville.

1995 Biological Changes in Human Populations with Agriculture. *Annual Review of Anthropology* 24:185–213.

1996 Unpublished data on file at Research Laboratories of Archaeology, University of North Carolina, Chapel Hill.

1997 *Bioarchaeology: Interpreting Behavior from the Human Skeleton.* Cambridge University Press, Cambridge.

Larsen, C. S., A. W. Crosby, M. C. Griffin, D. L. Hutchinson, C. B. Ruff, K. F. Russell, M. J. Schoeninger, L. E. Sering, S. W. Simpson, J. L. Takács, and M. F. Teaford

2000 A Biohistory of Health and Behavior in the Georgia Bight: 1. The Agricultural Transition and the Impact of European Contact. In *The Backbone of History: Health and Nutrition in the Western Hemisphere*, edited by R. H. Steckel and J. C. Rose. Cambridge University Press, Cambridge (in press).

Larsen, C. S., and D. E. Harn

1994 Health in Transition: Disease and Nutrition in the Georgia Bight. In *Paleonutrition: The Diet and Health of Prehistoric Americans*, edited by K. D. Sobolik, pp. 222–234. Southern Illinois University at Carbondale, Center for Archaeological Investigations, Occasional Paper No. 22.

Larsen, C. S., and G. R. Milner

1994 Bioanthropological Perspectives on Postcontact Transitions. In *In the Wake of Contact: Biological Responses to Conquest*, edited by C. S. Larsen and G. R. Milner, pp. 1–8. Wiley-Liss, New York.

Larsen, C. S., C. B. Ruff, and R. L. Kelly

1995 Structural Analysis of the Stillwater Postcranial Human Remains: Behavioral Implications of Articular Joint Pathology and Long Bone Diaphyseal Morphology. In *Bioarchaeology of*

the *Stillwater Marsh: Prehistoric Human Adaptation in the West-*
ern Great Basin, edited by C. S. Larsen and R. L. Kelly, pp.
107–133. Anthropological Papers No. 77. American Museum
of Natural History, New York.

Larsen, C. S., C. B. Ruff, M. J. Schoeninger, and D. L. Hutchinson
   1992 Population Decline and Extinction in La Florida. In *Disease*
         and Demography in the Americas, edited by J. W. Verano and
         D. H. Ubelaker, pp. 25–39. Smithsonian Institution Press,
         Washington, D.C.

Larsen, C. S., M. J. Schoeninger, D. L. Hutchinson, K. F. Russell, and
C. B. Ruff
   1990 Beyond Demographic Collapse: Biological Adaptation and
         Change in Native Populations of La Florida. In *Columbian Con-*
         sequences: Archaeological and Historical Perspectives on the
         Spanish Borderlands East, vol. 2, edited by D. H. Thomas, pp.
         409–428. Smithsonian Institution Press, Washington, D.C.

Larsen, C. S., M. J. Schoeninger, R. Shavit, and K. F. Russell
   1990 Dietary and Demographic Transitions on the Southeastern
         U.S. Atlantic Coast. *International Journal of Anthropology*
         5:333–346.

Larsen, C. S., M. J. Schoeninger, N. J. van der Merwe, K. M. Moore, and
J. A. Lee-Thorp
   1992 Carbon and Nitrogen Stable Isotopic Signatures of Human Die-
         tary Change in the Georgia Bight. *American Journal of Physical*
         Anthropology 89:197–214.

Larsen, C. S., R. Shavit, and M. C. Griffin
   1991 Dental Caries Evidence for Dietary Change: An Archaeological
         Context. In *Advances in Dental Anthropology*, edited by M. A.
         Kelley and C. S. Larsen, pp. 179–202. Wiley-Liss, New York.

Larsen, C. S., and D. H. Thomas
   1982 *The Anthropology of St. Catherines Island: 4. The St. Catherines*
         Period Mortuary Complex. Anthropological Papers of the Ameri-
         can Museum of Natural History 57:271–342.

   1986 *The Anthropology of St. Catherines Island: 5. The South End*
         Mound Complex. Anthropological Papers of the American Mu-
         seum of Natural History 63:1–46.

Larson, L. H.
   1957 The Norman Mound, McIntosh County, Georgia. *Florida An-*
         thropologist 10:37–52.

Larson, L. H., Jr.
   1980 *Aboriginal Subsistence Technology on the Southeastern Coastal*
         Plain During the Late Prehistoric Period. Riley P. Bullen Mono-
         graphs in Anthropology and History No. 2. Florida State Mu-
         seum, Gainesville.

Lawson, J.
1709 *A New Voyage to Carolina, Containing the Exact Description and Natural History of That Country.* London.
1960 *Lawson's History of North Carolina.* Garrett and Masie Publishers, Richmond.

Layrisse, M., C. Martínez-Torres, and M. Roche
1968 Effect of Interaction of Various Foods on Iron Absorption. *American Journal of Clinical Nutrition* 21:1175–1183.

Layrisse, M., and M. Roche
1964 The Relationship Between Anemia and Hookworm Infection. *American Journal of Hygiene* 79:279–301.

Lee, C.
1997 Paleopathology of the Hatchel-Mitchell-Moore Sites. *Bulletin of the Texas Archaeological Society* 68:161–178.

Lignereux, Y.
1997 Retrospective Diagnosis of Animal Tuberculosis on Archaeological Bones. Paper presented at the International Congress, The Evolution and Paleoepidemiology of Tuberculosis, Szeged, Hungary.

Little, E. A., and M. J. Schoeninger
1995 The Late Woodland Diet on Nantucket Island and the Problem of Maize in Coastal New England. *American Antiquity* 60:351–368.

Little, K. J., and C. Curren
1995 The Moundville IV Phase on the Black Warrior River. *Journal of Alabama Archaeology* 41:55–77.

Livingstone, F. B.
1973 *Data on the Abnormal Hemoglobins and Glucose-6-Phosphate Dehydrogenase Deficiency in Human Populations, 1967–1973.* Technical Reports No. 3. Museum of Anthropology, University of Michigan, Ann Arbor.

Loftfield, T. C.
1975 *Briefe and True Report . . . an Archaeological Interpretation of the Southern North Carolina Coast.* Ph.D. dissertation, University of North Carolina, Chapel Hill.
1985 Archaeological Testing and Excavations at 31On196, Permuda Island. Paper on file, North Carolina Office of State Archaeology, Raleigh.
1987 Excavations at 31On305, the Flynt Site at Sneads Ferry, NC. Vols. 1 and 2. Paper on file, North Carolina Office of State Archaeology, Raleigh.

Longin, R.
1971 New Method of Collagen Extraction for Radiocarbon Dating. *Nature* 230:241–242.

Lorant, S. (editor)
    1946   [sixteenth century] *The New World. The First Pictures of America.* Duell, Sloan & Pearce, New York.
Loucks, L. J.
    1976   *Early Alachua Tradition Burial Ceremonialism: The Henderson Mound, Alachua County, Florida.* M.A. thesis, University of Florida, Gainesville.
Lovell, N. C.
    1994   Spinal Arthritis and Physical Stress at Bronze Age Harappa. *American Journal of Physical Anthropology* 93:149–164.
Lukacs, J. R.
    1989   Dental Paleopathology: Methods for Reconstructing Dietary Patterns. In *Reconstruction of Life from the Skeleton,* edited by M. Y. Iscan and K. A. R. Kennedy, pp. 261–286. Alan R. Liss, New York.
MacCord, H. A., Sr.
    1986   *The Lewis Creek Mound Culture in Virginia.* Privately Printed, Richmond, Virginia.
MacCord, H. A., Sr., and O. D. Valliere
    1965   The Lewis Creek Mound, Augusta County, Virginia (44AU20), Part I. *Quarterly Bulletin of the Archaeological Society of Virginia* 20(2):37–47.
Marieb, E. N.
    1992   *Human Anatomy and Physiology.* 2nd edition. Benjamin/ Cummings, Redwood City, California.
Marquardt, W. H.
    1992   *Culture and Environment in the Domain of the Calusa.* Monograph No. 1. Institute of Archaeology and Paleoenvironmental Studies, University of Florida, Gainesville.
Marrinan, R. A.
    1993   Archaeological Investigations at Mission Patale, 1984–1991. In *The Missions of La Florida,* edited by B. G. McEwan, pp. 244–294. University Press of Florida, Gainesville.
Martin, D. L., A. H. Goodman, G. J. Armelagos, and A. L. Magennis
    1991   *Black Mesa Anasazi Health: Reconstructing Life from Patterns of Death and Disease.* Southern Illinois University at Carbondale Center for Archaeological Investigations Occasional Paper No. 14. Carbondale.
Martinez, C. A.
    1975   *Culture Sequence on the Central Georgia Coast, 1000 B.C.– 1650 A.D.* M.A. thesis, University of Florida, Gainesville.
Mascie-Taylor, C. G. N.
    1993   The Biological Anthropology of Disease. In *The Anthropology*

of Disease, edited by C. G. N. Mascie-Taylor, pp. 1–72. Oxford University Press, Oxford.

Mata, L., R. A. Kronmal, and H. Villegas
    1981   Diarrheal Disease: A Leading World Health Problem. In *Nutritional Problems in Modern Society,* edited by A. N. Howard, pp. 1–14. John Libbey, London.

Mathis, M. A.
    1986   The Flynt Site Ossuary (31On305) Excavation Summary. Paper on file, North Carolina Office of State Archaeology, Raleigh.
    1991   Broad Reach: A Unique Site or, The Truth about What We Missed. Paper presented at the 49th Annual Meeting of the Southeastern Archaeological Conference, Jackson, Miss.
    1993   Mortuary Processes at the Broad Reach Site. Paper presented at the 50th Annual Meeting of the Southeastern Archaeological Conference, Raleigh, N.C.

McEwan, B. G.
    1993   Hispanic Life on the Seventeenth Century Florida Frontier. In *The Missions of La Florida,* edited by B. G. McEwan, pp. 295–321. University Press of Florida, Gainesville.

McFalls, J. A., Jr., and M. H. McFalls
    1984   *Disease and Fertility.* Academic Press, Orlando.

McGrath, J.
    1988   Social Networks of Disease Spread in the Lower Illinois Valley: A Simulation Approach. *American Journal of Physical Anthropology* 77: 483–496.

Mensforth, R. P.
    n.d.   The Pathogenesis and Paleoepidemiology of Periosteal Reactions in Libben and Bt-5 Subadults. (unpublished ms. in the possession of the author.)
    1996   Observations on the Antiquity, Geographic Distribution, and Theoretical Significance of Violent Injuries, Scalping and Other Trophy-taking Behaviors among Archaic Hunter-gatherers of the Eastern United States. Paper presented at the 65th Annual Meeting of the American Association of Physical Anthropologists, Durham, North Carolina.

Mensforth, R. P., and C. O. Lovejoy
    1985   Anatomical, Physiological, and Epidemiological Correlates of the Aging Process: A Confirmation of Multifactorial Age Determination in the Libben Skeletal Population. *American Journal of Physical Anthropology* 68:87–106.

Mensforth, R. P., C. O. Lovejoy, J. W. Lallo, and G. J. Armelagos
    1978   The Role of Constitution Factors, Diet, and Infectious Disease in the Etiology of Porotic Hyperostosis and Periosteal Reac-

tions in Prehistoric Infants and Children. *Medical Anthropology* 2:1–59.

Metcalf, P., and R. Huntington
   1991   *Celebrations of Death: The Anthropology of Mortuary Ritual.* 2nd edition. Cambridge University Press, Cambridge.

Michals, L. M.
   1998   The Oliver Site and Early Moundville Phase Economic Organization. In *Studies in Moundville Archaeology*, edited by V. J. Knight, Jr., and V. P. Steponaitis, pp. 167–182. Smithsonian Series in Archaeological Inquiry, Smithsonian Institution Press, Washington, D.C.

Milanich, J. T.
   1994   *Archaeology of Precolumbian Florida.* University of Florida Press, Gainesville.

Milanich, J. T., and S. Milbrath (editors)
   1989   *First Encounters: Spanish Explorations in the Caribbean and the United States, 1492–1570.* University Press of Florida, Gainesville.

Miller, E.
   1994   Evidence for Prehistoric Scalping in Northeastern Nebraska. *Plains Anthropologist* 39:211–219.
   1996   The Effect of European Contact on the Health of Indigenous Populations in Texas. In *Bioarchaeology of Native American Adaptation in the Spanish Borderlands*, edited by B. J. Baker and L. Kealhofer, pp. 126–147. University Press of Florida, Gainesville.

Milner, G. R.
   1980   Epidemic Disease in the Postcontact Southeast: A Reappraisal. *Mid-Continental Journal of Archaeology* 5:39–56.
   1982   *Measuring Prehistoric Levels of Health: A Study of Mississippian Period Skeletal Remains from the American Bottom, Illinois.* Ph.D. dissertation, Northwestern University, Evanston.
   1983   The East St. Louis Stone Quarry Site Cemetery. *American Bottom Archaeology, FAI-270 Site Reports* 1. University of Illinois Press, Urbana.
   1991   Health and Cultural Change in the Late Prehistoric American Bottom, Illinois. In *What Mean These Bones?*, edited by M. L. Powell, P. S. Bridges, and A. M. W. Mires, pp. 52–69. University of Alabama Press, Tuscaloosa.
   1992   Disease and Sociopolitical Systems in Late Prehistoric Illinois. In *Disease and Demography in the Americas, Changing Patterns Before and After 1492*, edited by D. H. Ubelaker and J. Verano, pp. 103–116. Smithsonian Institution Press, Washington, D.C.
   1995   An Osteological Perspective on Prehistoric Warfare. In *Re-*

gional Approaches to Mortuary Analysis, edited by L. A. Beck, pp. 221–244. Plenum, New York.

1998 Archaeological Evidence for Prehistoric and Historic Intergroup Conflict in Eastern North America. In *Deciphering Anasazi Violence*, edited by P. Y. Bullock, pp. 69–91. HRM Books, Santa Fe.

Milner, G. R., E. Anderson, and V. G. Smith

1991 Warfare in Late Prehistoric West-Central Illinois. *American Antiquity* 56:581–603.

Milner, G. R., and V. G. Smith

1990 Ontonta Human Skeletal Remains. In *Archaeological Investigations at the Morton Village and Norris Farms 36 Cemetery*, edited by S. K. Santure, A.D. Harn, and D. Esary, pp. 111–148. Illnois State Museum Reports of Investigations 45, Springfield.

Milton, K.

1992 Comparative Aspects of Diet in Amazonian Forest-Dwellers. In *Foraging Strategies and Natural Diet of Monkeys, Apes and Humans*, edited by A. Whiten and E. M. Widdowson, pp. 93–103. Clarendon Press, Oxford.

Mires, A. M.

1982 *A Bioarchaeological Study of the Regional Adaptive Efficiency of the Caddo*. M.A. thesis, Department of Anthropology, University of Arkansas, Fayetteville.

Mitchem, J. M.

1989 *Redefining Safety Harbor: Late Prehistoric/Protohistoric Archaeology in West Peninsular Florida*. Ph.D. dissertation, University of Florida, Gainesville.

Mittler, D. M., and D. P. Van Gerven

1994 Developmental, Diachronic, and Demographic Analysis of Cribra Orbitalia in the Medieval Christian Populations of Kulubnarti. *American Journal of Physical Anthropology* 93:287–297.

Moggi-Cecchi, J., E. Pacciani, and J. Pinto-Cisternas

1994 Enamel Hypoplasia and Age at Weaning in Nineteenth Century Florence, Italy. *American Journal of Physical Anthropology* 93:299–306.

Monahan, E. I.

1994 *Bioarchaeological Interpretation of the Mortuary Practices at the Broad Reach Site, (31Cr218), Coastal North Carolina*. M.A. thesis, Wake Forest University, Winston-Salem.

1995 Bioarchaeological Analysis of the Mortuary Practices at the Broad Reach Site (31Cr218), Coastal North Carolina. *Southern Indian Studies* 44:37–69.

Monahan, E. I., and D. S. Weaver
   1996 Dental Health and Late Woodland Subsistence in Coastal
         North Carolina. Paper presented at the 65th Annual Meeting
         of the American Association of Physical Anthropology, Dur-
         ham, North Carolina.
Mooney, J.
   1890 The Cherokee Ball Play. *American Anthropologist* 3:105–132.
Moore, C. B.
   1897 Certain Aboriginal Mounds of the Georgia Coast. *Journal of
         the Academy of Natural Sciences of Philadelphia* 11:1–138. Re-
         printed 1998 in *The Georgia and South Carolina Coastal Expedi-
         tions of Clarence Bloomfield Moore*, edited by L. Larson, pp. 91–
         240. University of Alabama Press, Tuscaloosa.
   1907 Moundville Revisited. *Journal of the Academy of Natural Sci-
         ences of Philadelphia* 13:337–405. Reprinted 1996 in *The
         Moundville Expeditions of Clarence Bloomfield Moore*, edited by
         V. J. Knight, Jr., pp. 143–213. University of Alabama Press,
         Tuscaloosa.
Moore, J. F.
   1985 Archaeobotanical Analyses at Five Sites in the Richard B.
         Russell Reservoir, Georgia and South Carolina. In *Prehistoric
         Human Ecology Along the Upper Savannah River: Excavations at
         the Rucker's Bottom, Abbeville, and Bullard Site Groups*, assem-
         bled by D. G. Anderson and J. Schuldenrein, vol. 2, pp. 673–
         694. United States Department of the Interior National Park
         Service Archaeological Services Branch Southeast Regional
         Office, Atlanta.
Moorehead, W. K.
   1979 *Etowah Papers.* Charles G. Drake, Union City, Georgia.
Morris, I.
   1992 *Death-Ritual and Social Structure in Classical Antiquity.* Cam-
         bridge University Press, Cambridge.
Morse, D. F.
   1961 Prehistoric Tuberculosis in America. *American Review of Respi-
         ratory Diseases* 83:489–504.
   1967 Tuberculosis. In *Diseases in Antiquity*, edited by D. R. Broth-
         well and A. T. Sandison, pp. 249–271. C. C. Thomas, Spring-
         field.
   1969 Ancient Disease in the Midwest. *Illinois State Museum Reports
         of Investigations* No. 15, Springfield.
Moseley, J. E.
   1974 Skeletal Changes in the Anemias. *Seminars in Roentgenology*
         IX(3):169–184.

Mouer, L. D.

1983 A Review of the Archaeology and Ethnohistory of the Monacan Indians. In *Piedmont Archaeology,* edited by J. M. Wittkofski and L. E. Browning, pp. 21–39. Archaeological Society of Virginia Special Publication 10, Richmond.

Muller, J.

1997 *Mississippian Political Economy.* Plenum Publishing Corp., New York.

Murray, J. F., A. M. Merriweather, and M. L. Freedman

1956 Endemic Syphilis in the Bakwena Reserve of the Bechuanaland Protectorate. *Bulletin of the World Health Organization* 15:975–1039.

Murray, K.

1989 Bioarchaeology of the Parkin Site, Cross County, Arkansas. *Arkansas Archeologist* 27/28:49–61.

Musher, D. M., and J. M. Knox

1983 Syphilis and Yaws. In *Pathogenesis and Immunology of Treponemal Infection,* edited by R. F. Schell and D. M. Musher, pp. 101–120. Little, Brown & Co., Boston.

Myers, J. A.

1951 *Tuberculosis Among Children and Adults.* 3rd edition. C. C. Thomas, Springfield.

Myers, R. L., and J. J. Ewel

1991 *Ecosystems of Florida.* University of Florida Press, Orlando.

Neighbors, M. W., and T. A. Rathbun

1973 A Savannah II Burial from the Lewis Creek Site. Unpublished manuscript.

Nelson, B. A., D. L. Martin, A. C. Swedlund, P. R. Fish, and G. J. Armelagos

1994 Studies in Disruption: Demography and Health in the Prehistoric American Southwest. In *Understanding Complexity in the Prehistoric Southwest,* edited by G. Gumerman and M. Gell-Mann, pp. 59–112. SFI Studies in the Sciences of Complexity, Proceedings 16, Santa Fe.

Neumann, G. K.

1940 Evidence for the Antiquity of Scalping from Central Illinois. *American Antiquity* 5:287–289.

Newhouse, I. J., and D. B. Clement

1988 Iron Status in Athletes: An Update. *Sports Medicine Journal* 5:337–352.

Newman, M. T., and C. E. Snow

1942 Preliminary Report on the Skeletal Material from Pickwick Basin, Alabama. In *An Archaeological Survey of Pickwick Basin* in the Adjacent Portions of the States of Alabama, Mississippi, and Tennessee, edited by W. S. Webb and D. L. DeJarnette, pp. 397–507. Bureau of American Ethnology Bulletin 129. Smithsonian Institution, Washington, D.C.

Newsom, L. A.
1987   Analysis of Botanical Remains from Hontoon Island (8Vo202), Florida: 1980–1985 Excavations. *Florida Anthropologist* 40:47–84.

Newsom, L. A., and I. R. Quitmyer
1992   Archaeobotanical and Faunal Remains. In *Excavations on the Franciscan Frontier*, edited by B. R. Weisman, pp. 206–233. University Presses of Florida, Gainesville.

Nikiforuk, G., and D. Fraser
1981   The Etiology of Enamel Hypoplasia: A Unifying Concept. *Journal of Pediatrics* 98:888–893.

Norr, L.
1990   *Nutritional Consequences of Prehistoric Subsistence Strategies in Lower Central America.* Ph.D. dissertation, University of Illinois, Urbana-Champaign.

Norr, L., and D. L. Hutchinson
1998   Reconstructing Prehistoric Subsistence in South Florida (Abstract). *Florida Anthropologist* 51(3):163.

Oakley, C. B., Jr.
1971   *An Archaeological Investigation of Pinson Cave (1Je20).* M.A. thesis, Department of Anthropology, University of Alabama, Tuscaloosa.

O'Hear, J. W., and C. Larsen
1981   Burials. In *Archaeological Salvage Excavations at the Tibbee Creek Site (22Lo600) Lowndes County, Mississippi*, edited by J. W. O'Hear, C. Larsen, M. M. Scarry, J. Phillips, and E. Simons, pp. 127–152. Department of Anthropology, Mississippi State University, Starkville.

O'Leary, M. H.
1988   Carbon Isotopes in Photosynthesis. *Bioscience* 38:328–336.

Ortner, D. J.
1968   Description and Classification of Degenerative Bone Changes in the Distal Joint Surfaces of the Humerus. *American Journal of Physical Anthropology* 28:139–156.

1992   Skeletal Paleopathology: Probabilities, Possibilities, and Impossibilities. In *Disease and Demography in the Americas*, edited by J. W. Verano and D. H. Ubelaker, pp. 5–13. Smithsonian Institution Press, Washington, D.C.

Ortner, D. J., and M. F. Ericksen
1997   Bone Changes in the Human Skull Probably Resulting from

Scurvy in Infancy and Childhood. *International Journal of Osteoarchaeology* 7:212–220.

Ortner, D. J., E. H. Kimmerle, and M. Dietz
1999 Probable Evidence of Scurvy in Subadults from Archaeological Sites in Peru. *American Journal of Physical Anthropology* 108:321–331.

Ortner, D. J., and W. G. J. Putschar
1981 *Identification of Pathological Conditions in Human Skeletal Remains.* Smithsonian Contributions to Anthropology No. 28. Smithsonian Institution Press, Washington, D.C.

1985 *Identification of Pathological Conditions in Human Skeletal Remains.* Smithsonian Contributions to Anthropology No. 28. Smithsonian Institution Press, Washington, D.C.

Ortner, D. J., N. Tuross, and A. I. Stix
1992 New Approaches to the Study of Disease in Archaeological New World Populations. *Human Biology* 64:337–360.

Orton, S. T.
1905 A Study of the Pathological Changes in Some Mound Builder's Bones from the Ohio Valley, with Especial Reference to Syphilis. *University of Pennsylvania Medical Bulletin* 18:36–44.

O'Shea, J. M.
1984 *Mortuary Variability: An Archaeological Investigation.* Academic Press, New York.

O'Shea, J. M., and P. S. Bridges
1989 The Sargent Site Ossuary (25Cu28), Custer County, Nebraska. *Plains Anthropologist* 34-123:7–21.

Owsley, D. W.
1994 Warfare in Coalescent Tradition Populations of the Northern Plains. In *Skeletal Biology in the Great Plains. Migration, Warfare, Health and Subsistence,* edited by D. W. Owsley and R. L. Jantz, pp. 333–343. Smithsonian Institution Press, Washington, D.C.

Owsley, D. W., and H. E. Berryman
1975 Ethnographic and Archaeological Evidence of Scalping in the Southeastern United States. *Tennessee Archaeologist* 31:41–58.

Owsley, D. W., H. E. Berryman, and W. M. Bass
1977 Demographic and Osteological Evidence for Warfare at the Larson Site, South Dakota. *Plains Anthropologist Memoir* 13:119–131.

Owsley, D. W., and K. L. Bruweldheide
1997 Bioarcheological Research in Northeastern Colorado, Northern Kansas, Nebraska, and South Dakota. In *Bioarcheology of the North Central United States,* pp. 7–56. Arkansas Archeological Survey Research Series 49.

Pascoe, L., and W. K. Seow
　1994　Enamel Hypoplasia and Dental Caries and Australian Aborigi-
　　　　nal Children: Prevalence and Correlation Between the Two Dis-
　　　　eases. *Pediatric Dentistry* 16:193.

Pearson, C. E.
　1979　*Patterns of Mississippian Period Adaptation in Coastal Georgia.*
　　　　Ph.D. dissertation, University of Georgia, Athens.
　1984　Red Bird Creek: Late Prehistoric Material Culture and Subsis-
　　　　tence in Coastal Georgia. *Early Georgia* 12:1–39.

Peebles, C. S.
　1969　Moundville and Surrounding Sites: Some Structural Considera-
　　　　tions of Mortuary Practices II. *American Antiquity* 25:68–91.
　1971　Moundville and Surrounding Sites: Some Structural Considera-
　　　　tions of Mortuary Practices. In *Approaches to the Social Dimen-
　　　　sions of Mortuary Practices,* edited by J. A. Brown, pp. 68–91.
　　　　Society for American Archaeology Memoirs 25.
　1974　*Moundville: The Organization of a Prehistoric Community and
　　　　Culture.* Ph.D. dissertation, University of California, Santa
　　　　Barbara.
　1978　Determinants of Settlement Size and Location in the Mound-
　　　　ville Phase. In *Mississippian Settlement Patterns,* edited by
　　　　B. Smith, pp. 369–416. Academic Press, New York.
　1983a Moundville: Late Prehistoric Sociopolitical Organization in the
　　　　Southeastern United States. In *The Development of Political Or-
　　　　ganization in the Native North America,* edited by E. Tooker, pp.
　　　　183–201. American Ethnological Society, Washington, D.C.
　1983b Summary and Conclusions: Continuity and Change in a Small
　　　　Mississippian Community. In *Excavations in the Lubbub Creek
　　　　Archaeological Locality.* Vol. 1 of *Prehistoric Agricultural Com-
　　　　munities in West Central Alabama,* edited by C. S. Peebles, pp.
　　　　394–407. University of Michigan, Ann Arbor.
　1987a The Rise and Fall of the Mississippian in Western Alabama:
　　　　The Moundville and Summerville Phases, A.D. 1000 to 1600.
　　　　Mississippian Archaeology 22:1–31.
　1987b Moundville from 1000 to 1500 A.D. as Seen from 1840 to 1985
　　　　A.D. In *Chiefdoms in the Americas,* edited by R. D. Drennan
　　　　and C. A. Uribe, pp. 21–41. University Press of America,
　　　　Lanham.

Peebles, C. S., and S. M. Kus
　1977　Some Archaeological Correlates of Ranked Societies. *American
　　　　Antiquity* 42:421–448.

Peebles, C. S., and M. J. Schoeninger
　1981　Notes on the Relationship Between Social Status and Diet at
　　　　Moundville. *Southeastern Archeological Conference Bulletin*
　　　　24:96–97.

Peregrine, P. N.
   1992 *Mississippian Evolution: A World Systems Perspective.* Mono-
         graphs in World Archaeology No. 9. Prehistory Press, Madison.
Pfeiffer, S.
   1984 Paleopathology in an Iroquoian Ossuary, with Special Refer-
         ence to Tuberculosis. *American Journal of Physical Anthropol-
         ogy* 65(2):181–190.
Phelps, D. S.
   1983 Archaeology of the North Carolina Coast and Coastal Plain:
         Problems and Hypotheses. In *The Prehistory of North Carolina:
         An Archaeological Symposium,* edited by M.A. Mathis and J. J.
         Crow, pp. 1–52. North Carolina Division of Archives and His-
         tory, Raleigh.
Potter, S. R.
   1993 *Commoners, Tribute, and Chiefs: The Development of Algon-
         quian Culture in the Potomac Valley.* University Press of Vir-
         ginia, Charlottesville.
Powell, M. L.
   1983 Biocultural Analysis of Human Skeletal Remains from the Lub-
         bub Creek Archaeological Locality. In *Prehistoric Agricultural
         Communities of West Central Alabama,* vol. 2 (AD-A155 048/
         GAR), edited by C. S. Peebles, pp. 430–477. National Techni-
         cal Information Service, Washington, D.C. Distributed by the
         U.S. Army Corps of Engineers, Mobile District.
   1985 The Analysis of Dental Wear and Caries for Dietary Recon-
         struction. In *The Analysis of Prehistoric Diets,* edited by R. I.
         Gilbert, Jr., and J. H. Mielke, pp. 307–338. Academic Press,
         Orlando.
   1988 *Status and Health in Prehistory: A Case Study of the Moundville
         Chiefdom.* Smithsonian Institution Press, Washington, D.C.
   1990 On the Eve of the Conquest: Life and Death at Irene Mound,
         Georgia. In *The Archaeology of Mission Santa Catalina de
         Guale: 2. Biocultural Interpretations of a Population in Transi-
         tion,* edited by C. S. Larsen, pp. 26–35. Anthropological Papers
         of the American Museum of Natural History No. 68.
   1991a Endemic Treponematosis and Tuberculosis in the Prehistoric
         Southeastern United States: Biological Costs of Chronic En-
         demic Disease. In *Human Paleopathology: Current Syntheses
         and Future Options,* edited by D. J. Ortner and A. C. Aufder-
         heide, pp. 173–180. Smithsonian Institution, Washington, D.C.
   1991b Ranked Status and Health in the Mississippian Chiefdom at
         Moundville. In *What Mean These Bones?,* edited by M. L.
         Powell, P. S. Bridges, and A. M. W. Mires, pp. 22–51. Univer-
         sity of Alabama Press, Tuscaloosa.
   1992a Health and Disease in the Late Prehistoric Southeast. In *Dis-*

ease and Demography in the Americas, edited by J. W. Verano and D. H. Ubelaker, pp. 41–54. Smithsonian Institution Press, Washington, D.C.

1992b In the Best of Health? Disease and Trauma Among the Mississippian Elite. In *Lords of the Southeast: Social Inequality and the Native Elites of Southeastern North America,* edited by A. W. Barker and T. R. Pauketat, pp. 81–97. Archaeological Papers of the American Anthropological Association No. 3.

1994a Human Skeletal Remains from Ocmulgee National Monument. In *Ocmulgee Archaeology 1936–1986,* edited by D. J. Hally, pp. 116–129. University of Georgia Press, Athens.

1994b Treponematosis Before 1492 in the Southeastern United States of America: Why Call it Syphilis? In *L'origine de la Syphilis en Europe, avant ou après 1493?,* edited by O. Dutour, G. Palfi, J. Berato, and J.-P. Brun, pp. 158–163. Editions Errance, Paris.

1996a Health and Disease in the Green River Archaic. In *Of Caves and Shell Mounds,* edited by K. C. Carstens and P. J. Watson, pp. 119–133. University of Alabama Press, Tuscaloosa.

1996b Non-traumatic Skeletal Pathology at Koger's Island, Alabama. Paper presented at the 53rd Southeastern Archaeological Conference, Birmingham.

1998 Old Bones, New Perspectives: Paleoepidemiological Diagnosis of Infectious Diseases. Paper presented at the 97th Annual Meeting, American Association of Physical Anthropologists, Philadelphia.

Powell, M. L., P. S. Bridges, and A. M. W. Mires (editors)

1991 *What Mean These Bones?: Studies in Southeastern Bioarchaeology.* University of Alabama Press, Tuscaloosa.

Powell, M. L., and L. E. Eisenberg

1998 "Syphilis in Mound Builders' Bones": Treponematosis in the Prehistoric Southeast. Paper presented at the 67th Annual Meeting of the American Association of Physican Anthropologists, Salt Lake City, Utah.

Powell, M. L., and J. D. Rogers

1980 *Bioarchaeology of the McCutchan-McLaughlin Site.* Studies in Oklahoma's Past No. 5. Oklahoma Archaeological Survey, Norman.

1998 Chronological Trends in Moundville Health. In *Studies in Moundville Archaeology,* edited by V. J. Knight, Jr., and V. P. Steponaitis, pp. 102–119. Smithsonian Series in Archaeological Inquiry, Smithsonian Institution Press, Washington, D.C.

Quetel, Claude

1990 *History of Syphilis.* Johns Hopkins University Press, Baltimore.

Rafferty, J.

1986 Summary and Conclusions. In *Test Excavations at Two Wood-*

land Sites, Lowndes County, Mississippi, edited by J. Rafferty and M. E. Starr, pp. 135–139. Report of Investigations 3. Cobb Institute of Archaeology, Mississippi State University, Starkville.

Ramos, L. S.
1992 Classification of Mycobacteria by HPLC and Pattern Recognition. *American Biotechnology Laboratory* 10(8):26–32.

Rathbun, T. A.
1984 Skeletal Pathology from the Paleolithic through the Metal Ages in Iran and Iraq. In *Paleopathology at the Origins of Agriculture*, edited by M. N. Cohen and G. J. Armelagos, pp. 137–67. Academic Press, Orlando.
1986 The Contributions of Skeletal Biology to Southeastern Archaeology. In *Skeletal Analysis in Southeastern Archaeology*, edited by J. E. Levy, pp. 1–28. Publication No. 24. North Carolina Archaeological Council, Raleigh.

Rathbun, T. A., J. Sexton, and J. Michie
1980 Disease Patterns in a Formative Period South Carolina Coastal Population. *Tennessee Anthropological Association Miscellaneous Papers* 5:52–74.

Reichs, K. J.
1989 Treponematosis: A Possible Case from the Late Prehistoric of North Carolina. *American Journal of Physical Anthropology* 79:289–303.

Reitz, E. J.
1988 Evidence for Coastal Adaptations in Georgia and South Carolina. *Archaeology of Eastern North America* 16:137–158.

Research Laboratories of Archaeology
1996 NAGPRA Inventory of Human Skeletal Remains and Associated Grave Objects. On file, Research Laboratories of Archaeology, University of North Carolina, Chapel Hill.

Resnick, D., and G. Niwayama (editors)
1988 *Diagnosis of Bone and Joint Disorders*. 2nd edition. W. B. Saunders, Philadelphia.

Riggs, S. R., and M. P. O'Connor
1975 Evolutionary Succession of Drowned Coastal Plain-Barbuilt Estuaries. Paper presented at the Annual Meeting of the Geological Society of America, Salt Lake City.

Robbins, L.
1978 Yawslike Disease Process in a Louisiana Shell Mound Population. *Medical College of Virginia Quarterly* 14:24–31.

Roberts, C., and R. Dixon
1993 The Detection of *Mycobacterium tuberculosis* by PCR from Ancient Human Bone. Poster presented at the first Ancient Biomolecules Initiative conference, Cambridge.

258

References

Roberts, C., D. Lucy, and K. Manchester
   1994   Inflammatory Lesions of Ribs: An Analysis of the Terry Collection. *American Journal of Physical Anthropology* 95:169–182.
Roberts, C., and K. Manchester
   1995   *The Archaeology of Disease.* 2nd edition. Cornell University Press, Ithaca, New York.
Robey, D.
   1995   A Paleopathological Study of the Human Remains from the Roitsch Site. Paper presented at the 1995 Caddo Conference, Austin.
Rogers, J. D., and B. D. Smith (editors)
   1995   *Mississippian Communities and Households.* University of Alabama Press, Tuscaloosa.
Rose, J. C., B. A. Burnett, M. S. Nassaney, and M. W. Blaeuer
   1984   Paleopathology and the Origins of Maize Agriculture in the Lower Mississippi Valley and Caddoan Culture Areas. In *Paleopathology at the Origins of Agriculture*, edited by M. N. Cohen and G. J. Armelagos, pp. 393–424. Academic Press, Orlando.
Rose, J. C., and A. M. Harmon
   1989   Bioarcheology of the Louisiana and Arkansas Study Area. In *Archeology and Bioarcheology of the Lower Mississippi Valley and Trans-Mississippi South in Arkansas and Louisiana*, prepared by M. D. Jeter, J. C. Rose, G. I. Williams, Jr., and A. M. Harmon, pp. 323–354. Arkansas Archeological Survey Research Series No. 37, Fayetteville.
Rose, J. C., M. K. Marks, and L. L. Tieszen
   1991   Bioarchaeology and Subsistence in the Central and Lower Portions of the Mississippi Valley. In *What Mean These Bones?*, edited by M. L. Powell, P. S. Bridges, and A. M. W. Mires, pp. 7–21. University of Alabama Press, Tuscaloosa.
Rountree, H. C.
   1989   *The Powhatan Indians of Virginia: Their Traditional Culture.* University of Oklahoma Press, Norman.
   1993   The Powhatans and Other Woodland Indians as Travelers. In *Powhatan Foreign Relations*, edited by H. C. Rountree, pp. 21–52. University Press of Virginia, Charlottesville and London.
Salo, W. L., A. C. Aufderheide, J. E. Buikstra, and T. A. Holcomb
   1994   Identification of *Mycobacterium tuberculosis* DNA in a Pre-Columbian Peruvian Mummy. *Proceedings of the National Academy of Sciences* 91:2091–2094.
Sandford, M. K., G. Bogdan, D. S. Weaver, and L. Sappelsa
   1994   Possible Treponematosis from the Precolumbian Caribbean and Coastal North Carolina. In *L'origine de la Syphilis en Europe, avant ou après 1493?*, edited by O. Dutour, G. Palfi, J. Berato, and J. Brun, pp. 164–168. Editions Errance, Paris.

Sandford, M. K., G. Bogdan, G. E. Kissling, and D. S. Weaver
  1998   Treponematosis in the Prehistoric Caribbean, North Carolina
         Coast and Kentucky: Diagnostic Considerations. Paper pre-
         sented at the 67th Annual Meetings of the American Associa-
         tion of Physical Anthropologists, Salt Lake City, Utah.
Sarnat, B. G., and I. Schour
  1941   Enamel Hypoplasia (Chronologic Enamel Aplasia) in Relation
         to Systemic Disease: A Chronologic, Morphologic and Etio-
         logic Classification. *Journal of the American Dental Association*
         28:1989–2000.
Saunders, R.
  1988   *Excavations at 8NA41: Two Mission Period Sites on Amelia Is-
         land, Florida.* Miscellaneous Project Report Series No. 35.
         Department of Anthropology, Florida State Museum, Gaines-
         ville.
Saunders, S. R., and M. A. Katzenberg (editors)
  1992   *Skeletal Biology of Past Peoples: Research Methods.* Wiley-Liss,
         New York.
Scarry, C. M.
  1986   *Change in Plant Procurement and Production During the Emer-
         gence of the Moundville Chiefdom.* Ph.D. dissertation, Univer-
         sity of Michigan, Ann Arbor.
  1993a Agricultural Risk and the Development of the Moundville
         Chiefdom. In *Foraging and Farming in the Eastern Woodlands,*
         edited by M. C. Scarry, pp. 157–181. University Press of Flor-
         ida, Gainesville.
  1993b Variability in Mississippian Crop Production Strategies. In *For-
         aging and Farming in the Eastern Woodlands,* edited by M. C.
         Scarry, pp. 78–90. Ripley P. Bullen Series. University of Florida
         Press, Gainesville.
  1995   *Excavations on the Northwest Riverbank at Moundville: Investiga-
         tions of a Moundville I Residential Area.* Report of Investiga-
         tions 72. University of Alabama Museums Office of Archae-
         ological Services, Tuscaloosa.
  1998   Examining the Mundane: Domestic Life at Moundville. In
         Studies in Moundville Archaeology, edited by V. J. Knight, Jr.,
         and V. P. Steponaitis, pp. 63–101. Smithsonian Series in Ar-
         chaeological Inquiry. Smithsonian Institution Press, Washing-
         ton, D.C.
Scarry, C. M., and V. P. Steponaitis
  1992   Between Farmstead and Center: The Natural and Social Land-
         scape of Moundville. Paper presented at the 57th Annual Meet-
         ing of the Society for American Archaeology, Pittsburgh.
Scarry, J. F.
  1996   The Nature of Mississippian Societies. In *Political Structure*

and Change in the Prehistoric Southeastern United States, edited by J. F. Scarry, pp. 12–24. University Press of Florida, Gainesville.

Schlossberg, D. (editor)

1994   Tuberculosis. 3rd edition. Springer-Verlag, Berlin.

Schmorl, G., and H. Junghanns

1971   The Human Spine in Health and Disease. 2nd edition. Grune and Stratton, New York.

Schoeninger, M. J., and M. J. DeNiro

1981   Diagenetic Effects on Stable Isotope Ratios in Bone Apatite and Collagen. American Journal of Physical Anthropology 60:252.

1984   Nitrogen and Carbon Isotopic Composition of Bone Collagen from Marine and Terrestrial Animals. Geochimica et Cosmochimica Acta 48:625–639.

Schoeninger, M. J., M. J. DeNiro, and H. Tauber

1983   Stable Nitrogen Isotope Ratios of Bone Collagen Reflect Marine and Terrestrial Components of Prehistoric Human Diet. Science 220:1381–1383.

Schoeninger, M. J., and K. M. Moore

1992   Bone Stable Isotope Studies in Archaeology. Journal of World Prehistory 6:247–296.

Schoeninger, M. J., K. M. Moore, M. L. Murray, and J. C. Kingston

1989   Detection of Bone Preservation in Archaeological and Fossil Samples. Applied Geochemistry 4:281–292.

Schoeninger, M. J., L. Sattenspiel, and M. R. Schurr

1996   Transitions at Moundville: Diet, Habitation, and Health (Abstract). American Journal of Physical Anthropology Supplement 22:209.

Schoeninger, M. J., and M. R. Schurr

1998   Human Subsistence at Moundville: The Stable Isotope Data. In Studies in Moundville Archaeology, edited by V. J. Knight, Jr., and V. P. Steponaitis, pp. 120–132. Smithsonian Series in Archaeological Inquiry. Smithsonian Institution Press, Washington, D.C.

Schoeninger, M. J., N. J. van der Merwe, K. Moore, J. Lee-Thorp, and C. S. Larsen

1990   Decrease in Diet Quality Between the Prehistoric and Contact Periods. In The Archaeology of Mission Santa Catalina de Guale: 2. Biocultural Interpretations of a Population in Transition, edited by C. S. Larsen, pp. 78–93. Anthropological Papers of the American Museum of Natural History No. 68, New York.

Schultz, M.

1993   Initial Stages of Systematic Bone Disease. In Histology of Ancient *Human Bone: Methods and Diagnosis,* edited by G. Grupe and A. N. Garland, pp. 185–203. Springer-Verlag, Berlin, Germany.

Schultz, M., and C. S. Larsen
1997 Porotic Hyperostosis in Spanish Florida: Nature and Etiology of a Frequently Observed Phenomenon. *American Journal of Physical Anthropology* Supplement 24:206.

Schultz, R. J.
1972 *The Language of Fractures.* Williams and Wilkins Co., Baltimore.

Schurr, M. R.
1989 Fluoride Dating of Prehistoric Bones by Ion Selective Electrode. *Journal of Archaeological Science* 16:265–270.

Schurr, M. R., and M. J. Schoeninger
1995 Associations Between Agriculture Intensification and Social Complexity: An Example from the Prehistoric Ohio Valley. *Journal of Anthropological Archaeology* 14:315–339.

Schwarcz, H. P., and M. J. Schoeninger
1991 Stable Isotope Analyses in Human Nutritional Ecology. *Yearbook of Physical Anthropology* 34:283–321.

Scrimshaw, N. S.
1964 Ecological Factors in Nutritional Disease. *American Journal of Clinical Nutrition* 14:112–133.
1975 Interactions of Malnutrition and Infection: Advances in Understanding. In *Protein-Calorie Malnutrition,* edited by R. E. Olson, pp. 353–368. Academic Press, New York.

Scrimshaw, N. S., C. E. Taylor, and J. E. Gordon
1968 *Interactions of Nutrition and Infection.* World Health Organization Monograph 57. Geneva, Switzerland.

Sealy, J.
1986 *Stable Carbon Isotopes and Pre-Historic Diets in the Southwestern Cape Province, South Africa.* Cambridge Monographs in African Prehistory, Cambridge.

Sears, W. H.
1959 *Two Weeden Island Period Burial Mounds, Florida: The W. H. Browne Mound, Duval County; The MacKenzie Mound, Marion County.* Contributions of the Florida State Museum Social Sciences No. 5. University of Florida, Gainesville.

Sexton, J., and T. A. Rathbun
1977 Human Skeletal Remains from the Sea Palms and Lewis Creek Sites, Georgia. Unpublished manuscript.

Shapiro, G.
1990 Bottomlands and Rapids: A Mississippian Adaptive Niche in the Georgia Piedmont. In *Lamar Archaeology: Mississippian*

Chiefdoms in the Deep South, edited by M. Williams and G. Shapiro, pp. 147–162. University of Alabama Press, Tuscaloosa.

Shapiro, G., and B. G. McEwan

1992   *Archaeology at San Luis. Part One: The Apalachee Council House.* Florida Archaeology No. 6. Florida Bureau of Archaeological Research, Tallahasee.

Shearer, G., and D. H. Kohl

1994   Information Derived from Variation in the Natural Abundance of ^{15}N in Complex Biological Systems. In *Isotopes in Organic Chemistry: Heavy Atom Isotope Effects,* edited by E. Buncel and W. H. J. Saunders, pp. 191–237. Elsevier Science Press, Amsterdam.

Sheldon, C. T.

1974   *The Mississippian-Historic Transition in Central Alabama.* Ph.D. dissertation, University of Oregon, Eugene.

Simmons, S., C. S. Larsen, and K. F. Russell

1989   Demographic Interpretations from Ossuary Remains in Northern Spanish Florida. *American Journal of Physical Anthropology* 78:302.

Simpson, S. W., D. L. Hutchinson, and C. S. Larsen

1990   Coping with Stress: Tooth Size, Dental Defects, and Age-at-Death. In *The Archaeology of Mission Santa Catalina de Guale: 2. Biocultural Interpretations of a Population in Transition,* edited by C. S. Larsen, pp. 66–77. Anthropological Papers of the American Museum of Natural History No. 68, New York.

Smith, B. (translator)

1968   *Narratives in the Career of Hernando de Soto in the Conquest of Florida.* Reprint. Kallman Publishing Co., Gainesville. Originally published 1866, Bradford Club, New York.

Smith, B. D.

1987   The Archaeology of the Southeastern United States: From Dalton to de Soto, 10,500–500 B.P. In *Advances in World Archaeology,* edited by F. Wendorf and A. E. Close, vol. 5, pp. 1–91. Academic Press, New York.

1990   *The Mississippian Emergence.* Smithsonian Institution Press, Washington, D.C.

1992a Origins of Agriculture in Eastern North America. In *Rivers of Change,* edited by B. D. Smith, pp. 267–280. Smithsonian Institution Press, Washington, D.C.

1992b Prehistoric Plant Husbandry in Eastern North America. In *The Origins of Agriculture: An International Perspective,* edited by C. W. Cowan and P. J. Watson, pp. 101–119. Smithsonian Institution Press, Washington, D.C.

Smith, B. H.
1984 Patterns of Molar Wear in Hunter-Gatherers and Agricultural-ists. *American Journal of Physical Anthropology* 63:39–56.
Smith, B. N., and S. Epstein
1971 Two Categories of $^{13}C/^{12}C$ Ratios in Plants. *Botanical Gazette* 137:99–104.
Smith, M. O.
1995 Scalping in the Archaic Period: Evidence from the Western Tennessee Valley. *Southeastern Archaeology* 14:60–68.
1996a "Parry" Fractures and Female-directed Interpersonal Violence: Implications from the Late Archaic Period of West Tennessee. *International Journal of Osteoarchaeology* 6:84–91.
1996b Biocultural Inquiry into Archaic Period Populations of the Southeast: Trauma and Occupational Stress. In *Archaeology of the Mid-Holocene Southeast,* edited by K. E. Sassaman and D. G. Anderson, pp. 134–154. University Press of Florida, Gainesville.
Smith, M. T.
1987 *Archaeology of Aboriginal Culture Change in the Interior Southeast: Depopulation During the Early Historic Period.* University of Florida Press, Gainesville.
Snow, C. E.
1941 Possible Evidence of Scalping at Moundville. *Alabama Museum of Natural History Museum Paper* 15:55–59.
1942 Additional Evidence of Scalping. *American Antiquity* 4:398–400.
1948 Indian Knoll Skeletons of Site Oh2, Ohio County, Kentucky. *University of Kentucky Reports on Anthropology and Archaeology* 4:371–554.
South, S. A.
1962 *Exploratory Excavation of the McFayden Mound.* State Department of Archives and History, Raleigh.
1976 An Archaeological Survey of Southeastern North Carolina. *University of South Carolina Institute of Archaeology and Anthropology Notebook* 8:1–55.
Spielmann, K. A., M. J. Schoeninger, and K. Moore
1990 Plains-Pueblo Interdependence and Human Diet at Pecos Pueblo, New Mexico. *American Antiquity* 55:745–765.
Spigelman, M., and E. Lemma
1993 The Use of the Polymerase Chain Reaction (PCR) to Detect *Mycobacterium tuberculosis* in Ancient Skeletons. *International Journal of Osteoarchaeology* 3:137–143.
Steinbock, R. T.
1976 *Paleopathological Diagnosis and Interpretation.* Charles C. Thomas, Springfield, Illinois.

Steponaitis, V. P.
   1983   *Ceramics, Chronology and Community Patterns: An Archaeological Study at Moundville.* Academic Press, New York.
   1991   Contrasting Patterns of Mississippian Development. In *Chiefdoms: Power, Economy, and Ideology,* edited by T. Earle, pp. 193–228. Cambridge University Press, Cambridge.

Stodder, A. L. W.
   1994   Bioarchaeological Investigations of Protohistoric Pueblo Health and Demography. In *In the Wake of Contact: Biological Responses to Conquest,* edited by C. S. Larsen and G. R. Milner, pp. 97–107. Wiley-Liss, New York.
   1996   Paleoepidemiology of Eastern and Western Pueblo Communities in Protohistoric and Early Historic New Mexico. In *Bioarchaeology of Native American Adaptation in the Spanish Borderlands,* edited by B. J. Baker and L. Kealhofer, pp. 148–176. University Press of Florida, Gainesville.

Stodder, A. L. W., and D. L. Martin
   1992   Health and Disease in the Southwest Before and After Spanish Contact. In *Disease and Demography in the Americas,* edited by J. W. Verano and D. H. Ubelaker, pp. 55–73. Smithsonian Institution Press, Washington, D.C.

Strouhal, E.
   1991   Vertebral Tuberculosis in Ancient Egypt and Nubia. In *Human Paleopathology: Current Syntheses and Future Options,* edited by D. J. Ortner and A. C. Aufderheide, pp. 181–196. Smithsonian Institution Press, Washington, D.C.

Stuart-Macadam, P.
   1985   Porotic Hyperostosis: Representative of a Childhood Condition. *American Journal of Physical Anthropology* 66:391–398.
   1987   Porotic Hyperostosis: New Evidence to Support the Anemia Theory. *American Journal of Physical Anthropology* 74:521–526.
   1989   Porotic Hyperostosis: Relationship between Orbital and Vault Lesions. *American Journal of Physical Anthropology* 80:187–193.
   1992   Anemia in Past Populations. In *Diet, Demography, and Disease: Changing Perspectives on Anemia,* edited by P. Stuart-Macadam and S. Kent, pp. 150–170. Aldine de Gruyter, New York.

Swanton, J. R.
   1928   Social Organization and Social Usages of the Indians of the Creek Confederacy. *Forty-second Annual Report of the Bureau of American Ethnology,* pp. 25–472. Washington, D.C.
   1946   *The Indians of the Southeastern United States.* Bureau of American Ethnology Bulletin 137. Smithsonian Institution, Washington, D.C.

Tainter, J. A.
1980 Behavior and Status in a Middle Woodland Mortuary Population from the Illinois Valley. *American Antiquity* 45:308-313.

Taylor, G. M., M. Crossey, J. Saldanha, and T. Waldron
1996 DNA from *Mycobacterium tuberculosis* Identified in Medieval
Human Skeletal Remains Using Polymerase Chain Reaction.
Journal of Archaeological Science 23:789-798.

Thomas, D. H.
1987 *The Archaeology of Mission Santa Catalina de Guale: 1. Search
and Discovery.* Anthropological Papers of the American Museum of Natural History 63, part 2.
1989 *Archaeology.* 2nd edition. Holt, Rinehart and Winston, Fort
Worth.

Thomas, D. H, and C. S. Larsen
1979a *The Anthropology of St. Catherines Island: 2. The Refuge-
Deptford Mortuary Complex.* Anthropological Papers of the
American Museum of Natural History 56, part 1.
1979b *The Anthropology of St. Catherines Island: 4. The St. Catherines
Period Mortuary Complex.* Anthropological Papers of the American Museum of Natural History 57, part 4.

Tieszen, L. L.
1991 Natural Variations in the Carbon Isotope Values of Plants: Implications for Archaeology, Ecology, and Paleoecology. *Journal
of Archaeological Science* 18:227-248.

Tieszen, L. L., T. W. Boutton, K. G. Tesdahl, and N. A. Slade
1983 Fractionation and Turnover of Stable Carbon Isotopes in Animal Tissues: Implications for the $\delta^{13}C$ Analysis of Diet. *Oecolo-
gia* 57:32-37.

Tramont, E. C.
1990 *Treponema pallidum* (Syphilis). In *Principles and Practice of Infectious Diseases,* edited by G. L. Mandell, R. G. Douglas, Jr.,
and J. E. Bennett, pp. 1794-1808. Churchill Livingstone, New
York.

Trigger, B. G.
1978 *Handbook of the North American Indians.* Vol. 15, Northeast
(editor). Smithsonian Institution Press, Washington, D.C.
1989 *History of Archaeological Thought.* Cambridge University
Press, Cambridge.

Trimble, C. C.
1996 *Palaeodiet in Virginia and North Carolina as Determined by Stable Isotope Analysis of Skeletal Remains.* M.A. thesis, Department of Environmental Sciences, University of Virginia, Charlottesville.

Truesdell, S.
   1995   *Paleopathological and Paleoepidemiological Analysis of the Piggot Ossuary (31Cr14), Carteret County, North Carolina.* M.A. thesis, Wake Forest University, Winston-Salem.

Tuggle, W. O.
   1973   *Shem, Ham, and Japheth. The Papers of W. O. Tuggle*, edited by E. Current-Garcia and D. B. Hatfield. University of Georgia Press, Athens.

Turner, C. G., III
   1979   Dental Anthropological Indications of Agriculture Among the Jomon People of Central Japan: X. Peopling of the Pacific. *American Journal of Physical Anthropology* 51:619–636.

Turner, E. R., III
   1992   The Virginia Coastal Plain During the Late Woodland Period. In *Middle and Late Woodland Research in Virginia: A Synthesis*, edited by T. R. Reinhart and M. E. N. Hodges, pp. 97–136. Dietz Press, Richmond, Virginia.

Turner, K. R.
   1984   Health, Illness, and the People of Hoithlewaulee. In *Culture Change on the Creek Indian Frontier*, edited by G. A. Waselkov, pp. 48–61. Preliminary final report to the National Science Foundation, Grant Award #BNS-8305437.
   1986   Human Skeletal Remains: 22Lo860. In *Test Excavations at Two Woodland Sites, Lowndes County, Mississippi*, edited by J. Rafferty and M. E. Starr, pp. 131–134. Report of Investigations 3. Cobb Institute of Archaeology, Mississippi State University, Starkville.

Turner, T. B., and D. H. Hollander
   1957   *Biology of the Treponematoses.* World Health Organization, Geneva.

Tuross, N., M. L. Fogel, and P. E. Hare
   1988   Variability in the Preservation of the Isotopic Composition of Collagen from Fossil Bone. *Geochimica et Cosmochimica Acta* 52:929–935.

Tuross, N., M. L. Fogel, L. Newsom, and G. H. Doran
   1994   Subsistence in the Florida Archaic: The Stable-Isotope and Archaeobotanical Evidence from the Windover Site. *American Antiquity* 59:288–303.

Ubelaker, D. H.
   1974   *Reconstruction of Demographic Profiles from Ossuary Skeletal Samples.* Smithsonian Contributions to Anthropology No. 18. Smithsonian Institution Press, Washington, D.C.
   1989   *Human Skeletal Remains: Excavation, Analysis, Interpretation.* 2nd edition. Taraxacum, Washington, D.C.

1992 Porotic Hyperostosis in Prehistoric Ecuador. In *Diet, Demography, and Disease: Changing Perspectives on Anemia,* edited by P. Stuart-Macadam and S. Kent, pp. 201–217. Aldine de Gruyter, New York.

van der Merwe, N. J., and J. C. Vogel
1978 ^{13}C Content of Human Collagen as a Measure of Prehistoric Diet in Woodland North America. *Nature* 276:815–816.

Vaughn, M.
1992 Syphilis in Colonial East and Central Africa: The Social Construction of an Epidemic. In *Epidemics and Ideas: Essays on the Historical Perception of Pestilence,* edited by T. Ranger and P. Slack, pp. 269–302. Cambridge University Press, Cambridge.

Vogel, J. C., and N. J. van der Merwe
1977 Isotopic Evidence for Early Maize Cultivation in New York State. *American Antiquity* 42:238–242.

Vogel, J. O., and J. Allan
1985 Mississippian Fortification at Moundville. *Archaeology* 38:62–63.

Vogel, V. J.
1970 *American Indian Medicine.* University of Oklahoma Press, Norman.

Wada, E.
1980 Nitrogen Isotope Fractionation and its Significance in Biogeochemical Processes Occurring in Marine Environments. In *Isotope Marine Geochemistry,* edited by E. D. Goldberg, Y. Horibe, and K. Saruhaski, pp. 375–398. Uchida Rokakuho Publishing Co., Tokyo.

Wadsworth, G. R.
1992 Physiological, Pathological, and Dietary Influences on the Hemoglobin Level. In *Diet, Demography, and Disease,* edited by P. Stuart-Macadam and S. Kent, pp. 63–104. Aldine de Gruyter, New York.

Wakefield, E. C., and S. C. Dellinger
1940 Diseases of Prehistoric Americans of South Central United States. *CIBA Symposium,* 453–464.

Walker, K. J.
1992 The Zooarchaeology of Charlotte Harbor's Prehistoric Maritime Adaptation: Spatial and Temporal Perspectives. In *Culture and Environment in the Domain of the Calusa,* edited by William H. Marquardt, pp. 265–366. Monograph No. 1. Institute of Archaeology and Paleoenvironmental Studies, University of Florida, Gainesville.

Walker, J. M., and G. F. Miller
1992 Life on the Levee: The Late Woodland Period in the Northern

Great Valley of Virginia. In *Middle and Late Woodland Research in Virginia: A Synthesis*, edited by T. R. Reinhart and M. E. N. Hodges, pp. 165–186. Dietz Press, Richmond, Virginia.

Walker, P. L.

1985 Anemia Among Prehistoric Indians of the American Southwest. In *Health and Disease in the Prehistoric Southwest*, edited by C. F. Merbs and R. J. Miller, pp. 139–164. Arizona State University Anthropological Papers No. 34.

1986 Porotic Hyperostosis in a Marine-Dependent California Indian Population. *American Journal of Physical Anthropology* 69:345–354.

1989 Cranial Injuries as Evidence of Violence in Prehistoric Southern California. *American Journal of Physical Anthropology* 80:313–323.

Walker, P. L., and J. M. Erlandson

1986 Dental Evidence for Prehistoric Dietary Changes on the Northern Channel Islands, California. *American Antiquity* 51:375–383.

Walker, P. L., J. R. Johnson, and P. M. Lambert

1988 Age and Sex Biases in the Preservation of Human Skeletal Remains. *American Journal of Physical Anthropology* 76:183–188.

Wallace, R. L.

1975 *An Archeological, Ethnohistoric, and Biochemical Investigation of the Guale Aborigines of the Georgia Coastal Strand.* Ph.D. dissertation, University of Florida, Gainesville.

Walthall, J. A.

1980 *Prehistoric Indians of the Southeast.* University of Alabama Press, Tuscaloosa.

Ward, H. T., and R. P. S. Davis, Jr.

1991 The Impact of Old World Diseases on the Native Inhabitants of the North Carolina Piedmont. *Archaeology of Eastern North America* 19:171–181.

1993 *Indian Communities on the North Carolina Piedmont: A.D. 1000 to 1700.* Monograph Series 2. Research Laboratories of Anthropology, University of North Carolina, Chapel Hill.

1999 *Time Before History: The Archaeology of North Carolina.* University of North Carolina Press, Chapel Hill.

Ward, H. T., and J. H. Wilson, Jr.

1980 Archaeological Excavations at the Cold Morning Site. *Southern Indian Studies* 32:5–40.

Waselkov, G. A.

1987   Shellfish Gathering and Shell Midden Archaeology. In *Advances in Archaeological Method and Theory* 10, edited by M. B. Schiffer, pp. 93–210. Academic Press, Orlando.

1989   Seventeenth-Century Trade in the Colonial Southeast. *Southeastern Archaeology* 8:117–133.

1992   French Colonial Trade in the Upper Creek Country. In *Calumet and Fleur-de-Lys: Archaeology of Indian and French Contact in the Midcontinent,* edited by J. A. Walthall and T. E. Emerson, pp. 35–53. Smithsonian Institution Press, Washington, D.C.

Waselkov, G. A., J. W. Cottier, and C. T. Sheldon, Jr.

1987   Archaeological Excavations at the Early Historic Creek Indian Town of Fusihatchee. National Science Foundation grant proposal, Anthropology Program.

Watson, P. J.

1989   Early Plant Cultivation in the Eastern Woodlands of North America. In *Foraging and Farming: The Evolution of Plant Exploitation,* edited by D. R. Harris and G. C. Hillman, pp. 555–571. Unwin Hyman, London.

Weaver, D. S., M. K. Sandford, G. Bogdan, and G. E. Kissling

1998   Treponematosis in the Prehistoric Caribbean, North Carolina Coast, and Kentucky: Paleoepidemiological and Evolutionary Perspectives. Paper presented at the 67th Annual Meeting of the American Association of Physical Anthropologists, Salt Lake City.

Webb, S.

1995   *Palaeopathology of Aboriginal Australians: Health and Disease across a Hunter-Gatherer Continent.* Cambridge University Press, Cambridge, England.

Webb, W. S., and D. L. DeJarnette

1942   *An Archaeological Survey of Pickwick Basin in the Adjacent Portions of the States of Alabama, Mississippi, and Tennessee.* Bureau of American Ethnology Bulletin 129. Smithsonian Institution, Washington, D.C.

1948a *The Perry Site Lu°25,* Units 3 and 4, Lauderdale Co., Alabama. Alabama Museum of Natural History Museum Paper 25. University of Alabama, Tuscaloosa.

1948b *Little Bear Creek Site Ct°8,* Colbert County, Alabama. Alabama Museum of Natural History Museum Paper 26. University of Alabama, Tuscaloosa.

Webb, W. S., and C. E. Snow

1945   The Adena People. *Reports in Anthropology and Archaeology.*

Vol. 6. Department of Anthropology and Archaeology, University of Kentucky, Lexington.

Weinberg, E. D.

1992   Iron Withholding in Prevention of Disease. In *Diet, Demography, and Disease: Changing Perspectives on Anemia,* edited by P. Stuart-Macadam and S. Kent, pp. 105–150. Aldine de Gruyter, New York.

Weisman, B. R.

1992   *Excavations on the Franciscan Frontier: Archaeology at the Fig Springs Mission.* University of Florida Press, Gainesville.

1993   Archaeology of Fig Springs Mission, Ichetucknee Springs State Park. In *The Missions of La Florida,* edited by B. G. McEwan, pp. 165–192. University Press of Florida, Gainesville.

Welch, P. D.

1991   *Moundville's Economy.* University of Alabama Press, Tuscaloosa.

1998   Outlying Sites Within the Moundville Chiefdom. In *Studies in Moundville Archaeology,* edited by V. J. Knight, Jr., and V. P. Steponaitis, pp. 133–166. Smithsonian Series in Archaeological Inquiry. Smithsonian Institution Press, Washington, D.C.

Welch, P. D., and C. M. Scarry

1995   Status-related Variation in Foodways in the Moundville Chiefdom. *American Antiquity* 60:397–419.

White, T. D.

1991   *Human Osteology.* Academic Press, San Diego.

Whitney, W. F.

1886   Notes on the Anomalies, Injuries and Diseases of the Native Races of North America. *Annual Report of the Peabody Museum* 3:433–448. Boston.

Widmer, L., and A. J. Perzigian

1981   The Ecology and Etiology of Skeletal Lesions in Late Prehistoric Populations of Eastern North America. In *Prehistoric Tuberculosis in the Americas,* edited by J. E. Buikstra, pp. 99–113. Northwestern University Archaeological Program Scientific Papers No. 5. Evanston.

Widmer, R. J.

1988   *The Evolution of the Calusa: A Nonagricultural Chiefdom on the Southwest Coast of Florida.* University of Alabama Press, Tuscaloosa.

Wilkinson, R. G., and K. M. Van Wagenen

1993   Violence Against Women: Prehistoric Skeletal Evidence from Michigan. *Midcontinental Journal of Archaeology* 18:190–216.

Willcox, R. R.
   1972   The Treponemal Revolution. *Transactions of the St. John's Hospital Dermatological Society* 58:21–37.
Willey, G. R.
   1982   *Archaeology of the Florida Gulf Coast.* Reprint. Florida Book Store, Gainesville. Originally published 1949, Smithsonian Miscellaneous Collections, vol. 113, Smithsonian Institution Press, Washington, D.C.
Willey, G. R., and J. A. Sabloff
   1980   *A History of American Archaeology.* 2nd edition. W. H. Freeman, New York.
Willey, P., and T. E. Emerson
   1993   The Osteology and Archaeology of the Crow Creek Massacre. *Plains Anthropologist Memoir* 27:227–269.
Williams, H. U.
   1927   The American Origin of Syphilis. *Archives of Dermatology and Syphilology* 16(6):683–696.
   1932   The Origin and Antiquity of Syphilis: The Evidence from Diseased Bones. A Review with Some New Material from America. *Archives of Pathology* 13:779–814, 931–983.
   1936   The Origin of Syphilis: Evidence from Diseased Bones. *Archives of Dermatological Syphilis* 33: 783–787.
Williamson, M. A.
   1998   *Regional Variation in Health and Lifeways Among Late Prehistoric Georgia Agriculturalists.* Ph.D. dissertation, Purdue University, West Lafayette.
Wilson, D. E.
   1998   *Variations in the Skeletal Record of Prehistoric Treponematosis on the Gulf Coastal Plain.* Ph.D. dissertation, Department of Anthropology, University of Texas, Austin.
Wood, J. W., G. R. Milner, H. C. Harpending, and K. M. Weiss
   1992   The Osteological Paradox: Problems in Inferring Prehistoric Health from Skeletal Samples. *Current Anthropology* 33:343–358.
Wood-Jones, F.
   1910   Fractured Bones and Dislocations. In *The Archaeological Survey of Nubia Report for 1907–1908.* Vol. 2. *Report on the Human Remains,* edited by G. Elliot-Smith and F. Wood-Jones, pp. 293–342. National Printing Department, Cairo.
Woodruff, A. W.
   1982   Recent Work Concerning Anemia in the Tropics. *Seminars in Hematology* 19:141–147.
Worth, J. E.
   1995   *The Struggle for the Georgia Coast: An Eighteenth-Century Span-*

ish Retrospective on Guale and Mocama. Anthropological Papers of the American Museum of Natural History No. 75.

Yarnell, R. A.

1993   The Importance of Native Crops during the Late Archaic and Woodland Periods. In *Foraging and Farming in the Eastern Woodlands,* edited by C. M. Scarry, pp. 13–26. University Press of Florida, Gainesville.

Yarnell, R. A., and M. J. Black

1985   Temporal Trends Indicated by a Survey of Archaic and Woodland Plant Food Remains from Southeastern North America. *Southeastern Archaeology* 4:93–106.

Youmans, G. P.

1979   *Tuberculosis.* W. B. Saunders Co., Philadelphia.

Zahler, J. W., Jr.

1976   *A Morphological Analysis of a Protohistoric-Historic Skeletal Population from St. Simons Island, Georgia.* M.A. thesis, University of Florida, Gainesville.

Contributors

Patricia S. Bridges was an Associate Professor of Anthropology at Queens College and the Graduate Center, CUNY, until her untimely death from cancer at age 43 in February 1999. She had served as Chair of the Department of Anthropology at Queens College since 1994. As a graduate student at the University of Michigan, Bridges developed her research interest in skeletal markers of physical activities with her Ph.D. dissertation, *Changes in Long Bone Structure with the Transition to Agriculture: Implications for Prehistoric Activities.* In later publications on the osteological correlates of weapon use, skeletal evidence for warfare, gendered divisions of labor, and changing patterns of osteoarthritis in Archaic and Mississippian Native American populations of the Midwest and Southeast, Bridges cautioned against simplistic reconstructions of behavior based on specific skeletal features. She co-edited (with M. L. Powell and A. M. W. Mires) *What Mean These Bones? Studies in Southeastern Bioarchaeology* (University of Alabama Press, 1991). Shortly before her death, she completed an analysis of osteoarthritis in Woodland period populations in the Lower Illinois Valley.

Elizabeth Monahan Driscoll is a doctoral candidate in the Department of Anthropology at the University of North Carolina at Chapel Hill. She is interested in mortuary symbolism and the political economy of diet and health. Her research focuses on the bioarchaeology of native peoples of the coastal and piedmont regions of North Carolina during the Late Woodland and Mississippian periods.

Debra L. Gold is an Assistant Professor of Anthropology at St. Cloud State University. She received her Ph.D. from the University of Michigan (1999), where she developed an interest in using a bioarchaeological perspective to examine the emergence of social complexity in the prehistoric interior Mid-Atlantic and Southeast.

Dale L. Hutchinson is an Associate Professor of Anthropology at East Carolina University. He is interested in late prehistoric human adaptation and evolution, and his research includes dietary reconstruction, health and disease, and population dynamics in North and South America. One of his current projects focuses on coastal adaptation in North Carolina and south Florida.

Keith P. Jacobi is an Assistant Professor of Anthropology at The University of Alabama and Curator of Human Osteology at the Alabama Museum of Natural History. He has published articles on the health of Barbadian slaves at Newton Plantation and on the dental genetics of the historic Tipu Maya. Current areas of interest include Mississippian period warfare in northern Alabama, dental morphology and dental metrics at Moundville, health in Alabama as seen through skeletal remains from early nineteenth-century cemeteries, and the health of the historic Chickasaw.

Patricia M. Lambert is an Assistant Professor of Anthropology at Utah State University. Her research focuses on biological and behavioral responses to stress in prehistoric populations of California, North Carolina and Virginia, the Southwest, and north coastal Peru. She is particularly interested in prehistoric warfare and is currently at work on a volume examining the causes and consequences of warfare in hunter-gatherer societies of coastal southern California.

Clark Spencer Larsen teaches biological anthropology at the University of North Carolina, where he is the Amos Hawley Distinguished Professor. Most of his research focuses on precontact and contact era bioarchaeology in the American Southeast, but he has also undertaken projects in other localities in North America and Europe. He received his Ph.D. from the University of Michigan in 1980. He is the President of the American Association of Physical Anthropologists. He is the author of various articles and books, including *Bioarchaeology: Interpreting Behavior from the Human Skeleton,* published by Cambridge University Press.

Lynette Norr is an Assistant Professor of Anthropology and Affiliate of the Department of Geology and the Center for Latin American Studies at the University of Florida. As a doctoral student she established a bone stable isotope prep laboratory at the University of Illinois Department of Anthropology, where she conducted research on paleodiet and health status in lower Central America. Her dissertation was awarded the 1992 Society for American Archaeology Dissertation Prize. After a four-year postdoc in that same laboratory with Dr. S. H. Ambrose, she continues her paleodietary research in Latin America and in the southeastern United States at the University of Florida. Her current archaeological investigations along the Pacific coast of Panama examine Early Ceramic seasonal settlement and coastal subsistence and support an archaeological field school.

Mary Lucas Powell retired in 1997 from the position of Director/Curator of the William S. Webb Museum of Anthropology at the University of Kentucky, which she had held for eleven years. This change has permitted her to focus her professional energies on research into the "natural history" of tuberculosis and treponematosis in pre-Columbian New World populations. She has published numerous articles on health and disease in prehistoric Native American populations of the Midwest and Southeast. Her revised Ph.D. dissertation from Northwestern University was published as *Status and Health in Prehistory, A Case Study of the Moundville Chiefdom* by the Smithsonian Instutution Press (1988). In 1996 she began a new research focus on Late Classical/Medieval populations of the western Mediterranean and is currently the staff bioarchaeologist for a long-term excavation project at the site of Torre de Palma (1st–15th centuries A.D.) in eastern Portugal. In 2000, Powell will assume the editorship of the quarterly *Newsletter* and other publications of the Paleopathology Association, a scholarly organization with a worldwide membership of anthropologists, physicians, and other researchers interested in ancient disease and health.

Marianne Reeves is a doctoral candidate at the University of North Carolina at Chapel Hill. While maintaining an interest in the dental health of historic peoples of the Southeastern United States, she focuses her current research on dental defects in medieval Danish populations.

Lisa Sattenspiel is an Associate Professor of Anthropology at the University of Missouri-Columbia. Her main interests are in the geographic spread of infectious diseases, paleodemography, and human ecology. Dr. Sattenspiel's current research projects include a study of the influence of fur-trapping activities on the spread of the 1918–19 influenza epidemic through three central Canadian native communities (with Ann Herring) and a study of the interactions between social networks, childhood stress levels, and illness in a small Caribbean villages (with Mark Flinn).

Margaret J. Schoeninger is a Professor of Anthropology at the University of Wisconsin in Madison. After receiving her Ph.D. in anthropology from the University of Michigan, Dr. Schoeninger was a postdoctoral fellow in the Department of Earth and Space Science at the University of California at Los Angeles, where she worked with Dr.

Michael DeNiro developing methods for elucidating various archaeological problems based on stable isotope ratios of carbon and nitrogen. Her work since that time has emphasized the use of stable isotopes (carbon, nitrogen, and oxygen) in paleoecology, paleodiet, and paleonutrition.

Mark R. Schurr is an Assistant Professor of Anthropology at the University of Notre Dame. His research focuses on the archaeology of eastern North America (especially the Southeast and the Lower Great Lakes region). A childhood chemistry set fostered an early interest in chemistry, which eventually led to a B.S. in Chemistry and a continuing interest in archaeological chemistry, especially stable isotope analysis.

Leslie E. Sering is a graduate student in the Department of Anthropology at the University of Michigan. She is currently pursuing a Ph.D. in anthropology, with a focus in archaeology and complex societies. She has worked in the American Southeast and Mesoamerica on a variety of bioarchaeological projects.

David S. Weaver is a Professor of Anthropology at Wake Forest University. His work in bioarchaeology includes research on treponematoses, other aspects of paleopathology, and osteoporosis. He also has worked for almost 20 years on experimental regimes for osteoporosis, using nonhuman primates as models to investigate those treatments. With Italian and Austrian colleagues, he has recently begun work in human evolution as well.

Matthew A. Williamson is an Assistant Professor in the Department of Health and Kinesiology at Georgia Southern University where he is the Director of the Anatomy and Physiology Program. Dr. Williamson's primary interest is in the study of pathological lesions of the skeleton. He has coauthored a book chapter on this subject dealing with historic remains from the midwestern United States and is currently writing a coauthored chapter focusing on the reconstruction of the conflict between Native Americans and Europeans at the colonial period site of Ft. Laurens, Ohio. Dr. Williamson is also a consulting forensic anthropologist with works in progress on facial reconstruction, forensic taphonomy, and tissue rehydration.

Index